Common Pitfalls in the Evaluation and Management of Headache

Case-Based Learning

T0382649

Common Pitfalls in the Evaluation and Management of Headache

Case-Based Learning

Elizabeth W. Loder
The John R. Graham Headache Center, Brigham and Women's Faulkner Hospital; and
Department of Neurology, Harvard Medical School, Boston, MA, USA

Rebecca C. Burch
The John R. Graham Headache Center, Brigham and Women's Faulkner Hospital; and
Department of Neurology, Harvard Medical School, Boston, MA, USA

Paul B. Rizzoli
The John R. Graham Headache Center, Brigham and Women's Faulkner Hospital; and
Department of Neurology, Harvard Medical School, Boston, MA, USA

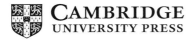

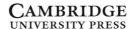

University Printing House, Cambridge CB2 8BS, United Kingdom

Cambridge University Press is part of the University of Cambridge.

It furthers the University's mission by disseminating knowledge in the pursuit of education, learning and research at the highest international levels of excellence.

www.cambridge.org
Information on this title: www.cambridge.org/9781107636101

First published 2014
Reprinted 2018

Printed in the United Kingdom by Print on Demand, World Wide

A catalog record for this publication is available from the British Library

Library of Congress Cataloging in Publication data
Loder, Elizabeth, author.
Common pitfalls in the evaluation and management of headache : case-based learning / Elizabeth W. Loder, Rebecca C. Burch, Paul B. Rizzoli.
   p. ; cm.
Includes bibliographical references and index.
ISBN 978-1-107-63610-1 (pbk.)
I. Burch, Rebecca C., author.   II. Rizzoli, Paul, author.   III. Title.
[DNLM: 1. Headache – diagnosis – Case Reports.   2. Headache – therapy – Case Reports. WL 342]
RC392
616.8′491 – dc23   2013049904

ISBN 978-1-107-63610-1 Paperback
Additional resources for this publication at
www.cambridge.org/9781107636101

· ·

We dedicate this book to the memory of Dr. John Ruskin Graham, an early pioneer in the field of headache medicine and founder of our Headache Center at the Brigham and Women's Faulkner Hospital in Boston. His work and ideals live on at the Graham Headache Center. We strive to uphold Dr. Graham's legacy of kindness, understanding, and expert care for those affected by headache disorders.

Contents

Preface

The *Illustrated Oxford Dictionary* defines a *pitfall* as "an unsuspected snare, danger, or drawback." This idea of dangers that are disguised or difficult to recognize is reflected in the word's second meaning, which is a "trap or snare," often a covered pit, into which unwary animals (or doctors?) might fall. Most doctors correctly realize that evaluation and treatment of headaches can be challenging. They know that most headaches are benign but fear missing the occasional serious cause of headache. Some believe that headache treatment is often unsuccessful and unrewarding.

To the extent that this aversion to headache exists, we think it is unfortunate. In our experience, headache diagnosis is mostly straightforward. Furthermore, headache medicine is often fascinating and gratifying. There are many unusual, intriguing types of headache as well as new and highly effective treatments for headache. We find that even "old-fashioned" treatments, correctly applied, can produce satisfying improvements for the right patient. As with any medical discipline, though, there *are* challenging aspects of headache medicine. Our purpose in writing this book is to make readers aware of the common and less obvious mistakes or pitfalls that we have encountered during our years in practice – as well as those we have observed in the practices of others.

There are many case-based neurology books available to practitioners who are interested in head pain, including several with an exclusive focus on headache.

This book differs from those in two ways. First, the cases in this book focus solely on challenging rather than routine aspects of headache diagnosis and treatment. Second, this book was written while the International Classification of Headache Disorders (ICHD) was being updated for just the third time since it was issued in 1988. As a result, all of the information in this book is current with the just-released ICHD-3 beta version of the classification. The ICHD-3 beta is available free of charge at the website of the International Headache Society (http://www.ihs-headache.org); you may wish to print it for easy reference while reading this book. We have not reproduced the diagnostic criteria verbatim but have instead summarized the clinical characteristics of each disorder, as specified in the latest version of the classification.

Among us, the three authors of this book have a combined experience of full-time Headache Medicine practice of almost half a century. PR and EL are seasoned veterans and bring many years of clinical experience to bear. In contrast, RB is in the early phase of her career; she has helped us focus on pitfalls and mistakes to which newcomers or non-headache specialists might be prone. We hope these dual perspectives make this a book that is useful to anyone who might see headache patients, from family practitioners to pain specialists. After all, who among us has so much experience that s/he cannot learn from the mistakes and near misses of others?

Acknowledgements

We offer our sincere thanks to Dr. Martin Samuels, the legendary and beloved chairman of the Department of Neurology at the Brigham and Women's and Brigham and Women's Faulkner Hospitals in Boston. His vision and backing led to the formation of the Division of Headache within the Brigham Department of Neurology – one of the first such divisions to be created within the Neurology Department of a leading US academic medical center. The Graham Headache Center, and by extension this book, would not exist without him.

We also thank Nicholas Dunton, our editor at Cambridge University Press, for inviting us to write this book. He tolerated with good humor the delay caused by the tardy release of the third version of the International Classification of Headache Disorders. We hope he feels the result was worth the wait! Our thanks also go to Kirsten Bot, assistant editor and publishing assistant, who was so helpful with the final phases of the book's production. We also thank our copy-editor, Anne Kenton, for her keen eye and attention to detail.

Elizabeth Loder, Rebecca Burch, Paul Rizzoli
July 2013

Chapter

1

Confusing one benign headache with another

Sometimes there is simply no mistaking which primary headache disorder is causing a patient's problem. In these lucky instances, a patient spontaneously provides a history so characteristic of a disorder that there can be no doubt about the diagnosis. In specialty headache practice, however, the patient who gives the doctor such a "silver platter" description of a headache problem is the exception and not the rule. Since the primary, nondangerous headache disorders are clinical diagnoses with, by definition, normal imaging and laboratory findings, the patient history is critical to making a diagnosis.

Unfortunately, as seasoned doctors know all too well, obtaining an accurate history can be difficult. This is particularly true for subjective symptoms such as headache, where patients are struggling to describe things like pain that cannot be directly observed or measured by the doctor. Then too, patients also are reporting symptoms that may come and go. Studies show that patient recall of headache frequency and features is low and deteriorates rapidly over time. A missed or delayed diagnosis of a primary headache disorder is unlikely to expose patients to life-threatening harm, but it does have consequences. For one thing, it may mean the patient does not have the benefit of new, highly effective treatments that work for some headache problems and not others.

In this chapter we deal with cases in which a patient with one of the "big three" common, nondangerous primary headaches – migraine, tension-type, or cluster headache – presented with ambiguous, overlapping features and was therefore mistakenly diagnosed. To minimize the chance of confusing these headaches, it is worth becoming familiar with the many ways in which the diagnostic features of common, nondangerous headaches can overlap or be missed. Far and away the most common pitfall is confusion about whether a patient has migraine or tension-type headache, so we'll start there.

Migraine or tension-type headache?

Case

A 34-year-old teacher was referred for consultation regarding recurrent headaches for the last five years. She was in good health and taking only occasional ibuprofen to treat the headaches. She estimated that headaches occurred on average twice a month, lasting a day or two at a time, and had not recently changed in character. They were bilateral, over her forehead, and sometimes accompanied by neck pain. She said that her job was stressful and wondered whether that might be causing the headaches. She missed a day of work every other month because of headaches, and reported she was seeking treatment because her missed work time had recently become "an issue" with her employer. Physical and neurologic examinations were normal except for mild tenderness on palpation over the posterior neck and upper trapezius muscles. She had previously been told that she probably had "tension headaches" and had been referred for physical therapy but did not find that treatment effective.

How can migraine be reliably distinguished from tension-type headache in this patient?

Careful evaluation of a full headache history is, in our experience, the most useful method of distinguishing between migraine and tension-type headache. In this case, the patient did not spontaneously report characteristic features of migraine such as nausea, vomiting, photo or phonophobia, or worsening with physical activity. On the other hand, we did not ask!

Table 1.1 lists migraine features that are contained in the diagnostic criteria for the disorder, along with examples of how these features can be missed or misinterpreted. The diagnostic criteria for migraine have not changed in the latest version (3-beta) of the International Classification of Headache Disorders (ICHD).

Table 1.1. Diagnostic features of migraine without aura: common pitfalls

"Silver platter" migraine features	"Not so obvious" migraine history
Duration of 4–72 hours	Duration uncertain because patient treats early or falls asleep. Shorter headaches often seen in children
Unilateral (often over the temple)*	Bilateral, posterior location of pain or prominent complaints of neck pain often lead to a diagnosis of tension-type headache, but neck pain occurs in almost three-quarters of migraine attacks
Throbbing*	Not all patients who otherwise have clear-cut migraine report throbbing pain; for many patients the throbbing quality of the pain is obvious only in fully developed, longer duration headaches, so patients who treat early or fall asleep may not experience this. Be alert for synonymous descriptions such as "pounding" or "with my heartbeat"
Moderate to severe pain intensity*	In migraine attacks that are treated or do not progress, pain may never reach severe intensity. Differences in pain reporting behaviors and pain perception among patients may affect patient ratings of pain intensity
Aggravated by or causing avoidance of physical activity*	Sedentary patients may not have noticed this feature of their headaches
Nausea and/or vomiting#	Vomiting is prominent in children with migraine, but often lessens as patients get older or headache frequency increases. Decreased appetite may be present instead
Photophobia and phonophobia#	Sensitivity to light or sound may become apparent only in headaches that have a chance to develop fully; these symptoms may not develop in milder *"forme fruste"* or treated attacks

* Only two of these four features are required for a diagnosis of migraine.
\# Only one of these two features is required for a diagnosis of migraine. At least five attacks meeting criteria are required before migraine without aura can be diagnosed.

Some diagnostic criteria for migraine are more useful than others when trying to decide between diagnoses of migraine and tension-type headache. A systematic review of diagnostic studies showed that the features most predictive of migraine as opposed to tension-type headache were nausea, photo and phonophobia. When present, a typical history consistent with migraine aura was, unsurprisingly, also highly predictive of a migraine diagnosis.

What benign headache disorder might account for this patient's headaches?

Taking the limited history at face value, this patient's presentation is compatible with a diagnosis of tension-type headache. It is tempting to think that the bilateral, posterior location of the headache and associated muscle tenderness clinch the matter. Migraine is, however, also in the differential. In fact, while tension-type headache is the most common type of headache in the general population, it is not the most common type of headache in patients whose headaches are troublesome enough to seek medical care. A wealth of good quality evidence suggests that once dangerous causes of headache have been ruled out, the likelihood is that patients consulting general physicians for troublesome headaches have migraine and not tension-type

headache. This is true even in patients like the one in our case who present with features such as muscle tension and neck pain and attribute their headaches to stress. Muscle tension and neck pain are common in both migraine and tension-type headache, as is aggravation of headaches by emotional stress or tension. In fact, migraine patients who have these overlap characteristics (particularly neck pain) are most likely to receive an incorrect diagnosis of tension-type headache.

In this case, further questioning revealed that the patient did have some loss of appetite with her headaches and she became mildly sensitive to light, features which support a diagnosis of migraine instead of tension-type headache.

Discussion

Research in primary care settings shows that most patients who seek care for troublesome headaches receive a diagnosis of tension-type headache. This is particularly likely to occur when patients report features that are assumed to be highly characteristic of tension-type headache – as the patient in our case did. For example, many physicians (and patients, too) assume that muscle pain or tenderness in the neck or shoulders is synonymous with tension-type headache. They may also assume the same thing in patients who

Table 1.2. Headache features and diagnosis of migraine

Clinical feature	Sensitivity of diagnosis of migraine (% of patients)	Specificity of diagnosis for migraine vs. tension-type headache (% of patients)	Likelihood ratio for diagnosis of migraine (95% confidence interval)	
			Positive	Negative
Nausea	82	96	23.2 (17.7–30.4)	0.19 (0.18–0.20)
Photophobia	79	87	6.0 (5.2–6.8)	0.24 (0.23–0.26)
Phonophobia	67	87	5.2 (4.5–5.9)	0.38 (0.36–0.40)
Exacerbation by physical activity	81	78	3.7 (3.4–4.0)	0.24 (0.23–0.26)
Unilateral	66	78	3.1 (2.8–3.3)	0.43 (0.41–0.45)
Throbbing or pulsating	76	77	3.3 (3.1–3.6)	0.32 (0.30–0.33)
Duration 4–24 hours	57	67	1.7 (1.5–2.0)	0.64 (0.58–0.71)
Duration 24–72 hours	13	91	1.4 (1.0–2.0)	0.96 (0.92–1.0)
Duration less than 4 hours	26	51	0.52 (0.44–0.61)	1.5 (1.3–1.6)

report high levels of psychologic or emotional tension. Faced with a clinical situation like the one described above, many physicians might consider sending the patient for physical therapy or prescribing a muscle relaxant, both treatments for tension-type headache.

The assumption that these symptoms are indicative of tension-type headache probably stems from the fact that the term "tension-type headache" suggests that "tension" of some sort – perhaps psychologic or muscle – may be the cause of headache. This is a diagnostic pitfall, however, since evidence to support these views is lacking. Although patients with tension-type headache do, as a group, have more pericranial tenderness than patients with migraine, muscle pain, especially neck pain, is nonetheless very common in migraine patients.

Electromyography (EMG) is not useful in distinguishing between the two disorders. Over a third of migraine patients report neck pain with at least some of their attacks. The neck pain can come before, during, or even after attacks; this variability in its time course makes it unlikely that neck pain is the "cause" of headache. Both migraine and tension-type headache patients have lower thresholds for experiencing pain with pressure on muscles than do people without headache; interestingly, the upper trapezius is the most common site of tenderness.

Similarly, elevated levels of psychologic and emotional distress are common in patients who seek medical care for stubborn headaches, and may in part reflect the impact of poorly controlled headaches on

their lives, rather than the other way around. It is certainly the case, however, that emotional stress is a commonly mentioned "trigger" of headache in both tension-type and migraine patients. In fact, as demonstrated in Table 1.2, there is considerable overlap of commonly reported triggers between migraine and tension-type headache. This underscores the surprisingly *low* diagnostic value of many triggers and other historical features commonly thought to be pathognomonic of one or the other disorder. Having patients keep a headache diary, such as the one illustrated in Table 1.3, should help in distinguishing between tension-type and migraine headaches when the diagnosis is uncertain.

In a large multinational study, over a thousand patients consulting physicians with a complaint of headache were asked to keep careful diaries of their headaches for up to six months. These records were then reviewed by headache experts, and the final diagnosis of headache type was compared with the diagnosis the treating physician had made at the patient's first visit. When physicians made a diagnosis of migraine, this diagnosis was correct in 98% of patients. When physicians diagnosed non-migraine headaches, such as tension-type headache, the diagnosis ultimately turned out to be wrong in 82% of patients. The predominant reason for misdiagnosis was having missed migraine. The authors of this study concluded that "These findings support the diagnostic approach of considering episodic, disabling primary headaches with an otherwise normal physical exam

Table 1.3. A headache diary that can help distinguish between migraine and tension-type headache

	Date	Date	Date	Date	Date
Just before the headache began, was there any disturbance of vision?	Yes OR No	Yes OR No	Yes OR No	Yes OR No	Yes OR No
Just before the headache began, did you have any weakness, numbness, or speech problems?	Yes OR No	Yes OR No	Yes OR No	Yes OR No	Yes OR No
What did the pain feel like?	Pounding, throbbing OR Steady, tightening, squeezing	Pounding, throbbing OR Steady, tightening, squeezing	Pounding, throbbing OR Steady, tightening, squeezing	Pounding, throbbing OR Steady, tightening, squeezing	Pounding, throbbing OR Steady, tightening, squeezing
Where was the headache located?	Right side of the head Left side of the head Both sides of the head	Right side of the head Left side of the head Both sides of the head	Right side of the head Left side of the head Both sides of the head	Right side of the head Left side of the head Both sides of the head	Right side of the head Left side of the head Both sides of the head
Did you experience nausea or vomiting with the headache?	Nausea OR Vomiting OR Both	Nausea OR Vomiting OR Both	Nausea OR Vomiting OR Both	Nausea OR Vomiting OR Both	Nausea OR Vomiting OR Both
Did the headache get worse with physical activity or keep you from being active?	Yes OR No	Yes OR No	Yes OR No	Yes OR No	Yes OR No
During the headache, were you bothered by light?	Yes OR No	Yes OR No	Yes OR No	Yes OR No	Yes OR No
During the headache, were you bothered by sound?	Yes OR No	Yes OR No	Yes OR No	Yes OR No	Yes OR No
At its worst, was your headache pain mild, moderate, or severe?	Mild OR Moderate OR Severe	Mild OR Moderate OR Severe	Mild OR Moderate OR Severe	Mild OR Moderate OR Severe	Mild OR Moderate OR Severe
How long did your headache last?	Less than 4 hours OR 4–72 hours OR Longer than 72 hours or constant	Less than 4 hours OR 4–72 hours OR Longer than 72 hours or constant	Less than 4 hours OR 4–72 hours OR Longer than 72 hours or constant	Less than 4 hours OR 4–72 hours OR Longer than 72 hours or constant	Less than 4 hours OR 4–72 hours OR Longer than 72 hours or constant

to be migraine in the absence of contradictory evidence."

In summary, once a diagnosis of a primary headache disorder has been made, it is appropriate for physicians to *think migraine*. Prospectively kept headache diaries are invaluable in making the diagnosis, as is a careful and probing history. Physicians should avoid placing too much emphasis on historical features such as pain location, muscle tension, psychologic stress, and headache triggers. In contrast, a history of nausea in conjunction with headaches is highly predictive of migraine.

Diagnosis

Migraine without aura.

Tip

Migraine often presents with features assumed to be highly characteristic of tension-type headache. Most patients consulting physicians for troublesome headaches have migraine and not tension-type headache.

Migraine with or without aura?

Case

An 18-year-old woman sought a second opinion because she had been told she should not use estrogen-containing contraceptives – "the pill" – due to her diagnosis of migraine with aura. Instead she was prescribed a progesterone-only pill but that had caused weight gain and irregular periods and she recently stopped it. She was not interested in an intrauterine device and did not think she would be able to use barrier methods reliably. Most of her friends were taking "regular birth control pills" continuously and thus did not have any withdrawal bleeding, and she wanted to do this too. The patient's headaches occurred only four or five times a year. She wondered if she might be able to use estrogen-containing oral contraceptives despite her headaches, since she did not want to get pregnant.

What important piece of information is still missing in this case?

It is not obvious that this patient's diagnosis of migraine with aura is correct. In fact, all we know is that she has headaches once every few months. In order to establish that she has migraine and/or aura, we need to know the details of her headaches and any accompanying features. In this case, the patient confirmed a diagnosis of migraine by describing unilateral, pounding headaches with nausea that last half a day when untreated and were severe enough to prevent her from usual activities, including her usual exercise routine. When asked if she has any warning signs, or other things that occur in association with her headaches, she mentioned that sometimes her vision was blurry prior to a headache. She added that occasionally "the pain is so bad I can't see." When questioned closely, she clarified this by saying that she actu-

Table 1.4. The Visual Aura Rating Scale (VARS)

Visual symptom characteristic	Risk score
Duration 5–60 minutes	3
Develops gradually over 5 or more minutes	2
Scotoma	2
Zig-zag line (fortification spectrum)	2
Unilateral (homonymous)	1
Maximum VARS score	10
Migraine with aura diagnosis	≥5

Adapted from: Eriksen *et al.* The Visual Aura Rating Scale (VARS) for migraine aura diagnosis. *Cephalalgia.* 2005;10:801–10, with permission.

ally could see just fine, but shut her eyes tightly because the pain was so bad. Even with further questioning she did not report additional associated symptoms.

Does this patient have migraine with aura?

Aura is a focal neurologic event, which means that it includes symptoms that can be attributed to dysfunction in a particular part of the brain. Aura symptoms can be visual, sensory, motor, or mixed. Visual aura is by far the most common form of aura. Most people who have any form of aura will, at least occasionally, *also* have visual aura. Common features of visual aura are the *scotoma*, an area of decreased visual acuity or visual loss (not seeing something that is there) or a positive visual phenomenon (seeing something that is not there) such as a zig-zag line. These areas of visual loss or distortion are surrounded by areas of normal vision. Figure 1.1 shows a typical scintillating scotoma drawn by a patient who has migraine with aura, who perceived that this scotoma was shimmering and pulsating. Often a scotoma will start as a small area in the center of the visual field, and then expand and move to the periphery of the visual field before fading away.

In migraine with aura, the aura typically precedes the headache; symptoms begin and fade away gradually and do not last longer than an hour. Symptoms also are unilateral (or, in the case of visual symptoms, homonymous – which means they occur in only half of the visual field). Once the aura begins to fade away, it is usually quickly followed by a headache. Sometimes aura can occur without a headache. Table 1.4 reproduces the Visual Aura Rating Scale, which is a method of diagnosing visual aura. This scale assigns points for the presence of certain aura symptoms; to diagnose

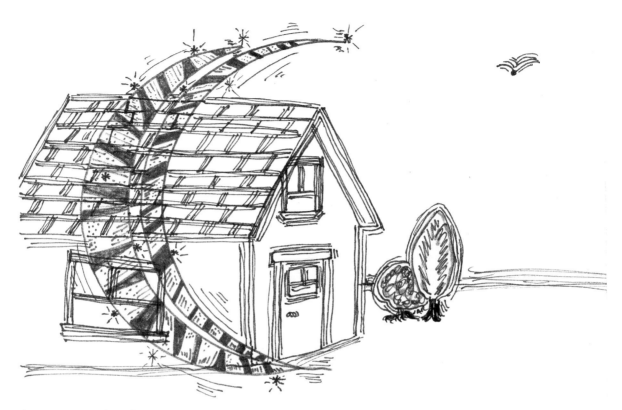

STARTED
10: PM

Figure 1.1 A typical scintillating migraine scotoma. Note the patient's attempt to convey the shimmering sensation of movement and vibration in the crescent-shaped, zig-zag visual phenomenon (fortification spectrum) that is drawn.

aura reliably requires a score of at least 5 of the possible 10 points.

Are estrogen-containing contraceptives contraindicated in women who have migraine with aura?

Migraine with aura is associated with an increased risk of ischemic stroke and so is the use of exogenous estrogens. The added risk of stroke with each of these things individually is quite small, but it is higher in the presence of additional risk factors, such as smoking or increasing age. Although it is difficult to place absolute numbers on these risks, authors of these studies note the increase in risk is likely to be multiplicative rather than additive. Because of these risks, guidelines from a number of authoritative groups, including the American College of Obstetrics and Gynecology, rec-ommend against the use of estrogen-containing contraceptives in women who are over 35 and have any type of migraine, or women who have migraine with aura, regardless of age.

Discussion

This patient's headaches met criteria for migraine but the visual events she described were not consistent with a diagnosis of aura. Thus, she has migraine without aura and the use of estrogen-containing contraceptives is not contraindicated. General visual blurring and visual sensitivity, while commonly reported by migraine patients, are not aura. The blurred vision described by this patient is better thought of as part of her headache prodrome. Prodromal events occur before a headache but are not focal neurologic events. Changes in mood, appetite, or concentration are commonly reported migraine prodrome symptoms.

Distinguishing between migraine aura and migraine prodromal or associated symptoms is important because evidence that migraine with aura increases the risk of stroke continues to mount.

Diagnosis

Migraine without aura.

Tip

Focal neurologic symptoms such as positive or negative visual phenomena or sensory disturbance are required for a diagnosis of migraine aura. Since essentially all patients with any sort of aura *also* have visual aura, it is only necessary to establish a history of visual aura in order to make a diagnosis.

Severe unilateral headaches in a man

Case

A 30-year-old man presented for management of cluster headache diagnosed by another physician. He reported an average of three headaches a month that tended to occur towards the end of the month: "They come in bunches. As soon as one is over I might get another one a day or so later." Headaches were located over his forehead bilaterally and he described them as throbbing, with occasional mild nausea. He was not sure how long headaches would last without treatment because for many years he had been using subcutaneous sumatriptan as soon as headaches began.

Is this history consistent with a diagnosis of cluster headache?

Not all elements of the history in this case fit with cluster headache. The bilateral nature of the pain is not typical of cluster headache, which is a strictly unilateral headache, usually located behind an eye. The throbbing nature of the pain is more typical of migraine than of cluster headache, in which the pain is usually described as sharp. The patient does report that headaches come "in bunches," but the period of several days between attacks is not typical of true cluster headaches, in which short headaches usually occur daily or even several times a day. The patient's response to sumatriptan is not helpful in clarifying the diag-

nosis, since sumatriptan is effective for the treatment of individual attacks of both migraine and cluster headache.

Additional questioning about the features and duration of individual headaches, as well as the pattern of attacks over time, can distinguish migraine from cluster headache. In this case, when questioned, the patient reported that as a child he would occasionally vomit with his headaches, and that they could last up to a day. Both of these features are more consistent with a diagnosis of migraine than with cluster headache.

Why was the diagnosis of migraine missed in this patient?

The criteria for diagnosing migraine are the same for men and women. Unfortunately, they do not fully reflect differences between the sexes in the clinical profile and presentation of migraine. Evidence from the American Migraine Prevalence and Prevention Study shows that, *on average*, men with migraine have fewer clinical features of migraine than women with the disorder. That is, men with migraine are less likely than women with migraine to report nausea, vomiting, photo or phonophobia. That does not mean they do not have these symptoms, but rather that they have *fewer* of these symptoms than women. Because doctors rely on these characteristic historical features to make the clinical diagnosis of migraine, men are at a disadvantage in receiving a correct diagnosis.

In this case, it seems likely that the patient's physician correctly recognized that cluster headache is more common in men and migraine is more common in women. She failed, though, to realize that neither headache type occurs exclusively in one sex.

Discussion

In addition to the fact that men with migraine report fewer migraine-associated features than women, there are other ways in which migraine may differ in men compared with women. For example, men with migraine report that, on average, their attacks are shorter, less severe, and less disabling than migraine attacks in women. Males with migraine also are not exposed to the potent migraine trigger of monthly changes in sex hormones as are females with the disorder, so there is no increase in migraine prevalence at puberty in males. This is in contrast to the situation in females, where migraine prevalence increases substantially at puberty and remains higher than the prevalence in men even into old age. This suggests that female hormones have an enduring effect on migraine susceptibility. In addition to this lifelong impact on disease risk, women with migraine also experience periodic increases in migraine attack frequency because of hormonal changes with the menstrual cycle.

Although the prevalence of migraine in men is lower than in women, migraine is an extremely common disorder in both sexes. By age 80, the cumulative incidence of migraine in men reaches almost 18% – meaning that almost one in five men will experience migraine during his lifetime. As high as this number is, though, it is certainly lower than the 44% lifetime cumulative incidence of migraine in women. Thus it is understandable that some physicians – and patients – view migraine as a "woman's disease." Unfortunately, the result is that when men seek care for their headaches, clinicians may be less likely to consider migraine as a diagnosis.

Diagnosis

Migraine without aura.

Tip

Migraine is more common in women than in men, but it is highly prevalent in both sexes. Diagnosis of migraine in men may be challenging because men with migraine have fewer typical migraine symptoms than do women.

Frequent, severe episodic headaches in a woman

Case

A 45-year-old woman had been treated for many years for a diagnosis of migraine. She treated individual headaches with 10 mg of oral rizatriptan. Headaches typically awakened her from sleep and were extremely severe, sometimes associated with nausea. They lasted two or three hours, so by the time the rizatriptan became effective the headache was almost over. For the last year her headaches had occurred nightly or every other night, although prior to that she would have headaches "only two or three months at a time and I could deal with that." With no break in her headaches she reported being sleep-deprived and anx-

ious. She was taking 160 mg of long-acting propranolol and 200 mg of topiramate daily. At the last visit she reported that the medications were ineffective and that she was "tired and can't think straight. I am about to lose my job."

Has this patient developed chronic migraine?

Chronic migraine is unlikely in this patient. Although daily, her headaches are short, usually lasting three hours or less. Another clue that this patient may not have migraine is that the headaches have not responded to aggressive treatment with the typically used migraine preventive treatments of propranolol and topiramate. Of course, not all patients with migraine improve with appropriate preventive treatment, but failure to respond to migraine-specific therapy may also suggest an alternative diagnosis. Most features of this patient's headaches are consistent with a diagnosis of cluster headache and not migraine. Additional questioning about the features and duration of individual headaches, as well as the pattern of attacks over time, can distinguish the two disorders (see Table 1.5).

In this case, the patient gave additional history which further clarified the diagnosis. For ten years before the onset of her daily headache she had just one or two bouts of daily or near-daily headache each year. Those periods of frequent headache lasted on average two months and seemed to come in the fall and spring of each year. Individual headaches have always been located behind the left eye and associated with left-sided nasal congestion and tearing of the left eye. Although they last only two to three hours, headaches are extremely severe, "like someone is stabbing me in the eye with a hot poker." The patient is restless and paces the floor during attacks. Her story is more consistent with episodic cluster headache that has now become chronic than with chronic migraine.

Why was cluster headache misdiagnosed in this patient?

The presentation of cluster headache is highly characteristic but the disorder is uncommon. In contrast to migraine, it is more frequent in men than in women. It is caused by dysfunction of central nervous system pain control mechanisms and has distinctive circadian and circannual features. Most physicians have never

Table 1.5. Distinguishing migraine from cluster headache

Pain features	Migraine	Cluster headache
Location	Often unilateral over the temple or forehead area but may be bilateral	Strictly unilateral; typically highly localized to behind one eye
Duration of attack	4–72 hours (adults)	15 minutes to 3 hours*
Frequency of attacks	Sporadic. Can "cluster" in bunches but rarely follow the distinctive pattern of true cluster headache	Attacks can occur once every other day up to eight times a day (for more than half of the time during an active cluster bout – headache frequency may increase or taper slowly at the beginning or end of a bout)*
Associated features	Nausea, vomiting, photo and phonophobia	Agitation or restlessness OR one of the following seven symptoms or signs must occur on the side of the headache: (1) eye redness or tearing; (2) nasal congestion or runny nose; (3) edema of the eyelid; (4) sweating of the forehead and face; (5) flushing of the forehead and face; (6) a feeling of ear fullness; (7) decreased pupil size or ptosis*
Sex ratio	Females > males	Males > females
Behavior during attack	Quiet; prefer to lie quietly in a dark room	Agitated, restless
Temporal features	Attacks typically occur at random and are not easily predictable	Attacks commonly occur at specific times of the day or night. Named for the way they "cluster" together occurring daily or almost daily for 2- to 3-month bouts. In episodic cluster headache these bouts are separated by periods of remission lasting at least a month; in chronic cluster headache remissions do not occur or are shorter than a month

* According to ICHD-3 beta, all of these criteria must be met in at least five attacks in order to make a diagnosis of cluster headache.

seen or treated a patient with cluster headache and may be especially likely to miss it in women, perhaps because women with cluster headache are more likely than men to have migrainous symptoms such as nausea. Diagnostic delay is common in any case, however, with one study showing that the median time from onset to symptoms was three years, with a range of one week to 48 years.

This patient's partial response to a triptan medication may also have contributed to confusion about the diagnosis, since many doctors think of triptans as "migraine medications." In fact, triptans are useful for treating individual attacks of cluster headache as well as migraine.

Discussion

Cluster headache is correctly diagnosed after the initial evaluation only 21% of the time. The most common incorrect diagnoses made in these patients are migraine (34%) and sinusitis (21%). Migraine and cluster can be differentiated on the basis of headache duration, frequency, seasonality, triggering factors, and pain behavior during a headache. The presence of autonomic features is usually part of the presentation of cluster headache but is not strictly necessary for diagnosis if the patient is agitated or paces during an attack. Aura is very rarely seen in cluster headache but should not rule out the diagnosis.

Preventive treatment of cluster headache differs from that of migraine. Typical migraine preventive drugs such as topiramate and propranolol are unlikely to be helpful for cluster headache. In this case the delay in accurate diagnosis has delayed institution of appropriate preventive treatment aimed at reducing or eliminating attacks of cluster headache. The mainstays of prevention for cluster headache are verapamil or lithium. There are no US Food and Drug Administration (FDA)-approved preventive treatments for cluster headache, but clinical experience shows that one or the other of these drugs, or occasionally the combination, brings the disorder under control for most patients.

The slow onset of action of oral triptans makes them a poor treatment choice for most patients with cluster headache. Subcutaneous sumatriptan, which patients can self-administer via an auto-injector, has a more rapid onset of action. It is the only triptan formulation that is FDA approved for treatment of cluster headache.

Diagnosis

Chronic cluster headache.

Tip

Cluster headache is more common in men but can also occur in women. It is often missed in both sexes.

Headache with disturbing visual perceptual alterations

Case

A 43-year-old woman reported she had experienced bad headaches since childhood. In response to the open-ended question "Does anything else happen with your headaches?" she tearfully related symptoms that "might sound crazy." At age 11 she awoke one morning and, while still lying in bed, realized that her hands did not feel "like they belonged to me." When she held them in front of her they looked long and twig-like, not like normal hands. These perceptions disappeared in a few minutes, but she then developed a severe, unilateral headache with vomiting. Over the years she has had many similar episodes of visual abnormality, all followed by severe headaches that meet criteria for migraine. Once while driving she noticed that a fence and the trees behind it appeared weirdly distorted in size and shape. This abnormality was limited to the left side of her visual field but was still present when she covered her left eye. The patient has discussed her headaches with other physicians, but not her visual symptoms, because of her fear that they might be interpreted as psychiatric in nature.

What conditions may be causing these symptoms?

Bizarre visual illusions and distortions that affect the apparent size, volume, shape, or position in space of objects are described with the term "metamorphopsia." Metamorphopsia is part of *Alice in Wonderland* syndrome, thought to be a particular sort of migraine with aura, but can also reflect structural eye disease (usually retinal) and has been reported in patients with idiopathic intracranial hypertension. Metamorphopsia is a common symptom in age-related macular degeneration or other diseases that affect the macula. Typically, patients will complain of "waves" or "bending" in objects known to be straight, such as doorframes or roof lines. Careful examination of the retina, as well as ancillary testing when necessary, including Amsler grids or fluorescein angiography, can usu-

ally identify non-aura disorders that might be causing metamorphopsia.

In this case, the symptoms were associated with migraine and occur in consistent temporal relation to the headaches. The patient was otherwise healthy, and Alice in Wonderland syndrome is the most likely diagnosis.

How should this patient be treated?

As is the case for more typical forms of aura, there are no clinically available treatments that will specifically treat the aura of Alice in Wonderland syndrome. (Intravenous ketamine reportedly aborts aura in about half of sufferers, but is not a practical approach to outpatient therapy.) Rather, treatment is aimed at reducing the number of migraine episodes using typical migraine preventive therapy, and also focuses treating the pain of any headache that accompanies the aura. Triptans and other vasoconstrictive agents are *not* contraindicated in this disorder or in migraine with more typical forms of aura.

Discussion

This unusual form of aura is called "Alice in Wonderland syndrome" because of its similarity to the experiences of Lewis Carroll's fictional Alice in Wonderland. It was first described in 1955. The visual abnormalities in Alice in Wonderland syndrome are more peculiar than those of typical visual aura. The visual disturbance may also be associated with alterations in the perception of time, or feelings of depersonalization or derealization, which seem to be what the patient in this vignette experienced during her first childhood episode. Figures 1.2 and 1.3 depict an illustration of the metamorphopsic visual distortions of this illness.

Alice in Wonderland syndrome is said to be more common in children than adults. In our experience this apparent difference in prevalence may stem from the reluctance of adults to describe symptoms they fear will result in stigmatization. Children may be less worried about this. In their 2008 book *Headache in Children and Adolescents*, Winner *et al.* report that "The children rarely seem frightened by these illusions and relate the experience in enthusiastic detail. Witnesses of the child's event will either remark that the child has an unusual, bemused look on the face or describe the child changing body positions so that they can 'get under a low ceiling.'"

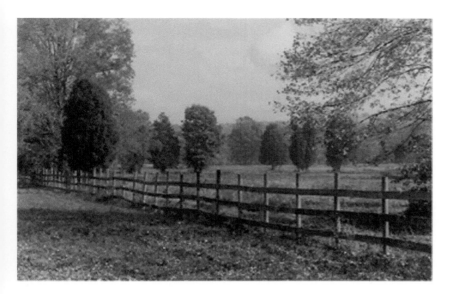

Figure 1.2 Normal vision.

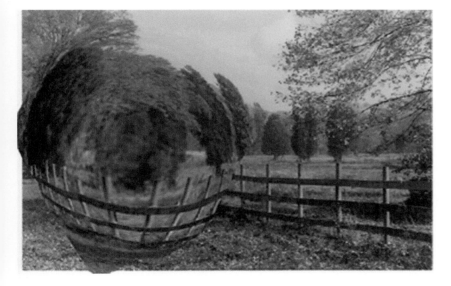

Figure 1.3 Metamorphopsia in left hemi-field of vision.

Diagnosis

Alice in Wonderland syndrome – commonly thought to be a form of migraine with aura.

Tip

Treatment for Alice in Wonderland syndrome does not differ from that of typical visual aura with migraine. It is important to recognize it because the diagnosis is reassuring for patients who may otherwise fear the symptoms mean they are "crazy."

"Cluster migraine"

Case

A 27-year-old woman reported frequent headaches characterized by retro-orbital pain, always on the right, up to four hours in duration but usually shorter because she had learned to treat the headaches immediately with sumatriptan. The pain could become severe quite quickly, and when the pain was at its worst it was a 10/10 and had a stabbing quality. With the most severe pain she also noticed tearing and redness of the right eye. When the pain was milder she preferred to be lying down, but at its worst, "it doesn't matter what I do, it just hurts." There was associated photophobia and some nausea but no aura. She had noticed that she had times when her headaches occur very frequently, up to twice a day, and other times when she would have several weeks without a headache. In the past she had been told she had "cluster migraines." One of her other physicians thought she had cluster headache and started verapamil, which had improved the frequency of headaches only mildly.

Are this patient's autonomic features helpful in making a diagnosis?

Autonomic features (lacrimation, conjunctival injection, forehead or facial sweating, miosis, ptosis, eyelid edema, rhinorrhea, or nasal congestion) are a defining characteristic of the headaches classified as trigeminal autonomic cephalagias (TACs), including cluster headache. The latest version of the headache classification, ICHD-3 beta, however, does not require that they be present in order to make a diagnosis of cluster headache if the patient has the characteristic restlessness or physical agitation that are seen in cluster headache. ICHD-3 beta has also added a sensation of fullness in the ear to the list of autonomic features that may be seen in cluster headache patients.

Headache-associated autonomic signs or symptoms are not unique to cluster headache or other TACs, however. They may be seen in association with migraine headaches as well. In one population-based study, one of four patients with migraine had unilateral autonomic symptoms with at least some attacks. One study also found that migraines occurring with unilateral autonomic symptoms were more severe than those occurring without. In a prospective study comparing patients recruited from a headache center with migraine headaches with those with cluster headache, 56% of patients with migraine had cranial autonomic symptoms with some of their headaches. Thus, the presence of autonomic features in this case does not necessarily indicate a diagnosis of cluster

headache, and is also compatible with a diagnosis of migraine.

Is "cluster migraine" an appropriate diagnosis in this patient?

The ICHD recognizes Cluster headache, one of the TACs, and Migraine as two separate categories of headaches. "Cluster migraine" is not a recognized term in any edition of the ICHD, including ICHD-3 beta, and this term often causes a great deal of confusion among patients and providers.

Migraine sufferers sometimes hear the term "cluster" and relate this to their experience of having intervals of frequent headaches interspersed with times when headaches are less frequent. In our experience, these changes in headache frequency are commonly the result of environmental factors such as changes in lifestyle (a move, a new job), stress, changes in sleep habits, or dietary changes. Intrinsic factors such as hormonal changes associated with menstrual periods may also contribute to cyclical changes in susceptibility to migraine. All of these things may lower the threshold for the development of migraine, resulting in an increase in headache frequency. Another phenomenon often leading to "runs" of migraine activity is rebound headache, in which withdrawal from symptomatic medications used to treat a previous headache leads to another headache.

The patient described in this case meets criteria for migraine without aura and not for cluster headache, which was described earlier in this chapter. The term "cluster migraine" is not a recognized diagnosis and should be avoided.

Discussion

Autonomic activation during headache is a function of the trigeminal autonomic reflex. This reflex occurs when nociceptive input from the trigeminal system, as occurs during headache, stimulates the trigeminocervical complex. This in turn stimulates the superior salivatory nucleus, which gives rise to autonomic fibers providing innervation to the head. Autonomic symptoms are most commonly seen in the TACs, but can also occur in migraine. Compared to cranial autonomic symptoms in TACs, the symptoms in migraine are more likely to be bilateral, mild or moderate in severity, and to occur inconsistently with headache attacks. Lacrimation is the autonomic symptom most commonly associated with migraines. In contrast, the autonomic symptoms associated with cluster headaches are unilateral 80% of the time and almost always ipsilateral to the headache when they are unilateral.

Distinguishing between "runs" of migraines and a bout of true cluster headache can occasionally be challenging. A very careful history should be taken with attention to headache duration, location of pain, other associated features such as phono or photophobia, and frequency. By ICHD criteria, migraine and cluster should not overlap. Accurate diagnosis can be difficult when treatment has eliminated features needed for diagnosis as, for example, might occur with treatment that shortens the duration of migraine headaches. In these cases, a description of typical *untreated* headaches can be very useful.

In contrast to migraine, cluster headache bouts are often distinctly seasonal, possibly because of headache triggering by changes in day length or seasonally related changes in circadian rhythms. This seasonal periodicity is uncommon in migraine. Within individual patients, the seasonality of cluster headache bouts may be stereotyped over many years. Some cluster headache patients are able to predict months in advance when a cluster bout will occur.

It can also be helpful to determine if the patient has headaches outside of the identified "cluster" periods. A patient with episodic cluster headache rarely has any headaches at all outside of their cluster periods or bouts, while patients with migraine will usually have occasional isolated headaches even during their "good periods." While this is a general rule, it is not always true, however, since an occasional patient with chronic cluster headache (defined as cluster headaches occurring for over a year without remission or with remission for less than one month) will experience occasional isolated headaches. The true cluster headache pattern, with periods of headaches occurring from one every other day to eight per day followed by complete remission periods, is almost never seen in migraine.

Diagnosis

Migraine without aura.

Tip

Migraine headaches can present with autonomic features in up to half of patients. "Cluster migraine" is a confusing term which should be avoided.

Stabbing headaches in a migraineur

Case

A 39-year-old woman presented to the office with a "new headache type." She had a long-standing history of episodic migraine without aura. Headaches had increased in frequency over the last three years. She attributed this to increased stress from having a second child four years ago and from increased responsibilities at work. Her migraines had gone from occurring about once a week to as many as three per week.

In the last four months, she had also developed severe stabbing or "shock-like" pains behind the eye, in the temple, or in the parietal area on either side. These lasted only a few seconds at a time but sometimes occurred in volleys of up to 10 or 20 closely spaced jabs of pain in the course of an hour. She had some days without this new type of pain but more typically the pain happened between one and ten times a day. She had seen her dentist last week for a routine checkup, and had been told her symptoms might be due to trigeminal neuralgia. There were no autonomic features and no provoking factors that she was able to identify. She continued to have her typical migraine without aura headaches and these had not changed in character or frequency. Her neurologic examination was normal.

What is the differential diagnosis of sharp, stabbing pain in a migraineur?

Several disorders can produce brief, stabbing head pain. The differential diagnosis is worth knowing because complaints of sharp, stabbing head pain are remarkably common. Possible causes include (1) a trigeminal or other neuralgia; (2) primary stabbing headache; or (3) one of two uncommon forms of ultra-short unilateral stabbing headache in the TAC family known as SUNCT (Short-lasting, Unilateral, Neuralgiform headache attacks with Conjunctival injection and Tearing) or SUNA (Short-lasting Unilateral Neuralgiform attacks with Autonomic features – with the autonomic features required for diagnosis being identical to those required for a diagnosis of cluster headache). Both SUNCT and SUNA produce pain that is similar in location to that of cluster headache but much shorter, in the range of 1–600 seconds.

Table 1.6. Clinical characteristics of primary stabbing headache

Pain occurs as a single stab or may be a series of stabs

Individual stabs last only a few seconds and may recur with irregular frequency

Stabs may be from one to many per day

Pain primarily occurs in the orbit, temple, or parietal areas, in the distribution of the first division of the trigeminal nerve

No accompanying symptoms, including no autonomic symptoms

The pain characteristics in this case are similar to those of trigeminal neuralgia, but trigeminal neuralgia typically does not switch sides or locations. Trigger zones, areas of the face or mucosa where stimulation reliably reproduces the pain, are frequently but not always seen in trigeminal neuralgia. This patient does not report a history of pain triggering. In the absence of autonomic features, a TAC such as SUNCT or SUNA is highly unlikely. Thus, the most likely etiology for the stabbing pain in this patient is primary stabbing headache. The clinical characteristics of primary stabbing headache are listed in Table 1.6.

Primary stabbing headache is more prevalent than either trigeminal neuralgia or SUNCT/SUNA and is very frequently seen in patients with migraine, where it is often located in the same area where the migraine pain is felt.

Does any further workup need to be done for this new headache type?

Secondary causes of stabbing headaches have been described in case reports, and include herpetic meningoencephalitis, ischemic stroke, acute thalamic hemorrhage, and meningioma. Posterior fossa lesions may present with SUNA- or SUNCT-like symptoms. In this case, the four-month duration of symptoms without worsening, the nonfocal neurologic examination, and the relative youth and good health of the patient are all reassuring. In our clinical experience, the development of stabbing headache in a migraineur often accompanies worsening of the primary headache. However, stabbing headaches presenting in older patients, with progressive worsening of symptoms, an abnormal neurologic examination, or failure to respond to appropriate treatment are all situations requiring a workup for secondary causes. If this patient had presented acutely with a new stabbing headache and associated neurologic symptoms, further evaluation would be warranted.

Discussion

Primary or idiopathic stabbing headache has been known by many names over the years, including "jabs and jolts" and "ice-pick" headaches. The pathophysiology is not well understood. It occurs in about 2% of the general population, but is even more prevalent in patients with other primary headache disorders. Up to 40% of migraineurs and 27% of patients with tension-type headache may have comorbid primary stabbing headache, and it has also been described in patients with hemicrania continua (one of the TACs). In these cases, the stabs tend to occur in the location most affected by the underlying primary headache type. The frequency of attacks can vary from a single stab a few times a year to up to 50 per day. In some cases the stabs start out infrequently and progress to volleys of stabs lasting minutes to hours. Stabbing headaches occurring outside the distribution of the trigeminal nerve have also been described with some regularity.

Classically, primary stabbing headache is considered an indomethacin-responsive headache and indomethacin is first-line treatment when treatment is indicated. If the stabs are infrequent, reassurance about their benign nature may be all that is needed. About 30% of patients may not improve with indomethacin. Case reports have also described improvement with gabapentin, celecoxib, and melatonin in those who did not respond to or could not tolerate indomethacin. Although not a phenomenon described in the literature, our clinical experience is that occasional stabbing headaches in migraineurs often improve with appropriate treatment of the migraine itself. This approach may spare the patient treatment with indomethacin, which like all anti-inflammatory drugs can have serious gastric side effects.

In this case, the patient's underlying migraine headaches were increasing in frequency due to environmental factors. Because of the increased frequency, she was started on amitriptyline for prevention of migraine. At her follow-up visit two months later, the migraines had returned to their previous weekly pattern and the stabbing headaches had completely resolved.

Diagnosis

Primary stabbing headache in the setting of migraine without aura.

Tip

Primary stabbing headache is commonly associated with migraine and does not necessarily require a workup for secondary headache if there are no accompanying neurologic features.

Chronic continuous headache with acute onset

Case

A 29-year-old right-handed female presented for evaluation of a "life-altering headache." There was no family history of migraine and she recalled no headache problems during high school or college. On September 8 (about four months prior to consultation), she had awakened with a headache that never resolved. She recalled nothing unusual around that time, specifically no serious physical or emotional trauma or illness that had been associated with the onset of headache. She did recall having a mild upper respiratory infection several days before the headache began. She described the headache as a pressure sensation behind the left eye, usually 3/10 in severity but reaching 5/10 at its worst, always present from the time she woke up in the morning to the time she went to sleep. This pain had been unremitting since onset. She had mild nausea with the headache but otherwise no associated symptoms or autonomic features and the headache did not wake her from sleep.

Evaluation had included a normal magnetic resonance angiogram and venogram of the brain; normal CT angiogram; normal lumbar puncture with opening pressure of 150 mm cerebrospinal fluid (CSF); normal routine laboratory studies; negative Lyme titers; and normal antinuclear antibody (ANA) level, thyroid-stimulating hormone (TSH) level, erythrocyte sedimentation rate (ESR), and C-reactive protein (CRP) level. She had been diagnosed with migraine but failed to improve with aggressive trials of typical migraine preventive drugs, except for a brief reduction in pain severity with a course of oral prednisone. She had initially been unable to work and had moved back in with her parents. Recently, however, she had returned to work after several months away because her disability

Table 1.7. Clinical characteristics of new daily persistent headache

Head pain for more than 3 months that is constant
Unremitting from onset or within 24 hours of onset
No completely characteristic features, although migrainous features such as photophobia, phonophobia, or nausea are frequently described
Female predominance with F:M ratio 1.4–2.5:1
Onset of pain is clearly remembered by the patient, although fewer than half of patients recall a triggering event

benefits had expired. She reported being frustrated by her symptoms and inability to plan activity.

What is the differential diagnosis in this case?

The differential diagnosis for unremitting headache with acute onset is lengthy. Most of the potential causes are secondary forms of headache in which the head pain is due to some underlying process. For this reason, an extensive workup for secondary causes of headache (as was done in this case) is necessary. In this case, the patient had appropriate testing but no secondary cause of headache had been identified.

A number of primary headache disorders can produce the clinical scenario of acute onset, unrelenting headache, and should be considered in this patient. These include hemicrania continua, chronic migraine, chronic tension-type headache, and new daily persistent headache (usually referred to by its initials of NDPH).

One highly characteristic feature of NDPH is that many patients (about half) recall the precise date when the headache started. This is so characteristic of the illness that the diagnostic criteria for NDPH state that the onset must be "distinct and clearly remembered." In our experience many patients also note the exact time of onset with great precision, for example "My headache began at 5:02 p.m. on September 8, 2003." Although the headache may pursue a "stuttering" course initially, it quickly becomes constant. In fact, diagnostic criteria require that the headache become constant within 24 hours of onset (see Table 1.7 for other clinical characteristics). When the onset of a refractory headache is so clearly recalled, and in the absence of abnormal tests or examinations, a diagnosis of NDPH is far more likely than another primary headache disorder.

What advice can be provided to the patient about the natural history of NDPH, and is any further workup required?

Many patients are relieved to be given a name for their condition. By the time a patient receives this diagnosis, they have usually had an extensive evaluation and some have developed a conviction that doctors have no idea what is wrong and have "given up." Clarification that the condition is recognized, classified, and studied can itself be reassuring. Patients are sometimes disappointed by the lack of good quality information about the natural history of the disorder, and by the lack of identified treatments for it. Providers often share their frustration!

The clinical features of NDPH are highly variable, and it can resemble migraine or tension-type headache. In the absence of validated treatments for NDPH, treatment is usually aimed at the phenotype of the particular patient's headaches. Thus, patients whose headaches have features of migraine, such as nausea, may be treated as this patient was, with drugs typically used for migraine. A few specific agents have been reported in the literature as benefitting small numbers of patients. These include the antiepileptic drugs topiramate and gabapentin, the tetracycline derivative doxycycline, corticosteroids, nerve blocks, and mexiletine.

Unfortunately, treatment of this disorder is often unsuccessful. It is still useful to follow the patient regularly and to consider periodically whether other evaluation is warranted. It may be useful, for example, to consider evaluation for an underlying sleep disorder. One other test to consider in patients who have not had it is a lumbar puncture. This can identify disorders of CSF pressure, which in our experience can mimic almost any form of primary headache, including NDPH. A good therapeutic relationship with a patient can also prevent them from trying unproven or dangerous therapies out of desperation.

Discussion

NDPH was first described in 1986 and is currently classified as one of the "other" primary headache disorders (other than migraine, tension-type, and the TACs, that is). It is a diagnosis used with some trepidation by most clinicians, since it is essentially a clinical description of the patient's presentation without clear evidence of any pathophysiologic explanation.

Table 1.8. Secondary causes to rule out in case of apparent new daily persistent headache

Vascular:
- Carotid or vertebral artery dissection
- Cerebral venous thrombosis
- Giant cell arteritis

Nonvascular:
- Disorder of CSF pressure, either high or low
- Meningitis
- Sphenoid sinusitis
- Intranasal (contact point) headache (pain caused by contact of intranasal structures such as nasal septum and nasal turbinate)
- Cervical facet disease
- Intracranial neoplasm or mass lesion
- Medication overuse headache

In addition to more commonly recognized causes of secondary headache that are described in Table 1.8, studies currently suggest two other possible pathophysiologic mechanisms for NDPH. The first is a localized inflammatory process of the central nervous system, perhaps precipitated by a viral illness of some kind. The second theory is that the headache might result from a connective tissue process that leads to joint laxity and cervical spine hypermobility. Some authors have suggested a typical physiognomy for NDPH patients, classically a tall, thin female with a long neck, joint laxity, and hypermobility in the cervical spine.

NDPH appears to be rare. In epidemiologic studies, patients with NDPH are usually grouped together with other people who have "chronic daily headache," and they account for about 10% or less of such patients in most studies. Early descriptions of NDPH emphasized that it was often self-limited and could remit after months to years. Most headache specialists, however, see patients in whom the disorder persists and is resistant to treatment. It is more common in females, with a sex ratio of about 2:1 and an earlier age of onset in females. Although initial reports of NDPH described headache with tension-type characteristics, recent case series suggest that more than half the time the headache may have associated migrainous features. Because of this, the ICHD-3 beta criteria for the disorder mention that the pain "lacks characteristic features, and may be migraine-like or tension-type like, or have elements of both." Similarly, no features are specified by the diagnostic criteria for the location of the headache or the quality of the pain.

As with the patient in this case, the onset of NDPH in many patients has been associated with trigger

Table 1.9. Suggested workup for apparent new daily persistent headache

Neuroimaging: brain MRI with and without gadolinium, MRV

Intra- and extracranial MRA

Lumbar puncture with opening pressure

Table 1.10. Clinical characteristics of hemicrania continua

- Unilateral, unremitting head pain lasting more than 3 months, with mild baseline pain but periodic exacerbations of severe pain
- During exacerbations
  Either: agitation or restlessness OR
  one of the following seven symptoms or signs must occur on the side of the headache:
  (1) eye redness or tearing;
  (2) nasal congestion or runny nose;
  (3) edema of the eyelid;
  (4) sweating of the forehead and face;
  (5) flushing of the forehead and face;
  (6) a feeling of ear fullness;
  (7) decreased pupil size or ptosis
- Response to indomethacin is complete at therapeutic doses

events, particularly a prior infectious, usually viral, illness, a stressful experience, or even an extracranial surgical procedure. It is difficult to evaluate whether these things are causally linked to headache or whether such events are recalled more easily by patients or clinicians who are eagerly searching for a cause of disabling, refractory headaches. In addition to any testing that is indicated by a particular patient's clinical presentation, Table 1.9 lists investigations that should be strongly considered to rule out head trauma or disorders of CSF pressure that can sometimes masquerade as NDPH.

Diagnosis

New daily persistent headache.

Tip

Acute onset of unremitting headache is characteristic of NDPH, but many secondary headaches present similarly. Although NDPH can have features of migraine, tension-type headache, or both, it is a distinct disorder.

Strictly unilateral headache

Case

A 46-year-old woman presented with a 20-year history of disabling headache that had not responded well to treatment. She had been diagnosed with chronic migraine due to severe headaches located on the right side of her head only. When queried specifically about associated symptoms of nausea, vomiting, photo and phonophobia, the patient endorsed only occasional mild nausea. She also reported "shadow headaches," by which she meant that in between episodes of severe headache she had continuous milder pain, also on the right side of the head. Her neurologic examination was normal, as was neuroimaging done in the last year.

She brought past medical records that documented prior unsuccessful treatment trials with a large number of preventive drugs for migraine, including botulinum toxin injections. The doses and duration of these trials appeared to have been adequate. Triptans were never effective for headache exacerbations, but large

doses of ibuprofen gave some relief. She had been told to discontinue this, however, because of worries that her daily use of the drug might be causing medication overuse headache. Her only other medication was over-the-counter pseudoephedrine, which she took for "a problem with my sinus on the right."

What additional question might clarify the diagnosis in this case?

It is understandable that a diagnosis of migraine has been made in this case. Migraine is the most common form of disabling headache in women of childbearing age, and it is often unilateral. Furthermore, it becomes chronic in some patients, who often have mild to moderate constant baseline pain with superimposed exacerbations of headache, just as this patient describes. When pressed, this patient also reported occasional nausea, another feature that may suggest migraine. It is easy to overlook the curious fact that her symptoms all appear to be right-sided. There is, however, an alternative diagnosis that is compatible with her continuous, unilateral headache: hemicrania continua, a primary headache with autonomic features.

The clinical criteria of hemicrania continua are listed in Table 1.10. In the new version of the headache diagnostic classification, it is now considered one of the trigeminal autonomic cephalgias (formerly it was considered with the "other" primary headaches). Like cluster headache and the other TACs, hemicrania continua is a side-locked, strictly unilateral headache with associated autonomic features. It differs from the other TACs, however, in that it is continuous. It is also uniquely responsive to a particular nonsteroidal anti-inflammatory medication, indomethacin. Response to this drug is required to make a firm diagnosis of hemicrania continua. (Unfortunately, this diagnostic requirement means that a definite diagnosis cannot be made in patients who present with a clinical picture compatible with hemicrania continua but cannot take or do not tolerate indomethacin.)

With the possibility of this alternative diagnosis in mind, the most useful additional question for the patient described in the case becomes "Have you ever had pain on the left side of the head?" In this case, the patient reports that she has never had left-sided pain. Further questioning revealed that this nasal congestion was right-sided, and that her husband had told her that her right eye was sometimes "droopy." Upon further discussion, the patient stated that these symptoms had never come up because no one had ever asked before.

What treatment should be tried next?

The patient's additional history makes a diagnosis of hemicrania continua likely, but a definite diagnosis requires a complete response to therapeutic doses of indomethacin. The reported effective dose of indomethacin in hemicrania continua ranges from 50 to 300 mg/day. This dosing regimen is also commonly used in patients with primary stabbing headache, another indomethacin-sensitive primary headache syndrome. Common practice is to begin with indomethacin 25 mg orally three times a day for three days; if the patient tolerates this but has no headache improvement the dose is increased to 50 mg three times a day for three more days, and again if no response to 75 mg three times a day for a further three days. The authors of ICHD-3 beta recommend that doses of up to 225 mg/day should be tried "if necessary."

There are no good treatment alternatives for patients who cannot use indomethacin. Patients may occasionally experience a partial, less complete response to other anti-inflammatory agents, but most patients who cannot tolerate indomethacin also have difficulty tolerating other anti-inflammatory drugs.

Discussion

This patient reported a long history of headaches diagnosed as migraine that have been refractory to appropriate treatment for migraine. This is a common story in patients who ultimately receive the diagnosis of hemicrania continua. Any history of side-locked,

continuous headache should prompt consideration of hemicrania continua, but this is especially true if the patient is partially responsive to nonsteroidal anti-inflammatory treatment.

The temporal pattern of hemicrania continua is low-grade baseline headache with occasional exacerbations. Patients may initially report only the more severe headaches and neglect to mention the lower-grade baseline headache because it is less bothersome to them. This is one reason hemicrania continua may be misdiagnosed as migraine. An additional clue to the correct diagnosis was the nasal congestion for which she took daily decongestants, which upon questioning was ipsilateral to the headache, as was the previously undisclosed ptosis. Patients with hemicrania continua may also report a sense of something being stuck in the eye, such as an eyelash or a piece of sand, sometimes called a "foreign body sensation." This is another symptom patients frequently do not report spontaneously.

When headache treatment fails, a number of possible explanations may be considered: (1) incorrect diagnosis; (2) exacerbating factors have been missed; (3) treatment has been inadequate; or (4) unrealistic expectations or comorbidity exist. In this case, additional and open-ended questioning about the headache history provided important clues to correct diagnosis and treatment.

Diagnosis

Hemicrania continua.

Tip

Hemicrania continua is easily confused with chronic migraine. Important characteristics, including accompanying autonomic features and the side-locked character of the pain, may not be volunteered by the patient.

Further reading

Migraine vs. tension-type headache

Calhoun AH, Ford S, Millen C, *et al.* The prevalence of neck pain in migraine. *Headache.* 2010;50(8):1273–7.

Diener HC, Pfaffenrath V, Pageler L, *et al.* Headache classification by history has only limited predictive value for headache episodes treated in controlled trials with OTC analgesics. *Cephalalgia.* 2009;29(2):188–93.

Fernandez-de-las-Penas C, Madeleine P, Caminero AB, *et al*. Generalized neck-shoulder hyperalgesia in chronic tension-type headache and unilateral migraine assessed by pressure pain sensitivity topographical maps of the trapezius muscle. *Cephalalgia*. 2010;30(1):77–86.

Jensen R. Pathophysiological mechanisms of tension-type headache: a review of epidemiological and experimental studies. *Cephalalgia*. 1999;19(6):602–21.

Smetana GW. The diagnostic value of historical features in primary headache syndromes: a comprehensive review. *Arch Intern Med*. 2000;160(18):2729–37.

Tepper SJ, Dahlof CG, Dowson A, *et al*. Prevalence and diagnosis of migraine in patients consulting their physician with a complaint of headache: data from the Landmark Study. *Headache*. 2004;44(9):856–64.

Wober C, Holzhammer J, Zeitlhofer J, Wessely P, Wober-Bingol C. Trigger factors of migraine and tension-type headache: experience and knowledge of the patients. *J Headache Pain*. 2006;7(4):188–95.

Diagnosing migraine with aura

Eriksen MK, Thomsen LL, Olesen J. The Visual Aura Rating Scale (VARS) for migraine aura diagnosis. *Cephalalgia*. 2005;10:801–10.

Migraine in men

Stewart WF, Linet MS, Celentano DD, Van Natta M, Ziegler D. Age and sex-specific incidence rates of migraine with and without aura. *Am J Epidemiol*. 1991;134(10):1111–20.

Stewart WF, Wood C, Reed ML, Roy J, Lipton RB, AMPP Advisory Group. Cumulative lifetime migraine incidence in women and men. *Cephalalgia*. 2008;28(11):1170–8.

Cluster headache in women

Rozen TD, Fishman RS. Female cluster headache in the United States of America: what are the gender differences? Results from the United States Cluster Headache Survey. *J Neurol Sci*. 2012;317(1–2):17–28.

Rozen TD, Fishman RS. Cluster headache in the United States of America: demographics, clinical characteristics, triggers, suicidality, and personal burden. *Headache*. 2012;52(1):99–113.

van Vliet JA, Eekers PJ, Haan J, Ferrari MD, Dutch RUSSH Study Group. Features involved in the diagnostic delay of cluster headache. *J Neurol Neurosurg Psychiatry*. 2003;74(8):1123–5.

Alice in Wonderland syndrome

Podoll K, Robinson D. *Migraine Art – The Migraine Experience from Within*. Berkeley, California, North Atlantic Books. 2009; 85–146.

Todd J. The syndrome of Alice in Wonderland. *Can Med Assoc J*. 1955;73(9):701–4.

Winner P, Lewis D, Rothner AD, eds. *Headache in Children and Adolescents*. Lewiston, NY, BC Dekker, 2008.

"Cluster migraine"

Barbanti P, Fabbrini G, Pesare M, Vanacore N, Cerbo R. Unilateral cranial autonomic symptoms in migraine. *Cephalalgia*. 2002;22(4):256–9.

Lai TH, Fuh JL, Wang SJ. Cranial autonomic symptoms in migraine: characteristics and comparison with cluster headache. *J Neurol Neurosurg Psychiatry*. 2009;80(10):1116–19.

Obermann M, Yoon MS, Dommes P, *et al*. Prevalence of trigeminal autonomic symptoms in migraine: a population-based study. *Cephalalgia*. 2007;27(6):504–9.

NDPH

Goadsby PJ. New daily persistent headache: a syndrome not a discrete disorder. *Headache*. 2011;51(4):650–3.

Robbins MS, Evans RW. The heterogeneity of new daily persistent headache. *Headache*. 2012;52(10):1579–89.

Rozen TD. New daily persistent headache: clinical perspective. *Headache*. 2011;51(4):641–9.

Young WB. Expert Commentary on New Daily Persistent Headache. *Headache*. 2011;51(4):654–6.

Hemicrania continua

Lipton RB, Silberstein SD, Saper JR, Bigal ME, Goadsby PJ. Why headache treatment fails. *Neurology*. 2003;60(7):1064–70.

Rossi P, Tassorelli C, Allena M, *et al*. Focus on therapy: hemicrania continua and new daily persistent headache. *J Headache Pain*. 2010;11(3):259–65.

Chapter 2

Mistaking primary headache for another condition

In Chapter 1, we discussed pitfalls that can lead to confusing one type of primary headache disorder with another. Primary, nondangerous headaches may also be confused with or incorrectly attributed to multiple other medical conditions. It is of course possible for patients to have two separate forms of headaches (e.g. allergy-related headache and migraine), but this situation is probably not as common as many doctors assume. Some medical conditions, for example hypertension, are commonly but mistakenly assumed to be frequent causes of headache. Other conditions, such as sinus disease or temporomandibular joint dysfunction, may exacerbate an underlying primary headache disorder but are less commonly its sole cause. And finally, for some disorders, such as Arnold Chiari malformations or pituitary lesions, it may be impossible to determine with certainty whether the primary headache is related to the structural lesion.

Most of the medical conditions incorrectly assumed to produce headache are common, and under the right circumstances all of them can be the true cause of headaches. Their prevalence, however, means that often their association with headaches is due to chance. This matters because assumptions of causality may lead to overly aggressive treatment of the disorder assumed to be causing the headaches. Such treatment will not only be ineffective for the headaches but may also lead to other side effects or problems. A good example is sinus surgery that is done in the mistaken belief that migraine headaches are due to sinus disease. We see many patients whose migraines continue to be a problem but who also suffer from persistent post-surgical pain or dysesthesias.

In this chapter, we highlight the pitfalls that can lead to an incorrect diagnosis of headache due to another condition when the actual problem is a primary headache such as migraine.

"Sinus headache"

Case

A 55-year-old man reported a history of headaches since age 15. These were initially intermittent but had gradually worsened over the last several years and become constant. The episodic headaches he had when he was younger had been unilateral; severe; lasted up to 24 hours; and were associated with photophobia, phonophobia, and nausea. He had been diagnosed with "cluster and vascular tension headache."

He had been referred to an otolaryngologist because of frequent episodes of bilateral facial pain and rhinorrhea. An MRI scan showed mild mucosal thickening (Figure 2.1) in the maxillary sinuses bilaterally, and he was told that his headaches were probably due to sinus disease. After several rounds of antibiotic treatment failed to produce improvement in headaches, he had undergone a total of seven surgical sinus procedures over the course of 20 years in an unsuccessful attempt to treat headaches.

At the time of consultation he reported bilateral pain over the maxillary sinuses and forehead area, as well as the posterior head and neck. He rated the pain as 5 or 6 on a 0–10 scale at baseline, with daily exacerbations up to 8 or 9 lasting five to six hours that were associated with photophobia, phonophobia, osmophobia, and nausea. The headache increased when he bent over and he noted a sensation of pressure and fullness in the maxillary regions bilaterally.

The patient's exacerbations of pain responded well to symptomatic treatment with sumatriptan, but trials of typical preventive medications for migraine did not reduce the frequency or intensity of headache.

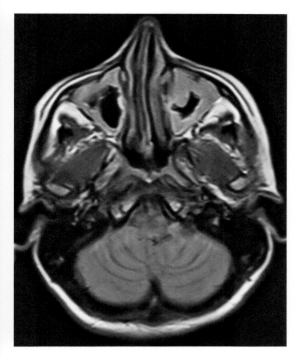

Figure 2.1 An MRI showing mucosal thickening in both maxillary sinuses. *Source:* http://commons.wikimedia.org/wiki/File:Brain_MRI_112010_rgbca.png.

Table 2.1. Clinical features of chronic vs. recurrent rhinosinusitis

Chronic rhinosinusitis	Recurrent acute rhinosinusitis
More than 3 months of a combination of purulent nasal drainage, nasal obstruction, facial pressure/pain, or reduced sense of smell AND Inflammation documented by direct observation or imaging	Four or more episodes per year of acute sinusitis with clearing of symptoms and findings in between

How is chronic sinus disease diagnosed?

The term *rhinosinusitis* is preferred to *sinusitis* because the middle turbinate is often involved in sinus disease. A clinical practice guideline from the American Academy of Otolaryngology – Head and Neck Surgery (AAOHNS) defines acute bacterial rhinosinusitis (ABRS) as up to four weeks of purulent nasal drainage, accompanied by nasal obstruction, facial pain/pressure/fullness, or both. Recurrent acute rhinosinusitis is diagnosed when four or more episodes of ABRS separated by symptom-free periods occur in one year. Chronic rhinosinusitis is defined as 12 weeks of two or more of the following symptoms: mucopurulent drainage, nasal obstruction/congestion, facial pain/pressure/fullness, or decreased sense of smell, as well as documented inflammation as evidenced by either purulent mucus or visible mucosal edema, nasal polyps, or radiographic imaging showing paranasal sinus inflammation. Table 2.1 lists criteria for distinguishing chronic rhinosinusitis from recurrent bouts of acute disease.

In this case we are not provided with enough information to be certain whether the patient's diagnosis of sinusitis was correct, but it seems reasonable to assume that the patient had at least recurrent acute bacterial rhinosinusitis if not chronic rhinosinusitis in addition to the primary headache syndrome.

Won't imaging clarify the diagnosis of sinusitis?

In this situation, diagnostic confusion is not usually resolved by diagnostic testing. It is important to note that there is considerable expert consensus that abnormalities on CT scan are not sufficient to make a diagnosis of rhinosinusitis. Some imaging abnormalities commonly assumed to indicate rhinosinusitis are not specific; for example, mucosal thickening may be seen in up to 40% of the asymptomatic population. Most expert guidelines suggest that a patient must meet clinical criteria for a diagnosis of sinusitis first, after which imaging is considered to be confirmatory rather than suggestive. Thus, abnormalities on sinus imaging or endoscopy that are consistent with sinusitis are not by themselves sufficient to assume that they are causing headache. CT is, however, particularly helpful in determining any anatomic abnormalities which may be exacerbating recurrent rhinosinusitis or chronic rhinosinusitis.

What sinus-related headaches do headache specialists recognize?

The International Classification of Headache Disorders (ICHD)-3 beta recognizes two types of headache related to sinus disease. The first is headache attributed to acute rhinosinusitis. The diagnostic criteria for this form of headache require clinical, endoscopic, or imaging evidence consistent with rhinosinusitis. In addition, however, some evidence of causality must be present in order to attribute any associated headache to the sinus abnormalities. Evidence that sinus abnormalities are causing headache can come in the form of a temporal relationship with the development of or any change in headache, or by exacerbation of the headache with pressure over the paranasal sinuses. If the physical sinus abnormalities are unilateral, an ipsilateral headache also stands as evidence of a causal relationship, according to these new criteria. Interestingly, the requirement that headaches be frontally located or accompanied by pain in the face, ears, or teeth has been removed from the new version of the classification.

ICHD-3 beta also recognizes headache attributed to chronic or recurring rhinosinusitis, commenting that while the association of headache with chronic sinusitis has been controversial, new evidence appears to support a connection. Imaging or endoscopic evidence of current or past infection or inflammation in the sinuses is required, along with at least two other things that support a causal connection. These can be either the development of or change in headache character that parallels the degree of sinusitis, the onset of headache in conjunction with the disorder, or exacerbation of the headache with pressure over the paranasal sinuses. As with headache attributed to acute sinusitis, a unilateral headache is also grounds to assume a causal connection when associated with ipsilateral imaging abnormalities.

The ICHD-3 beta appendix also includes proposed criteria for a diagnosis of headache attributed to disorder of the nasal mucosa, turbinates, or septum, for which evidence is limited. This headache is hypothesized to occur due to irritation or inflammation related to a hypertrophic or other process in the nasal cavity. It resolves fully after application of topical anesthetic or changes in severity in relation to gravitational or positional changes. Table 2.2 summarizes the clinical characteristics of headaches due to sinus or nasal disease.

Discussion

As with the patient in the vignette, migraine is commonly mistaken for a sinus problem. Patients may receive repeated courses of powerful antibiotics to treat the presumed sinus infection. Overuse of antibiotics is a serious public health problem, and can cause harm to individual patients as well. Sinus surgery performed in the mistaken belief that a patient with migraine has headaches due to sinusitis

Table 2.2. Clinical characteristics of headaches attributed to rhinosinusitis and disorders of the nasal cavity

	Sinus (rhinosinusitis) headache	Headache due to disorders of the nasal cavity
Pain location	Frontal headache radiating to face, ears, or teeth	If imaging or physical abnormalities are unilateral, headache should also be unilateral. Otherwise, no specific location is characteristic
Imaging	Direct or imaging evidence of changes consistent with chronic or acute sinusitis	Direct or imaging evidence of a hypertrophic or inflammatory process in the nasal cavity
Aggravating/ alleviating features	Headache develops or changes in conjunction with the clinical course of sinus inflammation	Pain often resolves with local application of anesthetic to the contact point region

can likewise have serious complications. We see many patients in our practice who have developed chronic pain problems or dysesthesias after having many sinus operations.

Many symptoms assumed to indicate a sinus origin of pain are not necessarily specific to rhinosinusitis and can be seen in migraine. These include a pain location in the face or area over the sinuses, changes in pain that correlate with the weather or seasons, and pain associated with rhinorrhea, sinus pressure, or nasal congestion. Fluctuations in barometric pressure associated with changes in weather are a frequently reported migraine trigger, for example, but are often interpreted as a trigger for sinus problems. Many patients who treat presumed "sinus headaches" with decongestants report that this treatment is modestly effective and assume that this proves the headaches are due to sinus problems. Decongestants, however, are vasoconstrictors and furthermore are often sold in combination with simple analgesics such as aspirin or acetaminophen. This combination of medications is, not surprisingly, sometimes helpful for migraine headaches and thus response to this treatment does not confirm the presence of sinus headaches. The majority of patients using these medications for presumed "sinus headache" will have an even better response to migraine-specific drugs. In one study, for example, the majority of self-diagnosed patients with "sinus headaches" experienced greater than 50% of reduction in pain with triptan use.

In the Sinus, Allergy, and Migraine study (SAM), 100 consecutive participants who responded to a questionnaire and believed that they had sinus headache were enrolled. After a detailed history and physical exam, only 3% were classified as having headache due to rhinosinusitis. The remainder met diagnostic criteria for migraine with or without aura (52%), probable migraine (23%), various forms of chronic migraine or other primary headaches (12%). In another study of almost 3000 patients with self- or physician-diagnosed "sinus headaches," 80% of the patients presenting with "sinus headaches" met diagnostic criteria for migraine with or without aura. It is thus abundantly clear that migraine is often mistaken for sinusitis.

Rhinosinusitis and migraine may also coexist, however, complicating the diagnosis. The majority of patients who attribute their headaches to sinus disease do have prior diagnoses of allergic rhinitis, acute rhinosinusitis, and (to a lesser extent) chronic rhinosinusitis, although the accuracy of those diagnoses is not clear. In the SAM study, a third of patients experienced chronic cranial autonomic symptoms whose exacerbations triggered migraine headaches, indicating to the authors that seasonal allergic rhinitis could at times trigger migraine.

Diagnosis

Migraine without aura and chronic rhinosinusitis.

Tip

A diagnosis of headache attributed to rhinosinusitis must be made clinically and then confirmed by imaging or endoscopy. Treatments such as antibiotics or surgery that are given for mistaken diagnoses of sinusitis expose patients to harm and prevent the use of more effective migraine-specific treatment.

Chronic headache after Lyme disease

Case

A 28-year-old woman with a prior history of episodic migraine presented for evaluation of a new and different type of headache, which she described as a constant, generalized pressure with a severity of 4/10 on a scale of 0–10. It was not associated with nausea but she was sensitive to light and noise. She still had her typi-cal, intermittent migraine headaches, which occurred on average once a week and responded well to sumatriptan. She was also taking six to eight tablets daily of a butalbital-containing medication to control her daily headache pain.

The patient suspected her new headache was a symptom of chronic Lyme disease. She lived in an endemic area and had noticed a tick bite four years ago. She was immediately and empirically treated with doxycycline. A friend, however, told her that Lyme disease often is not cured by short courses of antibiotic treatment and advised that she see a Lyme specialist. That physician had been treating her with regular high doses of vitamins and intravenous ceftriaxone through a percutaneous indwelling catheter. On review of systems, the patient had a large number of symptoms that she attributed to chronic Lyme disease.

Her neurologic examination was normal. A brain MRI and lumbar puncture were also normal. Cerebrospinal fluid (CSF) studies showed a normal protein and no antibodies to *Borrelia burgdorferi*.

How common is headache in patients with Lyme disease and is it likely that this patient's headaches were due to persistent neurologic infection?

Headache is common in patients with Lyme disease but by no means universal. About half of patients with new positive Lyme serology will report headache and headache is more common in patients with other symptoms of central nervous system and systemic involvement. In patients who only had positive CSF serology and headache, the headache features could resemble either migraine or tension-type headache.

Rarely, headache will be the only presenting feature of Lyme disease, which is usually not diagnosed until lumbar puncture shows characteristic CSF abnormalities of high protein, lymphocytic pleocytosis, and *Borrelia burgdorferi*-specific intrathecal antibodies.

It is, however, unlikely that this patient has persistent neurologic infection or headaches due to Lyme disease. She did not report the characteristic erythema migrans rash of Lyme disease and was treated promptly with appropriate antibiotic therapy for her tick bite. She has never had peripheral nervous system complications or CSF findings consistent with Lyme neuroborreliosis. Rather, her long-standing history of episodic migraine and daily use of combination

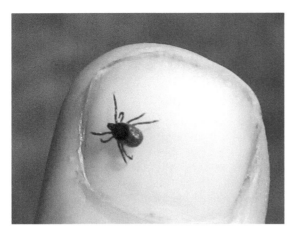

Figure 2.2 A deer tick of the sort that can transmit Lyme disease.

analgesics make medication overuse headache and chronic migraine far more likely diagnoses than Lyme disease.

What are the symptoms of chronic Lyme neuroborreliosis and how is it treated?

Chronic Lyme neuroborreliosis usually results from untreated or unsuccessfully treated Lyme disease which can become disseminated and affect the brain and nervous system. Neurologic complications usually appear a month or later after the tick bite. They include Bell's palsy, painful meningoradiculitis, or meningitis. The latter is a rare complication of Lyme disease, possibly more common in children, and often associated with papilledema. Late complications of Lyme neuroborreliosis can include cerebral vasculitis, progressive encephalitis, or encephalomyelitis. Lyme encephalitis characteristically produces evidence of nonspecific parenchymal involvement on neuroimaging. In the absence of parenchymal involvement, oral antibiotic treatment is usually considered satisfactory for this stage of the disease, although some patients may continue to have troublesome symptoms and require treatment with intravenous ceftriaxone or penicillin G.

Discussion

The spirochete *Borrelia burgdorferi*, which is transmitted to humans through the bite of deer ticks, is endemic in the United States. Infection risk is highest in wooded areas of New England, the northern Pacific coast, and the area around the Great Lakes.

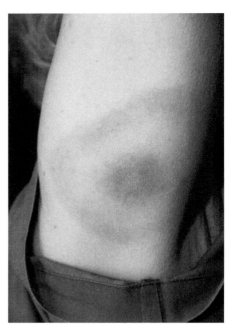

Figure 2.3 The characteristic erythema migrans rash of Lyme disease. *Source:* http://en.wikipedia.org/wiki/File:Erythema_migrans_-_erythematous_rash_in_Lyme_disease_-_PHIL_9875.jpg.

The diagnosis of early, uncomplicated disease is usually based on clinical features such as a history of tick exposure and the characteristic erythema migrans rash (Figures 2.2 and 2.3). Fever, headache, joint pains, fatigue, and other constitutional symptoms may occur. Serologic tests for Lyme disease are often negative in this early stage of the disease, and are not required for diagnosis: the erythema migrans rash itself is diagnostic. Most clinical guidelines agree that early infection responds well to short courses of oral antibiotics such as doxycycline.

Subjective symptoms that persist six months or more after treatment of Lyme disease are sometimes termed "post-Lyme disease syndrome." Headache is often a prominent symptom in such patients. However, it seems unlikely that the patient in this case ever had Lyme disease. Instead, she has a long history of episodic migraine, and her chronic headaches may be due to medication overuse or represent the development of chronic migraine. Most authorities agree that there is little good evidence that lengthy treatment with antibiotics improves outcomes in patients with post-Lyme disease syndrome. In fact, many harmful consequences of such prolonged treatment have been reported, including biliary damage as a result of prolonged use of ceftriaxone.

Diagnosis

Medication overuse headache; probable chronic migraine without aura.

Tip

Persistent Lyme disease is an unlikely cause of headache in patients who do not have objective findings of central nervous system involvement.

Headache in the setting of temporomandibular abnormalities

Case

A 42-year-old woman was seen in a headache clinic for evaluation of chronic headache. She reported having headaches since high school and described herself as someone who "always has headaches." The headaches were initially intermittent but had become daily over the last three years. They were worse in the mornings. She reported generalized head pain but the pain was most severe around the temples and jaw bilaterally. The pain was described as dull and achy and rated 4 on a scale of 0–10. When severe, the pain would become throbbing and was associated with photophobia, phonophobia, osmophobia, nausea, and sometimes vomiting. Stress, anxiety, and worsening jaw tension seemed to make the headaches worse, and they also seemed worse around her menstrual periods.

Recently the patient had become aware that she clenched her teeth constantly. After evaluation by a dentist she was diagnosed with displacement of the temporomandibular (TMJ) joint (Figure 2.4), a form of temporomandibular disorder (TMD). She also received diagnoses of bruxism and myofascial pain in the muscles of mastication. She was provided with a night guard to prevent nighttime bruxism, but her headaches persisted. She suspected that TMJ dysfunction was the cause of the chronic headache and had purchased several custom-made oral appliances from her dentist, aimed at reducing bruxism and improving her pain. Because the cost of these appliances was not covered by insurance, however, the patient had paid for them out of pocket. Her headaches continued, though, and surgery on the TMJ had been advised. However, before proceeding she wanted a second opinion.

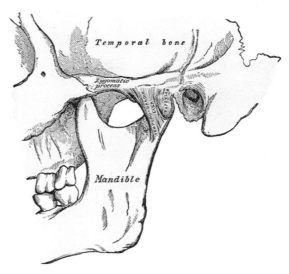

Figure 2.4 The temporomandibular joint. *Source:* http://en.wikipedia.org/wiki/File:Gray309.png.

How likely is this daily headache to be due to pathology of the TMD?

It can be difficult to make a diagnosis of headache attributed to TMD because many people grind or clench their teeth and occasional jaw pain is common. ICHD-3 beta requires that the diagnosis can only be made when there is clinical or radiologic evidence of pathology of the jaw or TMJ or associated structures. Furthermore, some evidence of causation is required in the form of development or change of the headache in conjunction with any pathologic changes, or exacerbation of pain by active or passive jaw movements or provocative maneuvers. If the joint pathology is unilateral, the headache pain must be ipsilateral to the site of the pathology.

A number of historical or examination features can be useful when trying to assess the possibility of TMD pathology. These include the presence of localized jaw pain or physical findings such as impaired jaw range of motion, joint sounds with movement (e.g. clicking), and muscle and joint tenderness to palpation.

In this case we are not provided with the details of the initial dental examination. On examination in the headache clinic, however, the patient did not give a clear history of pain development that correlated closely with demonstrated TMJ pathology. Furthermore, there was no impairment of jaw opening and minimal pain on palpation over the

25

Table 2.3. Clinical features of headache attributed to temporomandibular disorder

Imaging or clinical evidence of pathology in the TMJ or nearby structures or masticatory muscles

Evidence of a causal link between headache and this pathology, as demonstrated by onset or worsening of pain in association with the pathology, or worsening of pain with active or passive movements of the jaw or with provocative maneuvers including pressure on masticatory muscles or the TMJ

Table 2.4. Selected causes of postpartum headache

Primary causes:
  Migraine
  Other primary headaches

Secondary causes:
  Vascular:
    Ischemic stroke
    Hemorrhagic stroke, including subarachnoid hemorrhage
    Venous sinus thrombosis
    Reversible cerebral vasoconstriction (RCVS)
    Arterial dissection
    Vasculitis
    Hypertension/Posterior reversible encephalopathy
      syndrome (PRES)

  Nonvascular:
    Preeclampsia/eclampsia
    Idiopathic intracranial hypertension
    Post-dural puncture headache

temporomandibular joint. Many details of the patient's history seemed more compatible with a diagnosis of chronic migraine, such as the associated headache features of nausea, vomiting, and phono and photophobia. She was advised to postpone treatment of the TMJ and was treated with more aggressive preventive therapy for migraine. Her headaches became episodic and were more easily controlled with migraine-specific therapy.

Discussion

Jaw pain is common and many patients seen in specialty headache practice have already been evaluated and treated by a dentist for presumed TMJ pathology. It is difficult to estimate the true prevalence of TMDs. One large review suggested that they occur in roughly 10% of the population, mostly in middle-aged adults. Like migraine, they are more common in females than males. They may therefore coexist with migraine in many patients, but this does not mean they are a causal or contributing factor to headache problems. ICHD-3 beta criteria for a diagnosis of headache attributed to TMD are summarized in Table 2.3.

Diagnosis

Chronic migraine.

Tip

Familiarity with the presentation and findings in TMD as distinct from migraine can help prevent confusion when migraine masquerades as TMD.

Postpartum headache

Case

A 24-year-old woman developed acute headache six hours after a normal spontaneous vaginal delivery, for which she had epidural anesthesia. She had a history of episodic migraine with aura that had improved during the pregnancy.

After delivery she had the acute onset of a severe bifrontal headache, associated with nausea and blurred vision, which she identified as similar to her prior migraines but much more severe. The headache and nausea seemed to worsen when she was sitting up. Her neurologic examination showed mild diffuse hyperreflexia but was otherwise normal.

Because of the acute onset of headache an evaluation, including noncontrast head CT and MRI/MRA/MRV with contrast, was done and was negative. Urinalysis showed no proteinuria and her blood pressure was 132/85 mm Hg. A parenteral analgesic medication was administered. By the time the diagnostic testing was completed her headache had started to improve and she declined a recommended lumbar puncture.

What is the differential diagnosis of postpartum headache?

The differential diagnosis for postpartum headache is lengthy. Selected causes are listed in Table 2.4. They include both benign primary headaches such as migraine, and dangerous secondary causes of headache such as cerebral venous thrombosis. A detailed headache history and thorough neurologic examination can be helpful in differentiating between primary and secondary causes of headache, but a high suspicion of secondary causes is appropriate. Postpartum headaches that are similar to a patient's pre-existing headaches, particularly if the headaches persisted during pregnancy, are probably more likely to be benign. Likewise, a nonfocal neurologic examination is reassuring. In this case, the finding of hyperreflexia is of unclear significance. Furthermore, her report of an acute headache more severe than her usual headaches is concerning.

Should further diagnostic testing be done? If so, what?

Headache characteristics that should prompt workup for secondary headache in the postpartum period are similar to the "red flags" that warrant workup in other settings. These include a new headache or change in an established headache pattern, changes in mental status, new focal neurologic deficits, uncontrollable vomiting, or intractable headache. A history of primary headache disorder such as migraine is not always reassuring in the postpartum setting because migraine is associated with an increased likelihood of several dangerous causes of headache, including peripartum stroke, preeclampsia, and angiopathy or reversible cerebral vasoconstrictive syndrome.

Appropriate diagnostic investigation depends on the suspected cause of secondary headache. Imaging is frequently needed to assess for the possibility of intracranial vascular problems. A head CT and lumbar puncture can be performed to rule out intracerebral or subarachnoid hemorrhage, and MRA/MRV are appropriate to evaluate for vasculitis, vasoconstrictive syndromes, or cerebral venous thrombosis. Angiography may be needed when cerebral vasoconstriction or aneurysm are strongly suspected. An MRI of the brain with contrast may show meningeal enhancement in cases of post-dural puncture headache, and a lumbar puncture may show low opening pressure. If preeclampsia is suspected, monitoring for proteinuria, hyperreflexia, and hypertension is warranted.

In this case, the initial workup for causes of secondary headache was negative. Because the patient's headaches started to resolve after the MRI/MRA/MRV and this testing was negative, a lumbar puncture was deferred. She was monitored in the Mother and Baby Unit for an additional three days without recurrence of headache, and felt well at the time of discharge.

Discussion

About one-third of women experience headache in the postpartum period, and both primary and secondary postpartum headaches are more frequent in women with a prior history of migraine. Other factors associated with an increased risk of postpartum headache are known dural puncture, previous headache history, and multiparity.

Secondary causes are responsible for 25–50% of postpartum headaches; these are discussed elsewhere. Among the primary headache disorders that produce postpartum headache, recurrence of migraine is probably the most frequent. In one study of 1000 women with postpartum headache, migraine or another primary headache disorder was identified as the etiology in 75% of cases. Migraine may reappear within a week to one month after delivery and has been attributed to causes such as declining estrogen levels, sleep disruption, and stress.

Even when a diagnosis of migraine is made in a patient with postpartum headaches we believe it is prudent to avoid vasoconstrictive medications such as triptans because the postpartum period in migraineurs may be a situation of heightened susceptibility to the vasoconstrictive effects of triptans.

Diagnosis

Migraine without aura.

Tip

A high index of suspicion for dangerous causes of postpartum headache is appropriate, but the most common cause of postpartum headache in a known migraineur is migraine.

A middle-aged man with low-lying cerebellar tonsils

Case

A 49-year-old male was evaluated for frequent headache. He reported a family history of migraine. He had no history of childhood headache or of periodic symptoms related to migraine such as motion sickness. Headaches had begun in his mid 30s. They were infrequent and the pain was generalized and moderate in intensity. The headaches could last for days and generally did not respond to simple analgesics. They were attributed to sinusitis.

When the patient was in his late 30s the headaches became more severe and were associated with migrainous features such as nausea. He sought treatment and was diagnosed with migraine. He was prescribed

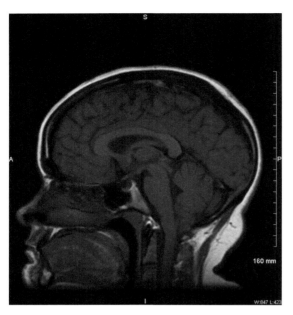

Figure 2.5 A sagittal T1 MRI image showing moderate tonsillar descent.

Table 2.5. Clinical and MRI characteristics of headache associated with Chiari malformation, type I

Headache that is occipital or suboccipital or precipitated by Valsalva maneuvers or lasts less than 5 minutes OR headache that has developed or changed in conjunction with a CM1 OR headache associated with posterior fossa dysfunction, indicated by lower cranial nerve or cervical spinal cord dysfunction or otoneurologic or brainstem symptoms such as dizziness, vertigo, oscillopsia.

Demonstration of a CM1 by MRI:
    ≥5 mm caudal descent of the cerebellar tonsils OR

    ≥3 mm caudal descent of the cerebellar tonsils plus posterior fossa crowding manifested by:
        compression of the posterolateral cerebellar CSF spaces
        reduced height of the supraocciput
        increased slope of the tentorium
        kinking of the medulla oblongata

Table 2.6. Clinical characteristics of cough headache

Headache precipitated *only* by coughing, straining, or Valsalva maneuvers
Sudden in onset
Location not specified
Lasts 1 second to 60 minutes

oral zolmitriptan 5 mg. This effectively aborted individual attacks of headaches but headache frequency increased and by his mid 40s the patient had two to three episodes of severe headaches weekly. In addition, he noted gradual onset of a constant low-grade head and posterior occipital pressure, which he described as "like a tourniquet" or tight band around his head and neck. The pain was not postural. There were no abnormalities on neurologic examination. An MRI of the head showed mild cerebellar tonsillar descent (Figure 2.5) into the foramen magnum.

The patient was seen by a neurosurgeon, who believed that his symptoms were related to a Chiari 1 malformation (CM1) and recommended surgery. The patient sought a second opinion from another neurosurgeon, who strongly advised against surgery and referred him for headache consultation.

At the time of his visit to the headache center the patient was experiencing three headache exacerbations weekly, each lasting one to two days, superimposed on the generalized tight sensation that was always present. The severe headaches were present when he awakened. They were described as throbbing, generalized, and associated with photophobia and nausea. The patient was taking frequent over-the-counter medications to treat his headaches and was occasionally using a butalbital combination medica-

tion prescribed by another physician. He was working but had been unable to exercise because of the headache. He had gained 30 pounds in the preceding year. His sleep was fragmented and he reported daytime somnolence. His neurologic examination was normal. A lumbar puncture showed a normal opening pressure and no CSF abnormalities.

How can headache attributed to a Chiari I malformation be diagnosed?

Headache related to a CM1 is characteristically located in the occipital region of the head and is intermittent rather than constant. It is often provoked by maneuvers or activities that temporarily raise CSF pressure, such as coughing or sneezing. It generally does not have features more characteristic of migraine or other primary headaches, such as associated nausea or photophobia. Table 2.5 lists the clinical and imaging features of this disorder.

CM1 is easily confused with cough headache, which is described in Table 2.6. Cough headache is a primary headache disorder in which headache is precipitated by cough or other Valsalva-type maneuvers, but is not associated with identifiable structural abnormalities. It is a diagnosis of exclusion, and should be made only after imaging has been done to assess for possible abnormalities of the posterior fossa.

Roughly 40% of patients who present with apparent "cough headache" in fact turn out to have CM1. Other reported secondary causes of headache precipitated by cough or Valsalva include carotid or vertebrobasilar diseases and cerebral aneurysms. Thus, neuroimaging plays an important role in differentiating secondary from primary causes of cough headache.

CM1 can also present as a more protean chronic headache, with or without exertional features, usually located in the posterior occipital or suboccipital regions. If associated with other neurologic signs and symptoms, the diagnosis is usually not particularly challenging. Often, however, headache is either the initial or only manifestation of the condition.

A diagnosis of symptomatic CM1 does not seem very likely in the patient described in this case, despite the documented cerebellar tonsillar descent. He does not describe headache in association with cough and his clinical presentation is more characteristic of migraine. Cerebellar tonsillar descent or "brain sag" can occur in patients with spontaneous intracranial hypotension, so a lumbar puncture is recommended in patients who have any cerebellar tonsillar descent to assess the possibility of a CSF leak.

What treatment should be recommended to this patient?

The patient likely had a past history of headaches compatible with a diagnosis of episodic migraine without aura. Unusual presenting features were the late age of onset and the initial nondescript features of the headache. Later, though, a more typical pattern of migraine emerged and his headache pattern was more easily recognizable as a transformation from episodic to chronic migraine. Although the posterior occipital neck pressure he reported might suggest a secondary headache cause such as CM1, there were few other features in the history or examination to suggest this diagnosis. Additionally, when carefully measured, the degree of tonsillar descent on the patient's MRI was less than 3 mm, meaning that he did not meet radiologic criteria for a CM1.

At times the historical features of a headache pattern do not allow a clear diagnosis to be made and further testing such as diagnostic neuroimaging may be warranted. If misinterpreted, however, imaging may confuse the situation further. This patient was advised that although it was possible the MRI findings were related to his headache, it was much more likely that this was an incidental finding and that he had a primary headache disorder for which medical management was indicated.

The patient improved with a brief course of oral steroids and discontinuation of daily analgesics. Amitriptyline and topiramate were added as preventive agents and a triptan drug was restarted for headache exacerbations. He was evaluated and found to have sleep apnea, for which treatment was started. At a follow-up visit, he considered his headaches well controlled on this regimen and had been able to resume daily exercise.

Discussion

A Chiari type 1 malformation is a cerebellar anomaly in which there is descent of the cerebellar tonsils to at least 3–5 mm below the foramen magnum. This abnormality often occurs alone but can also be associated with a spinal cord syrinx, hydromyelia, or hydrocephalus. Although generally considered to be a congenital lesion, symptoms often do not begin until adulthood. This delay may be due to altered CSF dynamics with aging or to changes in connective tissue that occur over time. Many people with documented cerebellar tonsillar descent – up to a third – are asymptomatic.

Descent of the cerebellar tonsils is a frequent incidental finding on MRI performed for other reasons. It is fairly common, with an incidence estimated to be around 0.5% of the population and a female to male ratio of 3:2. There is no clear correlation between the degree of cerebellar tonsillar descent and the clinical severity of headache. Thus, radiologic findings alone should almost never prompt surgical intervention. Rather, the clinical context of the findings must be carefully considered. Headache related to CM1 is often located in the occipital or suboccipital regions and is often worsened by cough Valsalva, postural change, or bending over.

MRI correlates of CM1 have been characterized based on large case series of affected patients. Herniation of the cerebellar tonsils 3–5 mm below a line drawn between the tip of the clivus and the rim of the foramen magnum is the most consistently used measurement to determine the diagnosis. Lesser amounts of descent are considered to represent merely tonsillar ectopia, and this is generally thought to be asymptomatic. Other MRI features may also be present, including elongation of the tonsils, caudal

Table 2.7. Classification of Chiari malformations

Malformation type	Description of congenital malformation
Type I	Elongation of the tonsils and the medial parts of the inferior lobes of the cerebellum into cone-shaped projections, which accompany the medulla oblongata into the spinal canal
Type II	Displacement of the parts of the inferior vermis, pons, and medulla oblongata together with elongation of the fourth ventricle (most cases are associated with spina bifida)
Type III	Herniation of the entire cerebellum into the cervical canal. This is associated with severe neurologic deficits
Type IV	Cerebellar hypoplasia

displacement of the brainstem and fourth ventricle, crowding of the posterior fossa with obliteration of the subarachnoid space, and bulbo-cervical kinking, an increased angle formed by the brainstem and cervical spine at their margin. Figure 2.5 illustrates some of these findings. The features of other degrees of Chiari malformation are described in Table 2.7.

Diagnosis

Chronic migraine; tonsillar ectopia.

Tip

The clinical context of headache occurring in the setting of low-lying cerebellar tonsils must be carefully considered. Caution is warranted in making a diagnosis of headache attributed to CM1, in order to avoid exposing patients to possible unnecessary surgery which can cause serious complications.

Cluster headache presenting as a dental problem

Case

A 49-year-old female was evaluated for a 20-year history of episodic left-sided headache. Headaches typically occurred daily for periods of one to two months during the spring every year, although she could go for several years without having any pain episodes. During her one- to two-month bouts of headache, she experienced headaches located behind the left eye. They were associated with tearing and the pain radiated to the left

cheek or teeth. The pain was described as sharp, stabbing, and excruciating: "definitely a 10/10, worse than childbirth." Individual episodes of pain lasted up to 30 minutes and usually occurred at night.

The patient had seen a dentist and undergone removal of her wisdom teeth with no benefit. She was then diagnosed with TMJ disorder and provided with a night guard. Her headache pattern seemed to improve after that, but the next year headaches recurred. Later she returned to the dentist. Several fillings were replaced and a suspected diseased tooth was removed. With each procedure she would seem to improve transiently before experiencing a return of her prior headache pattern. During a typical headache the patient paced the room, noting that it was better for her to walk than to remain in bed with a headache.

Her primary care physician had suggested that she might have cluster headache and referred the patient for evaluation. At the time of the neurologic evaluation she reported her headaches were unresponsive to treatment with opioid analgesics and her most recent bouts of headache had been separated by only six months. She was frustrated and commented: "I've been searching for an answer for 20 years. It's only on the left side."

What is the most likely diagnosis in this case?

This patient does meet diagnostic criteria for a diagnosis of episodic cluster headache. Despite this, an accurate diagnosis was not made until 20 years after her headaches began. Cluster headache is characterized by a severe unilateral orbito-temporal pain lasting from 15 minutes to 3 hours associated with ipsilateral autonomic features such as tearing, nasal congestion, eyelid edema, ptosis, or conjunctival edema.

Although cluster headache is more common in men, it does occur in females. Recent epidemiologic data suggest that the sex ratio is less lopsided than originally suspected. Currently the male:female ratio is estimated to be about 2:1.

Bouts of episodic cluster headache typically last 2–12 weeks and are separated by pain-free periods of at least 2 weeks but typically longer. Cluster headache is termed chronic when a remission is absent for a year or more or is present but of short duration, less than 14 days in length.

In this vignette, though the pattern meets criteria for a diagnosis of episodic cluster headache, the patient's bouts are becoming more frequent. It is possible that this is the beginning of a conversion from episodic to chronic cluster headache. It is not uncommon for physicians or patients to attribute the uncommon and unilateral pattern of cluster headache to local disease in the sinuses or teeth and direct inquiry to those disorders.

Was the dental work this patient had indicated?

It is unlikely that the dental work this patient had was in fact necessary. A dentist who is unfamiliar with the diagnosis of cluster headache can easily attribute cluster headache pain to a local dental process. The unilateral nature of the pain, as well as the fact that pain is often felt in the jaw area, means that patients frequently seek dental evaluation. Studies indicate that almost half of cluster patients will have visited a dentist for evaluation before the diagnosis of cluster headache is eventually made. Unfortunately, many undergo repeated, invasive dental procedures in an attempt to treat the pain. As with the patient described in this vignette, it can be years before an accurate diagnosis of cluster headache is made. This is unfortunate because medical therapy for cluster headache is often remarkably effective.

Discussion

For a variety of reasons, episodic cluster can be a challenging diagnosis and a delay in diagnosis from onset of symptoms of up to five years is described, though the delay may be longer in females with cluster. Episodic cluster will at times present to the dentist and the diagnosis can be missed. In one study just fewer than half of patients eventually diagnosed with cluster presented for dental evaluation as part of the initial evaluation of their pain and many of these patients received unnecessary or inappropriate dental management for their symptoms.

The current International Classification of Headache Disorders (ICHD) criteria for cluster include an orbital, supraorbital, and/or temporal localization for the pain. However, ipsilateral radiation of the pain to the face and teeth is not unusual in cluster. It is well documented that cluster may in part present with a midface localization or radiation of pain, and this is thought perhaps the main explanation for diagnostic confusion among dental practitioners.

A revision of the ICHD criteria for cluster to include this localization has been suggested as a possible step to mitigate the confusion.

Worsening or triggering of a cluster headache pattern after dental procedures has also been reported, explained in part by deafferentation of pain fibers in the region of the dental procedure leading to triggering of brainstem and spinal cord pain networks. The possibility that a dental procedure might precipitate a cluster attack further underlines the need to eliminate diagnostic confusion and avoid unnecessary procedures in these patients.

Given the pain severity and associated disability of cluster headache, it is important for dental personnel to recognize the features of this headache pattern; they may well be the first to see and diagnose the patient. Those in dentistry should redouble their efforts to render an accurate diagnosis and to avoid unnecessary and inappropriate dental treatments. Timely management in order to minimize patient disability is the goal.

Diagnosis

Episodic cluster headache.

Tip

Cluster headache is a unilateral pain disorder that is frequently mistaken for a dental problem. Familiarity with the characteristic pattern of cluster headache is important to avoid costly and unnecessary dental procedures.

An older woman with focal neurologic deficits but no headache

Case

A 71-year-old woman was seen in the emergency department. She reported that five hours ago, while reading a magazine, she suddenly developed a visual disturbance. She found the type on the magazine page blurry and could not make out the individual letters. She was able to see the face of her husband. After a few minutes she noticed a thin bright white line in the upper part of her visual field in the right eye. These symptoms continued for 20 minutes, when she developed numbness of her left cheek that gradually spread to the side of her nose and corner of her mouth. Her tongue was not numb. Five minutes later her husband noticed that she was unable to express herself and that her speech consisted of nonsense words. The visual changes lasted 40 minutes, the speech problems for 10 minutes and the numbness for an hour. She had no associated headache.

The patient had experienced a similar episode one month earlier. She had been seen in the emergency department and had a workup including brain imaging, Holter monitor, and carotid studies, all of which were negative. She was diagnosed with a transient ischemic attack and instructed to take 81 mg of aspirin daily. She had osteoarthritis and hypertension that was well controlled on lisinopril and was otherwise well. She was not a smoker and her cholesterol levels were normal.

In the past she had experienced periodic throbbing, unilateral headaches preceded by neurologic symptoms similar to those she had now. Her previous headaches had been diagnosed as migraine but she had not had any severe headaches for the last 20 years. After hearing about the patient's most recent event, the neurology resident on call diagnosed a second transient ischemic attack and was concerned that this had occurred despite aspirin therapy. She wondered whether the patient should be placed on additional antiplatelet therapy, a statin, or anticoagulated.

This patient had a negative workup a month ago. Should she be reinvestigated now or could this be a benign process?

The patient probably does not need additional testing or investigation for this second episode of transient neurologic deficits, but it is easy to understand the neurology resident's anxiety. The patient is in an age group where transient ischemic attacks and strokes are common. She also gives a clear history of neurologic deficits, although the reversible nature of her symptoms is more suggestive of a transient ischemic attack than a stroke. However, her symptoms have been fully evaluated with no suggestion of a thrombotic or embolic cause. In fact, this patient's symptoms are likely to be what the famous neurologist C. Miller Fisher termed "late-life migraine accompaniments."

Fisher's "rules" for the diagnosis of late-life migraine accompaniments (Table 2.8) are still useful clinically, and help to put the case of the patient in the vignette into clearer context.

Table 2.8. Clinical characteristics of "late-life migraine accompaniments" From C. Miller Fisher

- Most common aura is visual, followed by paresthesias, then aphasia/dysarthria, then (rarely) paralysis
- Symptoms usually build, one upon another
- There may be a spread or "march" of symptoms
- Progression from one symptom to the next is common
- ≥2 similar episodes required for confirmation
- Duration of each individual symptom is usually 15–25 minutes
- Symptoms may or may not be followed by headache
- Generally indicates a benign course
- Exclude other conditions. Requires normal imaging

What is the epidemiology of late-life migraine accompaniments, and should they be treated?

An analysis of data from the Framingham Study showed that migrainous visual accompaniments in late life are not rare. In over 2000 queried subjects, 1.23% reported migrainous visual symptoms. The majority of subjects reported stereotyped episodes and in over three-quarters of these subjects the episodes had begun after the age of 50. Well over half of people who experienced such episodes reported that the visual events occurred without headache, and the typical duration of an episode was 15–60 minutes. In contrast to a group of subjects who had been diagnosed with transient ischemic attacks, patients with late-life migraine accompaniments were far less likely to experience stroke subsequently. The authors of this study concluded that these events were not rare, were benign, and that "invasive diagnostic procedures or therapeutic measures are generally not indicated."

Although antiplatelet therapy such as low-dose aspirin is sometimes used in patients with transient ischemic attacks, there is no evidence to support its use in patients with late-life migraine accompaniments or other forms of aura. In the past some have advocated this approach on the assumption that decreased platelet aggregability might reduce the risk of subsequent ischemic events in such patients.

This practice is called into question, however, by a recent analysis of data from the Women's Health Study. In subgroup analyses of this randomized trial, women who had migraine with aura who had received 100 mg of aspirin every other day actually had a *higher* risk of subsequent myocardial infarction than women who had not received aspirin. Although these data come from subgroup analyses, and the risk was limited to women who had smoked or had hypertension, they do sound a cautionary note. In the absence of evidence that aspirin is helpful, and some suggestion of possible harm, we do not currently recommend treating patients with aura with aspirin therapy.

Discussion

Attacks of aura without migraine become more common as patients with migraine age. Most patients with late-life migraine accompaniments have a prior history of migraine and aura. In our practice we are reluctant to make a diagnosis of aura without migraine in the absence of a previous history consistent with migraine.

Headache expert Dr. William Young, writing about Dr. Fisher's masterful description of this clinically common phenomenon, has commented that "Once you learn of this symptom complex, you see it over and over again. It is easy to diagnose ... even obvious ... No one since has changed [Fisher's] clinical characterization, much less improved upon it. His writing is strange by today's standards, with his introduction, results section, and conclusion all mixed together, and much of the article is composed of illustrative cases. But once you slog through, you really will have the flavor of the condition, and when you are confronted with it, you are reassured, you reassure your patient, and common sense rules your management."

Diagnosis

Typical aura without headache (late-life migraine accompaniments or "acephalgic migraine").

Tip

Aggressive treatment or diagnostic investigation is not warranted in patients with a clinical scenario consistent with late-life migraine accompaniments. While antiplatelet therapy such as aspirin may be helpful for patients with transient ischemic attacks, there is no evidence to support its use in patients with late-life migraine accompaniments.

Prolonged aura

Case

A 36-year-old man with a 20-year history of migraine with typical visual aura presented in the emergency department. He reported that four hours previously he had one of his typical auras, including scintillations and a scotoma. After about an hour the scotoma gradually faded and he developed a right-sided headache that responded to treatment with zolmitriptan. The scintillations, however, have continued. In the past the visual symptoms associated with his headaches had never lasted longer than 40 minutes. Initial neurologic examination, including fundoscopy, was normal. The patient was sent for urgent ophthalmologic consultation, which showed no apparent ocular disease but did reveal an upper and lower quadrant right visual field deficit. A CT of the head with and without contrast showed no abnormalities. The patient was otherwise well and hematologic and chemistry tests were normal. About six hours after onset the visual symptoms resolved spontaneously. An MRI scan of the head done a month after the emergency department visit also proved to be normal.

The patient then disappeared from care, reappearing four years later. He reported that he traveled frequently for his work as a consultant. He had continued to have episodes of prolonged aura interspersed with episodes of typical visual aura lasting no longer than 40 minutes. On several occasions he had sought evaluation in emergency departments in different cities, where he had undergone several repeat CT scans, electroencephalogram (EEG), and lumbar puncture with no abnormalities found.

What is the likely diagnosis in this case?

This patient experiences aura symptoms that are completely characteristic of his typical visual aura with the exception of their duration. Such an occurrence naturally raises the suspicion of cerebral infarction, but testing in this case does not show evidence of ischemia. Unfortunately, the current ICHD-3 beta does not provide a diagnostic label for his episodes of prolonged aura. The criteria for typical visual aura specify that aura symptoms should not exceed 60 minutes. The criteria also include the diagnosis of "persistent aura without infarction" for cases where aura symptoms last longer than a week in the face of normal test results.

Patients whose auras fall between 60 minutes and a week, or who have repetitive attacks of aura with very short intervals of normality reside in a diagnostic "no man's land." Many terms have been used to describe this clinical situation, including "complicated migraine," "sustained visual aura," "persistent migraine aura," and "migraine aura status." Because most patients with prolonged aura have other attacks that fulfill criteria for some other form of aura, the authors of ICHD-3 beta recommend headaches in those cases should be coded to that other diagnosis. Otherwise, since they fulfill all but the duration criterion for a diagnosis of typical aura, they should be classified as probable migraine with aura, specifying the atypical feature (prolonged aura or acute-onset aura) in parentheses.

What is the differential diagnosis of prolonged aura?

The differential diagnosis of prolonged aura includes vertebrobasilar transient ischemic attack, carotid or vertebral dissection, cerebral vasculitis, reversible cerebral vasoconstrictive syndrome, occipital lobe epilepsy, or even cerebral venous thrombosis. In the case of this patient, those possibilities were eliminated by normal testing results. The passage of time without the development of additional problems also makes a dangerous explanation for his prolonged auras unlikely. Unfortunately, this patient's peripatetic lifestyle meant that he was subjected to repeat diagnostic testing to rule out dangerous diagnoses that might have accounted for his presentation.

Discussion

Persistent aura symptoms are not especially common but numerous case reports make it clear that they do occur. Persistent visual aura is often distressing for patients, who frequently report that they are either unable or afraid to drive. Figure 2.6 shows a drawing that illustrates visual abnormalities similar to those depicted by a 70-year-old man who suffered from repetitive attacks of aura for five weeks; looking at this it is not hard to understand how disabling persistent attacks of aura can be. In commenting on the patient's drawing, noted aura experts report that "Each repetition began with slowly undulating thick gray lines, which changed in a few minutes into a pinwheel of bright whirling color in his left visual field. Several minutes later this image slowed down and disappeared. After more than a week of suffering these hallucinations, he also developed brief attacks of 'electrical' paresthesias in his left hand. These were less frequent than the visual phenomena and alternated with them irregularly. Throughout his ordeal, he had a dull headache over his right eye." Because this is a relatively rare condition, there are no large clinical trials

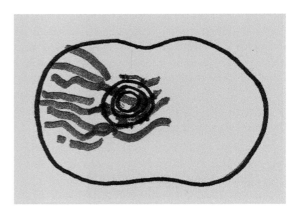

Figure 2.6 This drawing illustrates visual abnormalities of the kind described by a patient experiencing repeated attacks of visual aura. After Haas. Prolonged migraine aura status. *Ann Neurol.* 1982;11: 197–9. From www.drpaulrizzoli.com. Used with permission.

on which to base treatment recommendations. Case reports provide empirical support for trials of lamotrigine, acetazolamide, or valproic acid.

Diagnosis

Migraine with aura.

Tip

Aura symptoms that last longer than an hour but less than a week are difficult to classify. In patients who also have attacks of aura of typical duration, it is reasonable to assign a diagnosis of migraine with aura.

A middle-aged woman with vertigo and a history of migraine

Case

A 54-year-old woman was referred to the headache clinic by her primary care physician for possible migrainous vertigo. She had a history of migraine without aura in her 20s, which had largely abated after the birth of her last child in her late 30s. About three years ago she started having episodes of vertigo, lasting about two hours and initially occurring twice a month. When she had the vertigo, turning her head quickly exacerbated it. It did not seem to be provoked by any environmental factors such as dehydration. There was no headache associated with the vertigo, though she did note photo and phonophobia during some of the episodes.

Table 2.9. Clinical characteristics of migraine with brainstem aura

Aura must be followed within an hour by headache
Aura must occur with at least two brainstem symptoms, which include decreased level of consciousness, tinnitus, vertigo, dysarthria, diplopia, hypacusis, or ataxia
Each symptom can last 5–60 minutes, at least one symptom is unilateral, and at least one spreads gradually and/or at least two symptoms occur in succession

She had seen an otolaryngologist. Her examination, done at a time when she was not symptomatic, was normal. Specifically, a Dix–Hallpike maneuver did not provoke nystagmus. An MRI of the brain was normal. She was diagnosed with benign positional paroxysmal vertigo and started on meclizine, which was ineffective and made her tired. Her primary care physician thought the vertigo might be related to her history of migraine and referred her to the headache clinic.

Could this patient's vertigo be migrainous in origin?

The first two versions of the ICHD did not include criteria for migrainous vertigo or migraine-associated vertigo. ICHD-3 beta, however, lists criteria for vestibular migraine in the appendix, which is a place for candidate criteria for disorders that need further validation and testing. These criteria describe migrainous vertigo as the occurrence of moderate to severe vestibular symptoms lasting 5 minutes to 72 hours, where at least half of the episodes are associated with headache, visual aura, or photophobia and phonophobia. These symptoms must occur in a patient who meets diagnostic criteria for migraine.

It should also be noted that vertigo is listed as one of the brainstem symptoms characterizing "migraine with brainstem aura," formerly known as basilar or basilar-type migraine. These criteria are listed in Table 2.9. The classification notes that while there is some overlap between the two syndromes, most patients with vestibular migraine experience vertigo for longer than an hour. They also rarely experience vertigo in the same relationship to headache that is seen with typical migraine with aura, where the aura immediately precedes and is usually followed by headache. Instead, headache may not always occur in relation to vertiginous symptoms, and may coexist with rather than follow them. In addition, migraine with brainstem aura requires typical visual aura symptoms in addition to those believed to originate in the brainstem.

What treatments are available to this patient?

Until recently, research regarding treatment for vestibular migraine has been limited by the absence of clear, agreed-upon diagnostic criteria. There have been no randomized controlled trials of treatments for vertigo linked to migraine and high quality evidence to guide treatment is therefore lacking. One small and underpowered trial suggested benefit from zolmitriptan for acute treatment. Larger chart review or survey studies suggest that medications prescribed for migraine were generally effective in treatment of the vertigo in patients with both vertigo and migraine. Small interventional studies, typically open label, have evaluated beta-blockers, tricyclic antidepressants, calcium channel blockers, and antiepileptic drugs. One interventional study included a dietary modification that appeared to be beneficial for a subset of patients, although in our view such open-label results should be interpreted with caution.

Given the lack of a solid evidence base to guide treatment decisions, we typically start by treating vestibular migraine as we do any other form of migraine, with an emphasis on prevention if attacks are frequent. Specific preventive medications to be considered include propranolol, amitriptyline, and topiramate. Lifestyle modifications including adequate and regular sleep, maintaining good hydration, and a healthy diet are also emphasized. For treatment of acute episodes of headache or vertigo, a trial of triptans may be fruitful, even in patients without migrainous headache accompanying the episodes of vertigo. Sedative medications such as meclizine or benzodiazepines, often used in the treatment of vertigo of peripheral origin, are another option. Lastly, physical therapy or vestibular therapy might be considered.

Discussion

Vertigo is the sensation of rotational motion when the head and body are actually at rest. Patients often describe the feeling that they or the room are spinning; this sensation of movement distinguishes "vertigo" from "dizziness." Vertigo may occur spontaneously or may be triggered, often by a change in head position but also at times by visual triggers. Any of these types of vertigo may be accompanied by migrainous symptoms, whether headache or sensitivity to other sensory modalities, to suggest a diagnosis of vestibular migraine.

There is a wide variation in the duration of vertiginous symptoms, from minutes to days. The pathophysiology of vestibular migraine is not well understood, but an overlap between vestibular input and circuits involved in migraine seems likely. Both clinical and research interest in the topic has increase significantly over the last several years. The ICHD-3 beta notes that the temporal course of vestibular migraine rarely fits the pattern for typical aura (duration 5–60 minutes, immediately preceding headache) and therefore "episodes of vestibular migraine cannot be regarded as migraine auras."

Although the ICHD-3 beta has included these diagnostic criteria in order to stimulate further research aimed at validating the disorder, it is worth noting that other criteria for the diagnosis exist. Otolaryngologists may use the Neuhauser criteria. A diagnosis of definite migrainous vertigo by these criteria requires: (1) recurrent vestibular vertigo; (2) migraine according to the International Headache Society (IHS); (3) migrainous symptoms during at least two vertiginous attacks (migrainous headache, photophobia, phonophobia, or aura symptoms); and (4) vertigo not attributed to another disorder. Probable migrainous vertigo requires items 1 and 4 and another migrainous feature (migraine per IHS criteria, migrainous symptoms during vertigo, migraine triggers for vertigo, response to anti-migraine drugs).

Chronification of vertiginous symptoms is not as well described in the literature, but anecdotally we have occasionally seen patients evolve from episodic to chronic vertigo, seemingly in a process like that which occurs with headache. The symptoms may become less severe but more frequent or continuous over time, a phenomenon commonly seen with other migraine-associated symptoms such as photophobia. When the vertigo is not accompanied by headache or is not temporally associated with headache it is often unclear whether the vertigo is a migrainous symptom. In those cases we often empirically treat patients as if they have chronic migraine.

Diagnosis

Vestibular migraine.

Tip

A diagnosis of vestibular migraine may be considered for patients with a history of migraine when the vertigo is associated with other migrainous symptoms and other etiologies have been ruled out.

Further reading

Sinus disease

Eross E, Dodick D, Eross M. The Sinus, Allergy and Migraine Study (SAMS). *Headache*. 2007;47(2):213–24.

Schreiber CP, Hutchinson S, Webster CJ, *et al*. Prevalence of migraine in patients with a history of self-reported or physician-diagnosed "sinus" headache. *Arch Intern Med*. 2004;164(16):1769–72.

Lyme disease

Halperin JJ, Shapiro ED, Logigian E, *et al*. Practice parameter: treatment of nervous system Lyme disease (an evidence-based review): report of the Quality Standards Subcommittee of the American Academy of Neurology. *Neurology*. 2007;69(1):91–102.

Nord JA, Karter D. Lyme disease complicated by pseudotumor cerebri. *Clin Infect Dis*. 2003;37(2):e25–6.

TMD

LeResche L. Epidemiology of temporomandibular disorders: implications for the investigation of etiologic factors. *Crit Rev Oral Biol Med*. 1997;8(3):291–305.

Schiffman E. Diagnostic criteria for headache attributed to temporomandibular disorders. *Cephalalgia*. 2012;32(9):683–92.

Postpartum headache

Cardona L, Klein AM. Early postpartum headache: case discussions. *Semin Neurol*. 2011;31(4):385–91.

Klein AM, Loder E. Postpartum headache. *Int J Obstet Anesth*. 2010;19(4):422–30.

Chiari malformation

Grazzi L, Andrasik F. Headaches and Arnold-Chiari syndrome: when to suspect and how to investigate. *Curr Pain Headache Rep*. 2012;16(4):350–3.

Massimi L, Peppucci E, Peraio S, Di Rocco C. History of Chiari type I malformation. *Neurol Sci*. 2011; 32(Suppl 3):S263–5.

Mea E, Chiapparini L, Leone M, *et al*. Chronic daily headache in the adults: differential diagnosis between symptomatic Chiari I malformation and spontaneous intracranial hypotension. *Neurol Sci*. 2011;32(Suppl 3):S291–4.

Pascual J, González-Mandly A, Martín R, Oterino A. Headaches precipitated by cough, prolonged exercise or sexual activity: a prospective etiological and clinical study. *J Headache Pain*. 2008;9(5):259–66.

Taylor FR, Larkins MV. Headache and Chiari I malformation: clinical presentation, diagnosis, and controversies in management. *Curr Pain Headache Rep*. 2002;6(4):331–7.

Cluster presenting as a dental problem

Bahra A, Goadsby PJ. Diagnostic delays and mis-management in cluster headache. *Acta Neurol Scand*. 2004;109(3):175–9.

Balasubramaniam R, Klasser GD. Trigeminal autonomic cephalalgias. Part 1: cluster headache. *Oral Surg Oral Med Oral Pathol Oral Radiol Endod*. 2007;104(3): 345–58.

Bittar G, Graff-Radford SB. A retrospective study of patients with cluster headaches. *Oral Surg Oral Med Oral Pathol*. 1992;73(5):519–25.

Gross SG. Dental presentations of cluster headaches. *Curr Pain Headache Rep*. 2006;10(2):126–9.

Rozen TD, Fishman RS. Female cluster headache in the United States of America: what are the gender differences? Results from the United States Cluster Headache Survey. *J Neurol Sci*. 2012;317(1–2):17–28.

Shoji Y. Cluster headache following dental treatment: a case report. *J Oral Sci*. 2011;53(1):125–7.

Late-life migraine accompaniments

Fisher CM. Late-life migraine accompaniments as a cause of unexplained transient ischemic attacks. *Can J Neurol Sci*. 1980;7:9–17.

Kurth T, Diener H-C, Buring JE. Migraine and cardiovascular disease in women and the role of aspirin: subgroup analyses in the Women's Health Study. *Cephalalgia*. 2011;31(10):1106–15.

Wijman CA, Wolf PA, Kase CS, Kelly-Hayes M, Beiser AS. Migrainous visual accompaniments are not rare in late life: the Framingham Study. *Stroke*. 1998;29(8):1539–43.

Young WB. A knockout punch: C. Miller Fisher's migraine accompaniments. *Headache*. 2000;48:726–7.

Repetitive and prolonged migraine aura

Chen WT, Fuh JL, Lu SR, Wang SJ. Persistent migrainous visual phenomena might be responsive to lamotrigine. *Headache*. 2001;41:823–5.

Haan J, Sluis P, Sluis LH, Ferrari MD. Acetazolamide treatment for migraine aura status. *Neurology*. 2000;55:1588–9. http://www.migraine-aura.org/content/e25968/e26078/e26305/index_en.html.

Haas DC. Prolonged migraine aura status. *Ann Neurol*. 1982;11:197–9.

Vestibular migraine

Bisdorff AR. Management of vestibular migraine. *Ther Adv Neurol Disord*. 2011;4(3):183–91.

Furman JM, Marcus DA, Balaban CD. Vestibular migraine: clinical aspects and pathophysiology. *Lancet Neurol*. 2013;12(7):706–15.

Lempert T, Neuhauser H, Daroff R. Vertigo as a symptom of migraine. *Ann NY Acad Sci*. 2009;1164:242–51.

Neuhauser H, Leopold M, von Brevern M, Arnold G, Lempert D. The interrelations of migraine, vertigo, and migrainous vertigo. *Neurology*. 2001;56:436–41 .

Chapter 3

Missing dangerous causes of headache

In most patients with dangerous underlying causes of headache there are signs and symptoms that clearly point to the causal disorder. Typical features that suggest a dangerous or secondary cause of headache include fever, altered consciousness, or abnormal neurologic findings. One example of a rarely missed diagnosis is temporal arteritis presenting as a classic case of new-onset headache in an elderly person, accompanied by anemia, jaw claudication, and visible tortuosity of the temporal artery.

When such symptoms or signs are subtle or absent, however, dangerous causes of headache can be missed or mistakenly attributed to other disorders. Headache is also a common symptom of many illnesses. Patients may have more than one condition known to be associated with headache, making it difficult to assess causation.

Finally, a number of disorders can produce headaches that superficially resemble nondangerous causes of headache such as migraine or tension-type headache. Both of these headache types are common, so many patients presenting for evaluation of headache will have a prior history consistent with one of these benign headache syndromes. Migraine, for example, is a highly prevalent cause of severe headache, with a cumulative lifetime incidence of 44% in women and 18% in men.

A prior history of migraine or tension-type headache in a patient with a new or different form of headache is not necessarily reassuring, however. In fact, patients with a well-established history of benign headaches may be at especially high risk of having a dangerous cause of headache mistakenly attributed to their prior nondangerous headache disorder.

Cases in this chapter illustrate situations in which underlying medical or structural abnormalities responsible for headache were not recognized, and headache was mistakenly attributed to a nondangerous headache or other disorder.

New headache in an elderly woman

Case

A 75-year-old woman with no personal or family history of prior headache was referred to the headache center for consultation. She reported headaches over the last two months. The headaches began gradually but increased rapidly to the point where they were daily and constant. They were located over the top of her head and radiated to her forehead and face. The pain was variable: sometimes dull and sometimes a pressure sensation "like my head is going to fly off." The pain had been especially intense over the last two weeks. It ranged from 4 to 6 on a 0–10 pain scale. When asked, the patient said the headaches were associated with photo and phonophobia but she did not have nausea, vomiting, or worsening of headaches with physical activity or change of position.

The patient denied jaw claudication, visual disturbances, or associated autonomic symptoms. She reported that her sinuses felt "congested" and the headache temporarily improved when she sneezed. She was treating her headaches with over-the-counter acetaminophen plus phenylephrine. She had a 15 pound weight loss over the last year and reported that she has been told she is anemic. She was recently seen in the emergency department because of a severe headache, where a neurologic examination was normal and a CT scan of the head did not reveal any explanation for her headaches. At that visit, her systolic blood pressure ranged from 160 to 180 mm Hg. A diagnosis of headache due to poorly controlled hypertension was made and her blood pressure medication was adjusted.

A sinus CT was obtained on an outpatient basis when headaches did not improve despite better control of her blood pressure. The report she brought with her read as follows:

IMPRESSION:

1. Multifocal sinus disease, involving the bilateral anterior/posterior ethmoid air cells, sphenoid sinus, and left frontal sinus. This could account for the patient's headache.
2. No acute intracranial abnormality.

She was started last week on amoxicillin/clavulanic acid twice daily but her headaches continued.

What are the leading diagnostic possibilities and how would you proceed in evaluating them?

New-onset headache in an elderly person is a "red flag" situation that should prompt a careful search for an underlying causative condition. While hypertension or sinusitis may seem like plausible explanations for her problem, they do not entirely explain other worrisome features such as weight loss or anemia. Giant cell arteritis is an additional possibility that must be seriously considered in any patient over the age of 50 who presents with a new headache.

After consultation at the headache center, this patient had blood work and additional imaging performed. Results included a hematocrit of 30, an erythrocyte sedimentation rate (ESR) of 94 (normal 1–20), and a C-reactive protein (CRP) of 34.6 (normal 0–5). A magnetic resonance angiogram showed normal cerebral vessels and extensive mucosal thickening of the sphenoid sinus and ethmoid air cells with moderate mucosal thickening of the frontal sinus. The patient was continued on amoxicillin and clavulanic acid twice daily and 60 mg of prednisone was added each morning; a temporal artery biopsy was also performed. The patient's headaches resolved within two days and the temporal artery biopsy was positive for giant cell arteritis.

Why was the correct diagnosis delayed?

Somewhat surprisingly, this elderly patient had been seen by her primary care physician and in the emergency department with complaints of new headache but had not had either an ESR or CRP checked. Instead, her headaches were attributed to elevated blood pressure and later a possible sinus infection.

In hindsight, it seems clear that after these initial diagnoses were considered, the clinicians involved did not reflect on alternative causes for the patient's symptoms, a cognitive error known as premature closure. In one series of diagnostic errors, premature closure – failure to consider other diagnostic possibilities once a diagnosis had been identified that "fit the facts" – was the most common cause of missed diagnoses.

In this case the initial diagnoses only partially "fit the facts." Although the patient's blood pressure was indeed high in the emergency department, there were no other signs or symptoms consistent with a diagnosis of hypertensive encephalopathy. This makes it unlikely that her elevated blood pressure had occurred abruptly, which is the only setting in which hypertension is well validated as a cause of headache. Chronic hypertension is not commonly considered a cause of headache. Additionally, this patient's headaches did not improve even with better control of her blood pressure.

The CT scan shows extensive sinus disease, which might account for the patient's headaches – indeed, the radiology report suggests so – but antibiotic treatment did not produce improvement in her symptoms. Some sinus infections respond poorly to antibiotics, however, so sinusitis may in fact be contributing to this patient's symptoms, but it is far from being the only possible explanation. Diagnostic delay is not uncommon in giant cell arteritis. Predictably, delayed diagnosis is more common in patients like this one who do not present with "typical" features such as jaw claudication or visual disturbance.

Visual loss is the most feared complication of giant cell arteritis. Visual symptoms in combination with new-onset headaches would prompt most clinicians to consider a diagnosis of giant cell arteritis. However, visual problems are found in only a quarter to a third of patients at presentation. This patient did have headache, which is the most common initial symptom, found in almost 90% of patients. Unfortunately, this symptom alone was not enough to prompt consideration of giant cell arteritis in the presence of attractive competing explanations.

Discussion

The gold standard for diagnosis of giant cell arteritis is temporal artery biopsy. Most patients will also have elevated inflammatory markers. CRP may be more sensitive than the ESR, but either can be normal in the occasional patient with documented disease. Thus, most clinicians order both tests to improve diagnostic sensitivity.

The clinical presentation of giant cell arteritis is highly variable, and this can make diagnosis difficult. As was done in this case, steroid treatment should be initiated immediately if clinical suspicion of giant cell arteritis is high. Most experts agree that a few days of steroid treatment will not reduce the likelihood of a positive biopsy result. A normal temporal artery biopsy does not rule out a diagnosis of giant cell arteritis; false-negative biopsies can occur if unaffected portions of the artery (so-called "skip lesions") are sampled in the biopsy. In this patient's case, a high clinical index of suspicion for giant cell arteritis was present and the clinicians involved agreed that they would proceed with steroid treatment even if the biopsy were normal. She may well have coexistent sinus disease, too, and her clinicians planned to consult an otolaryngologist.

Diagnosis
Giant cell arteritis.

Tip
Many elderly patients have a large number of medical conditions that might plausibly cause or contribute to new-onset headaches. It is important to consider fully all possible explanations for headache rather than prematurely settling on the first diagnosis that appears to fit the facts of the case.

A young man with head pain, nausea, and fever

Case
A healthy 22-year-old man was seen in the emergency department for new-onset headaches. He was well until two weeks ago, when he began to experience intermittent severe left eye pain and head and face pain associated with fever, chills, nausea, and vomiting. The pain worsened with coughing, sneezing, or physical exertion. The headache was located over the vertex and occiput and the face pain in the V1 distribution. There was a history of an upper respiratory infection a week before onset of the headaches, but at the time of presentation the patient had no nasal or respiratory symptoms. Physical and neurologic examination revealed no abnormalities other than a slightly elevated temperature of 101 degrees Fahrenheit. A diagnosis of new-onset migraine was made and the patient

was treated with intravenous promethazine, with some symptomatic improvement.

Does this sound like migraine?
While some features of the patient's headaches are consistent with a diagnosis of migraine, other things, such as the fever and chills, are not. The headaches are of new onset and his pain is side-locked. All of these things suggest that further evaluation is warranted. In this case, a CT scan of the brain was ordered by the emergency department and performed as soon as the patient's pain had improved with treatment. The films showed an air/fluid level in the left sphenoid sinus. Laboratory tests done in the emergency department showed an elevated CRP of 12 and an ESR of 32.

In view of his new-onset headaches and history of fever and elevated inflammatory markers, the patient also has a lumbar puncture and is sent for blood cultures, and oral antibiotics are started. The cerebrospinal fluid (CSF) is clear, the opening pressure normal, and there is no pathogen growth at 48 hours. Blood cultures, however, grow *Haemophilus influenzae*.

What is the next step in management?
The positive blood cultures confirmed septicemia. The source of the infection was most likely the left sphenoid sinus, given the patient's prominent eye, head, and face pain and sinus abnormalities on CT scan. A careful search for sources of head and neck infection should start with a detailed ear, nose, and throat examination. In this case, an otolaryngologist noted pus in the left superior turbinate and confirmed the clinical impression of acute sphenoid sinusitis. The patient was treated with high-dose antibiotics and surgical debridement of the sphenoid sinus and recovered uneventfully.

Acute sphenoid sinusitis is not a common condition. It can be difficult to diagnose since typical signs and symptoms of sinusitis often are not present. For example, nasal congestion, discharge, or postnasal drips are not common in sphenoid sinusitis, which instead tends to present with headache and fever. The pain may be felt over the vertex, occiput, or in the periorbital region, and nausea is common. Pain is often worsened by coughing or physical exertion. It is easy to see how such a presentation could be mistaken for migraine, as it was in this case. Fortunately, however, diagnostic workup for secondary causes of headache

Table 3.1. Structures adjacent to the sphenoid sinus that may be affected by sphenoid disease

Cranial nerve 2
Cranial nerve 3
Cranial nerve 4
First division of cranial nerve 5
Second division of cranial nerve 5
Cranial nerve 6
Dura mater
Pituitary
Cavernous sinus
Internal carotid artery
Sphenopalatine ganglion
Sphenopalatine artery
Pterygoid canal and nerve

was pursued even after the preliminary diagnosis of migraine had been made.

Acute sphenoid sinusitis can be very serious, so aggressive treatment is warranted. The sphenoid sinuses lie within the sphenoid bone in the middle cranial fossa, adjacent to many critical structures (Table 3.1). These include the pituitary and the cavernous sinus. If infection spreads to the cavernous sinus or subarachnoid space, life-threatening complications can develop. The most common causative organisms are bacterial, especially staphylococcal or streptococcal infections, but fungal infections or Gram-negative infections can also occur.

What is the nociceptive innervation of the paranasal sinuses?

Sensation from the nasal mucosa and sinuses is transmitted through the first and second divisions of the trigeminal nerve with a very small contribution from the greater superficial petrosal branch of the facial nerve. In particular, the sphenoid and ethmoid sinuses are served by the posterior ethmoidal branch of the nasociliary nerve, which arises from the first division of the trigeminal nerve. This may account for the prominent occurrence of orbital and peri-orbital pain in cases of sphenoid sinusitis, since pain from the sinuses is usually referred to the corresponding dermatome.

In contrast, the maxillary sinus is innervated by the superior alveolar and infraorbital branches of the

second division of the trigeminal nerve, so mid-facial pain is more common with maxillary sinusitis. The frontal sinuses are innervated by the supraorbital and supratrochlear nerves of the first division of the trigeminal nerve.

Discussion

Some forms of sinusitis can be serious. This is especially true of sphenoid sinusitis. Untreated, infection can spread to involve the cavernous sinus or cause meningitis. Headache is the most common presenting symptom, and several case series suggest that the headache often awakens patients from sleep. Sphenoid sinusitis is also on the list of disorders that can produce sudden onset of extremely severe headache – so-called "thunderclap" headache – perhaps as a result of extension of infection through the wall of the sinus.

The location of the headache is variable: it is often over the vertex in addition to causing pain in the face or over the sinus region. Sensory changes in V1 or V2 or pus in the middle or superior turbinates on examination can help make the diagnosis, but these findings are not always present. X-rays or CT may show opacification of the sinus or thickening of the mucosa, but there is no clear correlation between the extent of opacification and the severity of illness. CT is probably somewhat better than MRI for the diagnosis of sinusitis, but either is probably sufficient for initial evaluation. In a review of 300 CT and MRI scans, the sphenoid sinus was visualized in all of the studies.

Diagnosis

Acute sphenoid sinusitis.

Tip

Acute sphenoid sinusitis can be missed when it mimics migraine by producing peri-orbital pain and nausea. It should be considered in any case of new-onset headache, particularly in the presence of fever or signs of inflammation with pain over the vertex of the head.

Weekend headache

Case

A 23-year-old woman had been seen multiple times over the last six months for complaints of headache. She had no prior history of headache although an aunt had migraine. She described the headaches as constant. When headaches began they mostly occurred on weekends or holidays but quickly became daily. Typically they were worst in the mornings and continued to be more severe on weekends. The pain was described as throbbing, and was rated on average 6 on a scale of 0–10.

Headaches were associated with dizziness, nausea, occasional vomiting, and, on two occasions, loss of consciousness. With both episodes of loss of consciousness she was taken to the emergency department. Testing included an MRI scan of the head, electrocardiogram, Holter monitor, and electroencephalogram, all of which were normal with the exception of occasional episodes of supraventricular tachycardia.

On both occasions she slowly improved during a short hospitalization for observation and was discharged with a diagnosis of chronic migraine. Treatment aimed at migraine had not been helpful, however. The patient reported modest, temporary relief from anti-inflammatory medications but none at all from triptans or a variety of preventive medications such as propranolol and topiramate.

Based on this patient's clinical presentation, what are some diagnostic considerations?

The patient's age and sex, the throbbing character of the headache, its duration and frequency, as well as associated features of nausea and vomiting all fit with a diagnosis of chronic migraine. It is also the case that many people with migraine report they are more likely to have headaches on weekends, holidays, vacations, or at other times of "letdown" from stress.

Other features of this patient's headache, however, did not fit with migraine: migraine is not typically associated with loss of consciousness, and it is rare for it to evolve so quickly to the chronic form of the disorder. Could this be new daily persistent headache which, as its name implies, presents as a constant headache? Perhaps, but the episodes of loss of consciousness still cannot be explained by that diagnosis.

In this case, the rapid evolution of the headache after onset, the unexplained episodes of loss of consciousness, and the lack of response to extensive trials of treatment aimed at migraine suggested that alternative diagnoses should be considered. In cases of difficult-to-diagnose headache, most experts agree that the crucial next step is "history, history, and more history."

Upon further questioning the patient confirmed that she had no prior history of headache. She worked as a technical editor and was able to do much of her work at home. As her headaches have worsened she had been spending more and more time at home and remarked that "I can't remember the last time I was in my office…the worse I get the more time I spend at home and the more time I spend at home the worse I seem to get." When asked about relatives with headache problems, the patient again mentioned her aunt. She added that she shared a house with her sister, who worked as a flight attendant. Her sister had recently also developed low-grade headache and nausea, but her headaches did not seem to be as severe.

Does the additional history change your mind about possible diagnoses?

The patient's offhand comment about getting worse as she spent more time at home was a clue to her diagnosis, as was the history of a similar illness in someone who lived with her. Headaches were initially most noticeable on weekends, when she was most often at home. As her illness progressed, she began to spend more time at home, at which point the headaches worsened and became daily.

All of these facts are consistent with a toxic environmental exposure in the home as a possible cause of headache. When her physicians learned that the patient's headaches began last October with the onset of cold weather they became suspicious about possible carbon monoxide exposure. On testing, the patient's carboxyhemoglobin level was 28% and her sister's was 18%. Inspection of their home showed a faulty furnace.

Carbon monoxide poisoning can be very difficult to diagnose when it results from chronic exposure to carbon monoxide from defective space heaters, kitchen stoves, or furnaces. The symptoms are nonspecific and easily attributed to other disorders such as migraine. In this case the patient's age, sex, and headache features, including the weekend occurrence of the headaches, all fit with a diagnosis of migraine.

Because migraine is so common in young women, it is a diagnosis that most physicians can easily call to mind. This is an example of a cognitive bias known as "availability bias," in which the differential diagnosis is strongly influenced by what is easily recalled. Here it was easy to assume that the weekend headaches reported by the patient were the typical "letdown" headaches of migraine, and not so easy to remember that at a more fundamental level they were related to absence from work – and exposure to the home environment – factors that might have reminded her doctors about environmental exposures that can produce headache.

Discussion

Carbon monoxide is odorless, so victims are not aware of exposure. It binds more tightly to hemoglobin than oxygen, with the result that oxygen delivery to the brain and other tissues is impaired. Diagnosis is based on finding a venous carboxyhemoglobin level above 10%.

Headache is the most common symptom of carbon monoxide poisoning and is thought to result from cerebral vasodilation in response to hypoxemia. Nausea and a general sense of malaise or other flu-like symptoms are also common. The higher the carboxyhemoglobin level and the more sustained the exposure, the worse the long-term outcome. Chronic encephalopathy can result with prolonged or very high level exposure.

Carbon monoxide poisoning is treated by removal from the exposure and with oxygen therapy; 100% oxygen is commonly administered for several hours. If carboxyhemoglobin levels are above 25%, guidelines recommend the use of hyperbaric oxygen at 2–3 atmospheres, if available. Hyperbaric oxygen rapidly increases the amount of oxygen that is dissolved in plasma and the half-life of carboxyhemoglobin is shortened from 4–5 hours in room air to about 20–25 minutes. There can be complications to hyperbaric treatment, including tension pneumothorax or cerebral edema. It is contraindicated in patients with chronic obstructive pulmonary disease.

One study found that roughly 15% of patients with headache who presented during the winter months to an urban emergency department had elevated carbon monoxide levels. Another study found that smoking a high number of cigarettes daily, use of a stove to heat living spaces, and similar illness in a family member were predictive of carbon monoxide poisoning, underscoring the value of a good environmental exposure history.

Diagnosis

Carbon monoxide intoxication.

Tip

Weekend headaches are a hallmark of migraine, but not all weekend headaches are migraine. Occult carbon monoxide poisoning can produce headache that is difficult to distinguish from migraine. In patients with refractory headaches occurring in winter and with similarly affected cohabitants, a high index of suspicion for carbon monoxide poisoning is appropriate.

A young woman with seizure and headache

Case

A 19-year-old woman with epilepsy was referred to the headache clinic for management of very severe headaches occurring after seizures. She was diagnosed with complex partial seizures two years ago and was undergoing treatment trials with antiepileptic drugs. Her seizures were less frequent with topiramate but still occurred about once every other month.

Following her seizures she experienced unilateral, throbbing, severe headache with photophobia, nausea, and vomiting. She rated the headaches as "10+" on a 0–10 pain scale and reported they could last up to a whole day. The pain was not relieved by ibuprofen. Because she and her epileptologist were primarily concerned about controlling seizures, the headaches had not been a focus of attention until recently.

Upon further questioning she admitted having occasional milder but similar headaches outside of the seizure episodes, often around her menstrual period. Her mother had "sick headaches" when she was younger.

What is the relationship between seizures and headaches?

The International Classification of Headache Disorders (ICHD) recognizes two forms of headache associated with epileptic seizures. The first, hemicrania epileptica, is diagnosed when headache is a primary manifestation of the seizure itself. The diagnostic criteria include headache lasting seconds to minutes, with features of migraine, developing synchronously with a partial epileptic seizure and resolving immediately after the seizure. The pain must be ipsilateral to the ictal discharge. This is a relatively uncommon phenomenon.

Much more common is post-ictal headache, which is diagnosed when a headache occurs after a seizure. The criteria include a headache with features of tension-type or migraine headache, developing within three hours after a partial or generalized epileptic seizure and resolving within 72 hours after the seizure. Prevalence estimates for post-ictal headache range from 25% to 50%.

Migralepsy, a disorder in which migraine is the putative trigger for an epileptic seizure, has been very rarely described and is a controversial diagnosis. Migraine and epilepsy share many features. Both are chronic neurologic disorders of long duration with episodic manifestations and exacerbations. Both disorders are characterized by paroxysmal "all or none" events.

While the exact pathophysiology of migraine without aura is unclear, it is generally accepted that migraine aura is associated with excessive cortical excitation, as is seizure activity. In migraine, cortical hyperexcitability is theorized to lower the threshold for cortical spreading depression, in which an orderly wave of neuronal depolarization travels across the surface of the cortex. This is followed by a period of depressed cortical activity as the neurons struggle to repolarize. Cortical spreading depression is generally accepted as the cause of migraine aura.

A number of similar molecular mechanisms are theorized to play a role in at least some cases of both disorders, such as abnormalities in ion channel function leading to increased glutamatergic tone. The possibility that migraine and epilepsy might share some underlying mechanisms is supported by epidemiologic evidence that shows the two disorders are comorbid. The prevalence of epilepsy is higher in migraineurs (1–71%) than in the general population (0.5–1%). Estimates of the prevalence of migraine in the epilepsy population range from 8.4% to 24%.

In this case, the patient has an established diagnosis of partial complex seizures, and the temporal relationship between the seizure and the resulting headaches is clear. A diagnosis of post-ictal headache is therefore appropriate. Based on her history of other similar headaches occurring in the absence of seizure, it seems likely that she has a diagnosis of migraine as well.

What treatment options are available?

In cases where headaches occur only after seizures, the most effective treatment is prevention of seizure episodes with antiepileptic therapies. If headaches also occur outside of seizure activity, an antiepileptic drug with evidence of efficacy for headache may be a good option. Antiepileptic drugs that may be effective for both seizures and migraine include topiramate and valproate. Evidence is less certain for gabapentin.

There is little evidence to guide the choice of symptomatic treatments for post-ictal headache. Case reports and clinic experience both support the practice of using migraine-specific therapies to treat patients whose post-ictal headaches have migrainous features. Anecdotally, some patients who have both migraine and post-ictal headaches note that their post-ictal headaches are more severe than their regular migraines.

If triptans or nonsteroidal anti-inflammatory drugs are not effective for post-ictal headache, this may be the rare situation in which the use of butalbital-containing drugs or opioid drugs is defensible. As with treatment of regular migraines, antiemetic treatment should be considered if nausea is a prominent accompaniment of the headache.

The patient in this case was treated with subcutaneous sumatriptan and oral prochlorperazine. This regimen was effective for most of her interictal and post-ictal headaches. At a follow-up visit she reported having a few very severe headaches for which this regimen was not effective and she was given a prescription for a butalbital-containing medication to use in those circumstances.

Discussion

Although epilepsy and headache may be comorbid conditions, they can usually be distinguished on clinical grounds alone. Because of this, electroencephalography (EEG) is not useful in the initial evaluation of patients with typical headaches. This is reflected in a practice parameter of the Academy of Neurology. EEG may be warranted in patients who have atypical visual aura where conditions such as occipital lobe epilepsy are being considered.

Headache as the sole manifestation of seizure is very rare, while headache occurring after a seizure with other manifestations is more typical. Post-ictal headache is relatively common, affecting up to half of patients with epilepsy. It may be more common in children. Despite being common, post-ictal headache is often overlooked. This may be because the headaches are not very severe, or may be because the seizure is more concerning and "overshadows" the subsequent headache. Because these headaches may be bothersome and refractory to minor analgesic treatments, however, they often warrant medical attention.

Diagnosis

Post-ictal headache; episodic migraine.

Tip

Post-ictal headache is common and can be severe. Failure to ask patients with epilepsy about post-ictal headache, and/or failure to recognize migrainous symptoms, may delay treatment.

Intermittent red eye and headache

Case

A 44-year-old woman reported intermittent redness and bulging of her right eye in association with headache. For five years, the episodes had occurred at least once a year and lasted for up to two weeks. During the episodes she had severe, 10/10 ipsilateral headache without migrainous features. Toward the end of the episodes her vision became blurry. She had been treated with antibiotic and steroid eye drops without benefit. Recently her symptoms had lasted longer than usual and while she was visiting a family member in the hospital a casual physician observer suggested she should seek emergency evaluation.

What are the possible causes of intermittent red eye and headache?

Redness of the eye can occur because of autonomic dysfunction, venous congestion, or an inflammatory condition. In this case, an inflammatory condition such as orbital cellulitis seems unlikely given the intermittent and unilateral nature of the symptoms and lack of association with other symptoms such as fever. Cellulitis is also unlikely to resolve spontaneously.

Cluster headache can present with a unilateral red eye and ipsilateral pain, but by definition the individual attacks cannot last for longer than three hours. Some patients with chronic cluster headache do develop a low-grade constant background discomfort in the orbital and temporal area, but the severe nature of the pain in this case is not consistent with that possibility.

Intermittent acute angle-closure glaucoma is another possibility, but it does not typically last for two weeks: the duration of a typical episode of angle-closure glaucoma is only 30 to 60 minutes. It is usually associated with other symptoms such as halos around lights. This patient has reported only blurry vision. Additionally, this patient does not report exposure to provocative agents that are associated with the development of acute angle-closure glaucoma, such as a dark or dim environment, prolonged near work, or sneezing.

Proptosis is not a feature of either cluster headache or glaucoma. A mass lesion of the orbit or retro-orbital area is a possibility but it is unlikely that would produce intermittent proptosis and redness. Cavernous sinus thrombosis could produce these symptoms, but it does not usually remit and recur.

What is the next step in evaluation of this patient?

The intermittent bulging and congestion of the eye suggest the possibility of a vascular lesion and the need for further imaging of the cerebral vessels. On examination during an episode, this patient had right proptosis, ptosis, and slightly decreased right visual acuity as well as dilated episcleral vessels. The optic discs were normal but the right retina showed some venous engorgement. A carotid cavernous fistula was suspected after the patient mentioned that she could "hear my heartbeat" when the eye was bulging.

A magnetic resonance angiogram did not show a fistula but the right cavernous sinus was enlarged. Conventional cerebral angiography confirmed a right carotid cavernous fistula.

Discussion

Carotid cavernous fistulas can cause eye pain, visual loss, and proptosis, probably due to marked orbital and cerebral venous congestion. In this case, the diagnosis of a carotid cavernous fistula was suggested by the recurrent and remitting nature of the episodes in combination with suspicious findings on examination, particularly the ocular bruit that was audible to the patient.

In carotid cavernous fistulas there is abnormal communication between the carotid artery and the cavernous sinus, usually through dural branches of the internal or external carotid artery. These fistulas can result from trauma, but the cause of non-traumatic fistulas is not known.

Elevated pressure in the cavernous sinus can produce substantial venous congestion in the orbit, with resulting visual loss. While small fistulas may seal over, larger and more symptomatic lesions are generally treated with endovascular techniques to close the connection.

Diagnosis

Carotid cavernous fistula.

Tip

A red, bulging eye accompanied by headache is not consistent with a primary headache disorder and requires further workup.

A young woman with morning headaches

Case

A 24-year-old female reported new-onset bilateral, frontal, and retro-orbital headache onset every morning that resolved later in the day. There were no associated symptoms. There was no prior history of headache. Her neurologic examination was normal. She was diagnosed with sinus headache and advised to try over-the-counter decongestants.

The headaches improved but then returned about three months later and were more intense. She returned to her doctor, who wrote in the chart that there were "no neurologic abnormalities." A computed tomographic scan of the head was ordered and she was referred for neurologic evaluation.

Is it appropriate to order imaging in this case?

Headache is common and usually benign, especially when there are no associated abnormalities and the neurologic examination is normal. If such patients meet criteria for one of the primary headache disorders such as migraine or tension-type headache, further evaluation is unlikely to be fruitful. In these circumstances the chance of finding a clinically meaningful abnormality on neuroimaging has been estimated at about 0.1%. Instead of imaging, reassurance

and management for the presumed benign condition is appropriate.

In this case, though, a diagnosis of sinus headache was made in the absence of any obvious symptoms of sinusitis. The patient is at an age where migraine commonly begins, but she does not have typical features of migraine such as nausea or sensitivity to light or noise. Despite initial improvement, her headache problem is progressing. Neuroimaging thus seems appropriate to evaluate the possibility of underlying explanations for headache.

A brain CT showed a lesion and early papilledema was noted on funduscopic examination by the neurologist. Brain MRI showed a 4 cm enhancing lesion in the left posterior fossa with significant mass effect on the cerebellum and the adjacent brainstem, and partial compression of the fourth ventricle. The patient was admitted for further evaluation and ultimately diagnosed with a medulloblastoma.

This seemed like a benign headache. What was missed?

This was a new-onset headache that did not clearly meet criteria for any primary headache. Although the initial visit note indicated that there were no neurologic abnormalities, no funduscopic examination was documented in the record. Thus, it is not at all clear that the neurologic examination was normal. Had a careful funduscopic examination been done, papilledema might have been detected and the diagnosis of medulloblastoma made sooner. It also seems likely that the initial improvement in the headache led to a false feeling of reassurance.

Discussion

Headache is present at some point in up to 50% of brain tumor patients, but it is rarely the presenting symptom. Nonetheless, doctors worry about cases like this one, in which a patient presenting with headache and no other features turns out to have a deadly brain tumor.

The response to cases like this should not be to image indiscriminately all patients with new-onset headache. Even in patients with new-onset headache the prior probability of a dangerous cause of headache is low when there are no associated symptoms – this particular case notwithstanding – and most imaging findings will be "incidentalomas" that do not change clinical care.

Rather, this case underscores the importance of a thorough neurologic examination, including a funduscopic examination, in every patient with new-onset headaches. It also illustrates the value of follow-up visits and clinical monitoring. Although the underlying tumor causing this patient's headaches was missed at the first visit, appropriate testing was done when she returned to report that she was worse.

Careful monitoring of the clinical course of headaches is a suitable way to gather more information about a headache problem where the diagnosis is not clear. This "watchful waiting" strategy avoids the harms and costs that come from over-testing while minimizing the likelihood that an important problem will be overlooked.

Diagnosis
Medulloblastoma.

Tip
Omitting the funduscopic examination in the evaluation of headache can lead to errors in diagnosis. A careful examination of the optic fundi is an essential part of the physical examination of every patient presenting with headaches.

More morning headaches

Case
A 58-year-old obese man with a history of episodic migraine since his teens presented for evaluation of subacute onset chronic headache about one year ago. The headache was holocephalic, moderate to severe in intensity, pounding, associated with mild photophobia and phonophobia, and worse with activity. There was no aura. He woke up with a headache every morning and sometimes awakened from sleep with a headache as well. He described his sleep as broken, and said he had been "a snorer" his whole life. His girlfriend noticed periodic apneas over the last two years. After nights when he didn't sleep well, his headaches were usually worse. A brain MRI was normal. Treatment with multiple abortive and preventive migraine medications for a diagnosis of presumed migraine was only

of mild benefit. He was significantly limited in his daily activities.

What are possible diagnoses for this headache presentation and what testing would you consider?
This patient has a history of a previous primary headache disorder, episodic migraine, and transformation from the episodic to the chronic form of the disorder might be one explanation for his daily headaches. Both snoring and sleep-disordered breathing are risk factors for progression of migraine.

Headache that is present every morning and more severe than at other times of day is commonly reported in many severe chronic headache disorders. It does not clearly point to a particular diagnosis. However, nocturnal hypoxia could also produce morning headache and can be seen in association with sleep apnea syndrome. This seems to fit with the report of apneic episodes during sleep.

An overnight polysomnogram in this patient showed moderate obstructive sleep apnea. He was started on continuous positive airway pressure therapy (CPAP) and within one week his daily headaches had resolved. He continued to have occasional intermittent migraine headaches.

Discussion
Obstructive sleep apnea is often associated with headache and is a risk factor for transformation of migraine from episodic to chronic. All patients with chronic headache or headache upon awakening should be questioned about symptoms of obstructive sleep apnea, such as frequent nighttime awakenings, witnessed apneas by bed partners, unrefreshing sleep, daytime somnolence, and irritability (Table 3.2). Certain risk factors for obstructive sleep apnea are also easily assessed in a routine office visit, including elevated body mass index (BMI), retrognathia, and presence of a large neck circumference. Some patients do not have full apneas, but may have nocturnal hypoxic episodes that could contribute to headache as well.

Obstructive sleep apnea and nocturnal hypoxic episodes are evaluated with a polysomnogram, which includes continuous oxygen saturation monitoring. Referral to a sleep specialist or for a polysomnogram should be considered in any patient who reports

Table 3.2. Features associated with obstructive sleep apnea

Morning headaches

Snoring

Daytime somnolence

Irritability

Unrefreshing sleep

Obesity

Large neck circumference

Poorly controlled hypertension

symptoms of obstructive sleep apnea, or has several risk factors for obstructive sleep apnea in addition to refractory headache. Preliminary studies suggest that most patients with headaches and obstructive sleep apnea have improvement of the headaches when the disorder is effectively treated.

This patient had a known primary headache disorder, which might have predisposed him to having headaches in response to another stimulus, in this case obstructive sleep apnea. However, treatment with migraine therapy did not completely resolve the headache. When he received treatment for obstructive sleep apnea he reverted to his previous pattern of episodic migraine. This illustrates the importance of looking for other potential causes or aggravating factors of headache in patients with known primary headache disorders whose headaches change in character.

Diagnosis

Obstructive sleep apnea causing progression from episodic to chronic migraine.

Tip

Obstructive sleep apnea can be a cause of difficult-to-treat chronic headaches and headaches often respond well to treatment of apnea.

A middle-aged man with side-locked headache

Case

A 35-year-old man had a five-year history of episodic left-sided headache that was side-locked (i.e. did not shift sides). The headache had been severe at times and was difficult to control. Although there was no family history of migraine or other chronic headaches the patient was thought to have migraine. A brain MRI scan showed a small pituitary adenoma without anatomic compression or extension. The patient reported no endocrine symptoms. The patient was advised that the finding was very unlikely to be the cause of his headache and additional trials of treatment for migraine were attempted.

Three years later the patient developed severe, chronic headache and was unable to work. A repeat MRI showed an increase in the size of the adenoma although there was still no evidence of extension or compression. Careful questioning elicited symptoms consistent with early acromegaly: an increase in shoe and glove size and hypertrophy of the gums. After neurosurgical evaluation he was offered surgical removal of the adenoma through a trans-sphenoidal approach. One month after surgery he was almost headache-free and planning to return to work.

Should the patient initially have been advised that the MRI finding was unrelated to the headache pattern?

Probably not, since headache is surprisingly common among patients with pituitary tumors. In fact, it is the presenting feature in 40–70% of cases. It does not seem to be related to the size of the tumor. In one small cohort of patients who had pituitary tumors and troublesome headaches, almost half had improvement in headaches following surgery, suggesting a causal relationship. However, 15% of patients reported worsening of headaches following surgery. Headache alone is generally not considered a sufficient indication for surgery because of this uncertainty.

What are the characteristics of headaches in people with pituitary tumors?

One study evaluated the phenotypic characteristics of 84 patients with pituitary adenomas. Headache was side-locked in 88% of cases, and over half described the pain as throbbing. In fact, the majority had headaches with many of the features of migraine. The presence of migrainous features was associated with a family history of migraine. Perhaps people with a genetic predisposition to migraine are also more likely to develop headache in the presence of a pituitary tumor.

Thus, in contrast to the general rule that headaches due to brain tumors have features of tension-type headache, headache associated with pituitary lesions more often fits criteria for episodic or chronic migraine.

Other headache patterns described with pituitary lesions include cluster headache, SUNCT (Short-lasting, Unilateral Neuralgiform headache attacks with Conjunctival injection and Tearing), or primary stabbing headache. No specific tumor type is associated with a specific headache type. Interestingly, only a few pituitary headaches meet the official criteria for intracranial neoplasm headache or pituitary hypersecretion headache, and thus revisions to the classification have been proposed. Almost half of patients will report severe disability due to headache.

Discussion

Pituitary headache may be more severe than typical migraine and when unilateral may often be side-locked. Less commonly, pituitary headache may mimic cluster or other more rare forms of primary headache. Pituitary headache may also be chronic and disabling. Growth hormone (GH)- or prolactin-secreting pituitary tumors are more likely to be associated with headache than nonsecreting tumors. The lack of association between headache and tumor size, volume, or compression suggests that traction is not the most likely mechanism of headache. The pathophysiology of these headaches is more likely to reflect the hormonal activity of the tumor than its physical characteristics.

Significant headache relief has been reported in some instances after treatment with somatostatin analogs, for example octreotide, in GH-producing tumors, or dopamine agonists, for example cabergoline or bromocriptine, in prolactinomas.

Diagnosis

Headache associated with growth hormone-secreting pituitary adenoma.

Tip

Pituitary tumors are a common incidental finding on neuroimaging for headache, and it is difficult to determine whether they are the cause of headache. When unilateral the headache is often side-locked, a historical feature that may indicate the headache is more likely to be due to a non-migraine process.

Fatal migraine

Case

A 53-year-old man with a long history of migraine with visual and dysphasic aura died following a two-month attack of constant, severe left-sided headache. The headache was associated with a persistent visual defect typical of his previous visual aura, as well as hemiplegia, and was assumed to be simply a particularly long episode of his usual migraine.

Can migraine be lethal?

We are cheating a bit here, because this case is not a patient from our practice. Rather, it was reported almost 130 years ago by Féré, a resident of the famous French neurologist Jean-Martin Charcot. Bousser and Welch point to this as "the first case of lethal migrainous stroke" but note that "in the absence of autopsy, the precise cause of death is unknown." The term "fatal migraine" occasionally appears in the neurologic literature, usually referring to cases in which an apparent attack of migraine aura persists and culminates in death from stroke. Obviously, it is always difficult in such cases to know whether the headache in question was an early symptom of the stroke, or whether the stroke was caused by the headache.

How might migraine aura lead to stroke?

The way in which an attack of migraine aura might cause stroke is not definitely known. A leading possibility is that an infarct might be caused by cerebral hypoperfusion due to migraine aura. Decreases in cerebral blood flow are known to occur in the setting of aura, but typically are not sufficient to produce ischemic symptoms. Migraine with aura is a common, long duration condition, and sufferers may have hundreds of auras over a lifetime. Yet true migrainous infarction is rare. In unusual circumstances, however – such as volume depletion or hypercoagulability – perhaps the hypoperfusion that occurs during aura is amplified and sufficient to produce a stroke.

Other theories are that migraine with aura is associated with other stroke-causing conditions such as patent foramen ovale or cerebral artery dissection. It is also possible that vasoconstrictive treatments used for individual attacks of migraine may occasionally produce stroke. Still another explanation is that migraine is associated with the presence of vascular risk factors such as endothelial dysfunction that raise stroke risk. Finally, the increased susceptibility to cortical spreading depression that is a hallmark of the migraine-prone brain may also act more generally to boost susceptibility to brain ischemia.

Discussion

Current diagnostic criteria in ICHD-3 beta allow a diagnosis of "migrainous infarction" only in patients known to have migraine with aura. The stroke must develop during a typical aura, and imaging must show a defect in the relevant brain location. Other explanations for stroke must be excluded with a careful workup. Several cases have been reported in which patients met criteria for migrainous infarction but later proved to have unusual explanations for stroke, including cardiac myxoma and cerebral aneurysms.

Unsurprisingly, a large proportion of true migrainous infarcts occur in the occipital lobe, which fits with the fact that most auras are visual and arise from that part of the brain. In addition to cases of true migrainous infarction, there are numerous case reports of long lasting aura symptoms that resolve without subsequent stroke. A technique known as magnetic resonance diffusion with apparent diffusion coefficient maps has been used to distinguish between long-lasting aura and true migrainous infarction.

For historical interest, let us close with yet another case from the past: this patient is a 47-year-old man with a long history of migraine with typical visual aura. His visual auras always consist of a left scintillating scotoma, which develops gradually, fades away within 20 minutes, and is followed by a headache that meets criteria for migraine. One day he had a typical attack of visual aura but the visual abnormality did not resolve and he was left with a permanent upper left quadrantic defect. Your thoughts?

The case is that of a real person, a pathologist by the name of Frank Mallory (attributed to Polyak and reported by Bousser and Welch). He had migraine without aura and at age 47 experienced a persistent upper left quadrantic defect that arose during a typical visual aura. When he died 30 years later an autopsy revealed a calcarine infarct.

Diagnosis

The first vignette is consistent with a diagnosis of migrainous infarction and death, but 130 years later and in the absence of autopsy results, this diagnosis of "fatal migraine" cannot be confirmed.

Tip

True migrainous infarction is rare, and careful evaluation is needed to distinguish it from other causes of stroke or persistent aura without stroke.

Severe headache in a new mother

Case

A 28-year-old woman developed acute headache six hours after a forceps-assisted vaginal delivery for which she had epidural anesthesia. She had a history of episodic migraine with aura that she ordinarily treated with sumatriptan. Her headaches had not improved during pregnancy but she treated them only with acetaminophen and bed rest.

Eight hours after delivery the patient reported a severe bifrontal headache with nausea and blurred vision. This was similar to her prior migraines but much more severe. Her neurologic exam showed mild diffuse hyperreflexia but was otherwise normal. Urinalysis showed no proteinuria and her blood pressure was 132/82 mm Hg. The patient reported that she had been expecting a bad headache after delivery and asked to be treated with sumatriptan.

Would you give this patient sumatriptan?

The patient is no longer pregnant so fears about unintended effects on the baby are not a reason to avoid the use of sumatriptan. Sumatriptan is also considered compatible with breast-feeding by the American Academy of Pediatrics, so plans to nurse the baby likewise are not a contraindication to its use.

Headache occurs in about a third of women during the postpartum period and is more common in those with a prior history of migraine. In fact, in one study of 1000 women with postpartum headache the cause was migraine or another primary headache over three-quarters of the time. This patient had a history of migraine and furthermore her headaches had not improved substantially during pregnancy. This is consistent with epidemiologic evidence that women who have migraine with aura are less likely to experience pregnancy-related improvement of headaches than women who do not have aura.

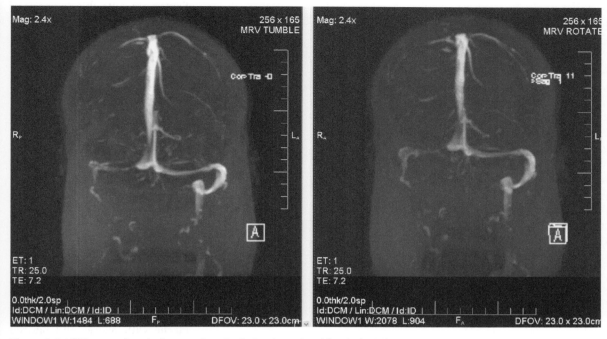

Figure 3.1 MRV images of cerebral venous thrombosis showing reduced flow in the right transverse sinus.

It is easy to understand how all of these things suggested that the patient's headache was a migraine and that sumatriptan would be an appropriate way to treat it. The patient was given sumatriptan but her headache did not improve. In fact, she became increasingly groggy and confused and several hours after a second dose of sumatriptan she had a generalized seizure.

Could this be something other than migraine?

It no longer seems particularly likely that the patient's headache was due to migraine. Although a diagnosis of migraine "fits the facts," this seems another case in which the cognitive error of premature closure might have occurred. Other less common causes of headache in the postpartum period also might "fit the facts."

For example, preeclampsia can occur in the post-partum period, and may be more common in patients with a history of migraine, especially migraine with aura. The patient's blood pressure was higher than might be expected in the postpartum setting, and she had hyperreflexia on examination. Now she has had a seizure. Could this be eclampsia?

The differential diagnosis of postpartum headache is long, however, and several other disorders could reasonably explain the findings in this case. Causes of secondary postpartum headache can be divided into vascular causes (stroke, venous sinus thrombosis, arterial dissection, vasculitis, reversible cerebral vasoconstrictive syndrome), and nonvascular causes (preeclampsia/eclampsia, idiopathic intracranial hypertension, post-dural puncture headache). Notably, seizures occur in almost 40% of patients with cerebral venous thrombosis, making that a top diagnostic possibility along with eclampsia.

The patient in this case was treated emergently with intravenous magnesium and phenytoin, and had an MRI, MRA, and MRV looking for vascular abnormalities. MRV confirmed transverse sinus thrombosis (Figure 3.1). The patient was begun on low-molecular-weight heparin and oral warfarin.

Discussion

The biggest risk of cerebral venous thrombosis occurs during the third trimester of pregnancy and the month following delivery. Headache is the most common symptom, occurring in about 90% of cases. In one series, roughly a third of patients had headaches with migrainous features, which underscores the challenge of distinguishing the early headaches of cerebral venous thrombosis from those of migraine.

Headache in cerebral venous thrombosis is presumably due to increased intracranial pressure from abrupt cerebral venous congestion. Papilledema is also a common finding. About a third of patients with cerebral venous thrombosis experience an intracranial hemorrhage. Headaches can persist for some time after cerebral venous thrombosis is treated.

Guidelines from the American Heart Association and American Stroke Association encourage testing for prothrombotic conditions such as factor V Leiden, protein S, or protein C deficiency in women who have had cerebral venous thrombosis, and recommend the use of low-molecular-weight heparin throughout future pregnancies.

Acute-onset severe headaches, particularly those associated with focal neurologic signs, are suggestive of vascular etiologies. In this clinical scenario, even in a patient with a history of benign headaches, extensive workup is often warranted. In this case, it is unlikely that the patient was directly harmed by sumatriptan, but that would not be true if her headache had been due to some other common causes of postpartum headache, such as reversible cerebral vasoconstrictive syndrome. The use of vasoconstrictive drugs such as the triptans or ergots could produce stroke in those cases.

Diagnosis

Cerebral venous thrombosis.

Tip

Although postpartum migraine is common, up to a quarter of postpartum headaches are due to other causes, including serious vascular problems that could be worsened by vasoconstrictive medications. For this reason, it is generally prudent to avoid triptans or ergots in the treatment of early postpartum headache.

Further reading

Temporal arteritis

Ezeonyeji AN, Borg FA, Dasgupta B. Delays in recognition and management of giant cell arteritis: results from a retrospective audit. *Clin Rheumatol.* 2011;30(2):259–62.

Graber ML, Franklin N, Gordon R. Diagnostic error in internal medicine. *Arch Intern Med.* 2005;165(13): 1493–9.

Poole TR, Graham EM, Lucas SB. Giant cell arteritis with a normal ESR and CRP. *Eye* 2003;17(1):92–3.

Sphenoid sinusitis

Digre KB, Maxner CE, Crawford S, Yuh WTC. Significance of CT and MR findings in sphenoid sinus disease. *AJNR Am J Neuroradiol.* 1989;10:603–6.

Lew D, Southwick FS, Montgomery WW, Weber AL, Baker AS. Sphenoid sinusitis. A review of 30 cases. *N Engl J Med.* 1983;309(19):1149–54.

Proetz AW. The sphenoid sinus. *BMJ.* 1948;2:243–5.

Carbon monoxide poisoning

Balzan MV, Agius G, Galea Debono A. Carbon monoxide poisoning: easy to treat but difficult to recognise. *Postgrad Med J.* 1996;72:470–3.

Heckerling PS. Occult carbon monoxide poisoning: a cause of winter headache. *Am J Emerg Med.* 1987;5(3):201–4.

Heckerling PS, Leikin JB, Maturen A, Perkins JT. Predictors of occult carbon monoxide poisoning in patients with headache and dizziness. *Ann Intern Med.* 1987;107(2): 174–6.

Post-ictal headache

Förderreuther S, Henkel A, Noachtar S, Straube A. Headache associated with epileptic seizures: epidemiology and clinical characteristics. *Headache.* 2002;42(7):649–55.

Ito M, Nakamura F, Honma H, *et al.* A comparison of post-ictal headache between patients with occipital lobe epilepsy and temporal lobe epilepsy. *Seizure.* 1999;8(6): 343–6.

Jacob J, Goadsby PJ, Duncan JS. Use of sumatriptan in post-ictal migraine headache. *Neurology.* 1996;47(4): 1104.

Rogawski MA. Migraine and epilepsy – shared mechanisms within the family of episodic disorders. In: Noebels JL, Avoli M, Rogawski MA, Olsen RW, Delgado-Escueta AV, editors. *Jasper's Basic Mechanisms of the Epilepsies [Internet],* 4th edition. Bethesda, MD, National Center for Biotechnology Information (US). 2012.

Scher AI, Bigal ME, Lipton RB. Comorbidity of migraine. *Curr Opin Neurol.* 2005;18(3):305–10.

Carotid cavernous fistula

Miller NR. Dural carotid-cavernous fistulas: epidemiology, clinical presentation, and management. *Neurosurg Clin N Am.* 2012;23(1):179–92.

Medulloblastoma

Ang C, Hauerstock D, Guiot MC, *et al.* Characteristics and outcomes of medulloblastoma in adults. *Pediatr Blood Cancer.* 2008;51(5):603–7.

Chan AW, Tarbell NJ, Black PM, *et al.* Adult medulloblastoma: prognostic factors and patterns of relapse. *Neurosurgery.* 2000;47(3):623–31; discussion 631–2.

Leary SE, Olson JM. The molecular classification of medulloblastoma: driving the next generation clinical trials. *Curr Opin Pediatr.* 2012;24(1):33–9.

Malheiros SM, Franco CM, Stávale JN, *et al.* Medulloblastoma in adults: a series from Brazil. *J Neurooncol.* 2002;60(3):247–53.

Obstructive sleep apnea

Bigal ME, Lipton RB. Modifiable risk factors for migraine progression. *Headache.* 2006;46(9):1334–43.

Bigal ME, Lipton RB. What predicts the change from episodic to chronic migraine? *Curr Opin Neurol.* 2009;22(3):269–76.

Neau JP, Paquereau J, Bailbe M, *et al.* Relationship between sleep apnoea syndrome, snoring and headaches. *Cephalalgia.* 2002;22(5):333–9.

Pituitary headache

Giustina A, Gola M, Colao A, *et al.* The management of the patient with acromegaly and headache: a still open clinical challenge. *J Endocrinol Invest.* 2008;31(10):919–24.

Levy MJ, Matharu MS, Meeran K, Powell M, Goadsby PJ. The clinical characteristics of headache in patients with pituitary tumours. *Brain.* 2005;128(Pt 8):1921–30.

Melmed S, Casanueva F, Cavagnini F, *et al.* Consensus statement: medical management of acromegaly. *Eur J Endocrinol.* 2005;153(6):737–40.

Stroke in the setting of migraine

Bousser MG, Welch KMA. Relation between migraine and stroke. *Lancet Neurol.* 2005;4:533–42.

Féré C. Note sur un cas de migraine ophtalmique à accès répétéssuivis de mort. *Rev Med (Paris).* 1883;3:194–201.

Kurth T, Chabriat H, Bousser MG. Migraine and stroke: a complex association with clinical implications. *Lancet Neurol.* 2012;11:92–100.

Polyak S. *The Vertebrate Visual System.* Chicago, IL, University of Chicago Press, 1957.

Cerebral venous thrombosis

Breteau G, Mounier-Vehier F, Godefroy O, *et al.* Cerebral venous thrombosis 3-year clinical outcome in 55 consecutive patients. *J Neurol.* 2003;250:29–35.

Saposnik G, Barinagarrementeria F, Brown RD Jr., *et al.*; on behalf of the American Heart Association Stroke Council and the Council on Epidemiology and Prevention. Diagnosis and management of cerebral venous thrombosis: a statement for healthcare professionals from the American Heart Association/American Stroke Association. *Stroke.* 2011;42(4):1158–92.

Pitfalls in diagnostic testing: imaging and lumbar puncture

Many causes of headache can be identified based on the history and physical examination. Patients who clearly meet criteria for a primary headache disorder generally do not need additional diagnostic testing. In some cases, however, there is clinical suspicion of a possible alternative diagnosis and testing is needed to "rule out" a sinister cause of pain. In the majority of these situations, clinical suspicion centers on possible structural or mechanical explanations for headaches. For this reason, a good case can be made that imaging tests and lumbar puncture (LP) are the most important diagnostic tools in headache medicine, with a correspondingly large number of mistakes that can be made and adverse events that can occur.

We all accept that failure to order a needed test, misinterpreting test results, or lack of follow-up of worrisome test results can lead to avoidable harm. We are less accustomed to thinking about the possibility of harm from ordering unnecessary tests, or other test-related harms that are more difficult to quantify. These include the iatrogenic anxiety that can be produced by false-positive test results and the long-term health risks of testing, such as the risk of cancer from test-related radiation.

This chapter reviews cases in which imaging tests or LP were overused, underused, or misused, as well as situations in which complications occurred as a result of testing. A common thread in all of these cases is that the decision to order a test and the interpretation of test results must be considered in the context of the individual patient and the specific clinical situation. Test results that do not fit the clinical picture should prompt careful reevaluation of the situation. Recognition of adverse events from testing and the appropriate management of test-related complications are also important aspects of headache management.

Refractory migraine in the emergency department

Case

A primary care physician received a nighttime call from an emergency department physician about a patient of hers, a 20-year-old woman, who had intermittent severe headaches. These occurred on average twice a month and met criteria for migraine. They typically responded well to oral sumatriptan. On occasion, though, the patient awakened with a well-established headache and prominent vomiting and was unable to keep her oral medications down. She then sought treatment in the emergency department, as she had this time.

Her records showed a total of six emergency department visits over the last three years for similar headaches. The emergency department physician reported that the patient's neurologic examination was normal, and the results of past testing, including three CT scans of the head, one MRI study, and an LP, had been normal.

What additional testing is needed?

The answer is "none." Severe, poorly controlled pain is a medical emergency and an appropriate reason to seek emergency care. Nothing about this patient's situation, however, suggests a dangerous underlying cause of headache or points to the need for additional testing. This patient meets criteria for migraine. She has had previous emergency department visits for similar headaches. Vomiting is a common accompaniment of her headaches, and her consequent inability to keep down oral medication is the main reason she is seeking care now.

It is unlikely that another CT scan of the head or other testing will identify anything that will alter her management. Furthermore, the radiation risks of diagnostic imaging are not negligible. They are highly dependent on age, with younger people being at higher risk than adults. The authors of a recent review of the risks of diagnostic CT scans concluded that "In summary, there is direct evidence from epidemiologic studies that the organ doses corresponding to a common CT study … result in an increased risk of cancer. The evidence is reasonably convincing for adults and very convincing for children."

A more reasonable plan would be to forgo additional diagnostic testing and treat the patient with subcutaneous sumatriptan. If this is effective and well tolerated, she could be given a prescription for a sumatriptan auto-injector so that she can give herself subcutaneous injections of the medication when oral treatment is not possible. As we mention elsewhere in this book, patients who have a history of prominent vomiting in association with migraine often benefit from having such a non-oral "rescue" treatment option available.

Can the radiation risks of a single head CT be quantified?

Yes. Radiation doses are measured in units of ionizing energy absorbed per unit of body mass. The radiation dose varies depending upon the type of imaging procedure, the number of scans obtained during the procedure, the equipment used, and other factors. Radiation doses from CT scans are much greater than doses from conventional X-rays. The estimated radiation dose from a typical CT scan of the head, for example, is 340 millisieverts. The radiation dose from a single CT scan of the head may seem small, but there is good research evidence that even exposures in this range are associated with a statistically significant increase in the lifetime risk of cancer. These risk estimates have not been extrapolated from studies of higher-dose exposures, but are instead based on long-term follow-up of groups with similar exposures. The estimated lifetime attributable risk of subsequent brain cancer as a result of a single CT scan of the head at age 20, for example, has been estimated at roughly 0.01%. At age ten, the risk is 0.02%. For an individual patient the risks are low, but on a population level it is estimated that diagnostic radiation exposure may account for 1.5–2% of all cancers.

Discussion

It is not uncommon to encounter patients with headache who have had multiple imaging procedures, including many that involve exposure to ionizing radiation. Repeated, probably unnecessary, scans are ordered when physicians and patients are frustrated about a lack of response to treatment and fear something might have been missed. In other cases, the results of previous scans may not be easily available, with the result that physicians are unaware of previous testing. The risk of unneeded testing may be especially high in the emergency department since physicians are often unfamiliar with the patient and fear missing serious causes of headache. In ordering diagnostic tests, though, the possible adverse effects of testing must be weighed against the likely benefits to the patient. In this case, the balance of benefit to harm for any additional testing is not favorable.

Diagnosis

Migraine.

Tip

The potential adverse health effects of radiation exposure should be taken into consideration when ordering diagnostic testing for headache.

A young woman with stable headaches

Case

A 22-year-old woman sought treatment for twice-monthly headaches that began four years ago. Her most severe headaches were throbbing, located behind the right or left temple, and associated with nausea and photophobia. They typically responded to treatment with an over-the-counter combination medication that contained acetaminophen, aspirin, and caffeine. Occasionally treatment was ineffective and she missed a day of work. Her neurologic examination, including funduscopic examination, was normal and she had no other medical problems and was taking no medications except for headache.

A friend of hers had similar headaches that respond well to almotriptan. The patient requested a prescription for that medication. She also requested an MRI scan of her head, saying "I don't think my headaches are caused by something serious, but you never know. I would feel better if I had a normal scan."

The physician diagnosed migraine, ordered an MRI scan, and prescribed almotriptan.

A month later the patient returned for a follow-up visit to review her MRI results. She reported that almotriptan had worked well for the only headache she had since her last visit. The MRI shows no mass lesion or other abnormalities but the radiologist's report described a small arachnoid cyst in the posterior fossa. Despite an explanation that this finding was unlikely to be related to her headaches, the patient was not reassured. She later called to request referral to a neurosurgeon and to obtain a copy of her scan for a second opinion.

Were there medical reasons to scan this patient?

The patient in this vignette met diagnostic criteria for migraine. Her condition had been stable for several years. A practice parameter from the American Academy of Neurology discourages the use of diagnostic imaging or other testing in these circumstances. This is because the prevalence of meaningful abnormalities in this clinical situation is low, on the order of approximately 0.2%, with an upper 95% confidence limit of approximately 0.6%. It is difficult to argue that a brain scan was medically necessary in this patient. Most clinicians have been faced with patients like this one who do not have a medical reason for testing but who request it nonetheless in order to allay anxiety.

Does testing reassure patients?

Only one study has examined this question in patients with headache. In that study the investigators measured baseline depression and health anxiety levels in patients with chronic daily headache and then randomized them to receive or not receive an MRI scan of the head. The results showed that patients who received a scan were less worried about their health at three months compared to those who had not received a scan. By a year, however, there were no differences in anxiety between the two groups. The group that had received a scan, though, had lower overall medical costs than the group that had not been scanned.

All of the patients in that study had normal test results, however, so the findings do not apply to situations like this one, in which patients undergo testing and are found to have so-called "incidentalomas"

– that is, test results showing abnormalities that are unlikely to be clinically significant.

Although this study suggested short-lived reductions in anxiety in patients with chronic daily headache who underwent testing, similar studies in other conditions have not clearly shown that testing reassures patients. In a systematic review of five controlled trials in a variety of conditions, four of five studies did not find that patients were reassured. The authors concluded that "the results point in the direction of diagnostic tests making hardly any contribution to the level of reassurance." They suggested that "a clear explanation and watchful waiting" might make testing unnecessary and commented that "if diagnostic tests are used, it is important to provide adequate pre-test information about normal test results."

When diagnostic imaging is indicated, should patients be warned of the possibility of incidental findings?

Discussing possible testing outcomes with the patient *before* test results come back may be advisable. This is because patients may have well-established beliefs about the seriousness of their symptoms that make it difficult for them to believe and be reassured by normal or clinically irrelevant test results. The authors of one study suggested that "providing an explanation about the meaning of normal test results before testing may weaken patients' preconceived ideas about their illness and provide a context to help patients make sense of the test result." The authors tested this hypothesis in a randomized trial among patients with chest pain referred for a stress test. Patients who participated in a discussion of what it would mean if they had normal test results were more likely to report feeling reassured at one and three months, and fewer were taking cardiac drugs at one month.

Based on this evidence, in our practice we make a point of discussing possible test results with patients *before* we send them for testing. This includes a discussion of the possibility that small abnormalities may be identified that do not have any diagnostic or treatment implications.

Discussion

Many doctors feel that patients will not be reassured about the benign nature of their condition without proof from testing that nothing is wrong. It is not uncommon for physicians to acquiesce to patient requests for tests that may not be necessary. Despite their good intentions testing can cause unintended adverse effects, including a paradoxical increase in anxiety when results deviate from normality. Ordering a test may reinforce the patient's belief that something is wrong. Some tests involve exposure to radiation, which may increase the risk of later cancers. Test results of uncertain significance may set in motion yet more diagnostic testing or lead to treatment that causes harm, a situation known as the "medical cascade." Unnecessary testing contributes importantly to healthcare costs. It is also possible that patients will continue to feel anxious and worried even after they receive normal test results.

Diagnosis

Migraine.

Tip

There is limited evidence to support the view that diagnostic testing reassures patients who are anxious about the cause of their headaches. It may be difficult to reassure patients whose test results reveal minor abnormalities of no clinical relevance.

A young man with constant headaches

Case

A 19-year-old man sought medical treatment for constant, low-grade headaches with superimposed episodes of more severe headache several times a week. He reported a history of carsickness and intermittent headaches dating back to childhood. Many members of his family, including his mother and a sister, had severe episodic headaches and had been diagnosed with migraine. When he was a child the patient's headaches occurred on average twice a month, but about a year ago they had gradually worsened and become constant. Severe exacerbations of headache were described as global; throbbing; and associated with photo and phonophobia, nausea, and vomiting. These episodes of more severe headaches seemed to be brought on by emotional stress and had been responsive to both triptans and nonsteroidal anti-inflammatory medications such as aspirin. The patient was not experiencing difficulties in school or daily

activities as a result of the headaches and was able to exercise if the headaches were low grade.

A complete review of systems was negative and the patient had no prior history of medical problems. His general and neurologic examinations were normal. The physician did not believe that further diagnostic testing was indicated. The patient was advised to begin a low dose of amitriptyline as a preventive medication and continue using a triptan to treat severe headaches.

Were there medical reasons to scan this patient?

This young man's headaches met diagnostic criteria for chronic migraine. He had experienced a change in headache pattern – something that might be considered a "red flag" historical feature – but the transformation from episodic to chronic headache occurred a year ago and was gradual. Furthermore, his neurologic examination was normal. Additional reassuring historical features are the strong family and personal history of migraine and the carsickness, which is often viewed as a childhood precursor of migraine.

Patients like this are familiar to anyone who works in a specialty headache clinic; in fact, this clinical pattern of early childhood onset of migraine headaches with the gradual development of daily or near-daily headache is an extremely common clinical scenario. There is little in this patient's clinical presentation to suggest that initial imaging should have been recommended.

At the patient's first follow-up visit, he reported substantial improvement in his headaches with the amitriptyline, and almotriptan worked well for those that did occur. The patient's parents, however, were very concerned about his headaches and requested neuroimaging. The physician ordered an MRI scan of the head, which showed a right parietal mass. Additional workup identified this as a low-grade astrocytoma.

How do you reconcile this finding with the fact that neuroimaging is not recommended in cases of stable headache that meet criteria for migraine?

This is certainly a startling finding. A single case like this can have a disproportionate effect on a physician's beliefs about diagnostic testing. Had this finding been undetected at the initial headache evaluation and come to light later on, it is likely that the family would have considered that an important diagnosis had been delayed or missed. Low-grade astrocytomas are slow-growing glial tumors that occur most frequently in younger people. Since they can undergo malignant transformation, treatment of some type is usually recommended and prolonged survival is possible. It seems likely that the fortuitous discovery of this patient's tumor improved his long-term outcome.

Should an event like this change your practice? Since it is never possible to be certain a patient doesn't have something seriously wrong, shouldn't we image everyone with headache?

There is no right or wrong answer to these questions; rather, they are something that individual doctors must decide for themselves. We believe that physicians should think very carefully before adopting an indiscriminate approach to testing in order to reduce liability risks. Medical ethics experts have pointed out that defensive testing "essentially transfers test utility from the patient (for care) to the physician (for self-protection)." This is in conflict with the physician's professional obligation to put the patient's interests ahead of his or her own. Since diagnostic testing can expose patients to harm, ordering tests that are not indicated also is in conflict with the physician's ethical obligation to "first do no harm."

Finally, it is not clear that such an approach really does reduce the risk of a malpractice lawsuit, since numerous studies show that the likelihood patients will file a malpractice suit has little to do with actual malpractice or the extent of harm suffered. Extensive reliance on testing is probably more common among less capable physicians. One study of test-ordering behavior among neurologists found that older doctors, those who felt more confident in their diagnoses, and those who were board certified ordered fewer tests.

Discussion

Physicians can be strongly influenced by unusual or especially dramatic cases, and falsely perceive them to be more common than they are. Such cases tend to stick in the memory and are easily recalled. This is sometimes called "availability bias" because these diagnoses are easily "available." It is not difficult to imagine that this particular case, in which a serious problem was found in a patient who had little indication for scanning, might reinforce a doctor's belief that "everyone should be scanned because otherwise you might miss something."

"Defensive medicine" refers to the practice of ordering tests that are not medically indicated in order to protect the physician from an accusation of medical malpractice if rare but serious disorders are missed; in other words, situations such as the case described in this vignette. It would be difficult, perhaps impossible, to convince a jury that the headaches experienced by a patient such as this one were really due to migraine, especially in hindsight and with an abnormal test result. Should the possibility of rare, serious disorders lead doctors to order extensive diagnostic testing "just in case?"

Several features of this case suggest that the tumor was unrelated to the patient's headache problem and represented an incidental imaging finding. This patient's history is consistent with long-standing migraine that began at a time when he could not have had a brain tumor. It is also unlikely that a tumor like this would present as episodic migraine followed by transformation to a chronic pattern. Finally, his headaches improved with treatment aimed at migraine. Taken as a whole, it seems far more likely that the tumor, at the time it was detected, was asymptomatic. In fact, further history in this patient is that although he had transient improvement in headaches once the tumor was removed, headaches returned rapidly after surgery and resumed a chronic pattern. He reestablished care in the headache center for management of his chronic migraine.

Thus, we do not think that this case stands as evidence that all patients should be scanned in order to avoid missing rare events. Rather, it is a reminder that "uncommon events occur uncommonly" but can produce an outsized impact that may tend to sway us from our principles.

Diagnosis

Chronic migraine; incidental low-grade astrocytoma.

Tip

It is not practical, possible, or desirable to image all patients with headache. We recommend that doctors stick to their principles and image only when indicated.

Severe, sudden headache while mowing the lawn

Case

A 44-year-old woman presented to the emergency department one hour after the sudden onset of an extremely severe, generalized headache. The headache occurred while she was mowing the lawn on a warm summer day. There was associated nausea and mild photophobia but no phonophobia, and the pain was so severe she didn't want to move. She denied any aura prior to the headache. She had a remote history of migraine in her 20s but no significant headaches recently. She reported that this headache was very different from her previous migraines.

What is the clinical term used to describe the sudden onset of extremely severe headache, and what is the differential diagnosis?

The sudden onset of extremely severe headache is referred to as "thunderclap headache." The classic clinical scenario is a headache that reaches maximal intensity within seconds or minutes of onset. Thunderclap headache is a clinical presentation rather than a diagnosis, and the list of entities that can cause it is extensive (see Table 4.1). The experience is so dramatic that it is often likened to being hit by lightning (perhaps a more illustrative image than a peal of thunder!)

Both primary and secondary disorders can cause thunderclap headache. The best known and most-feared cause of thunderclap headache is subarachnoid hemorrhage, and initial workup appropriately focuses on this possibility. Other causes include intracerebral hemorrhage, reversible cerebral vasoconstrictive syndrome (RCVS), arterial dissection, stroke, and cerebral venous thrombosis. This long list of possible vascular sources means that a good rule of thumb in formulating a differential diagnosis for thunderclap headache

Table 4.1. Selected causes of thunderclap headache

- **Primary**
  - Primary thunderclap headache
  - Exertional headache
  - Cough headache
  - Headache associated with sexual activity
- **Secondary**
  - Reversible cerebral vasoconstrictive syndrome (RCVS)
  - Subarachnoid hemorrhage
  - Intracerebral hemorrhage
  - Cerebral venous thrombosis
  - Arterial dissection
  - Stroke
  - Pituitary apoplexy
  - Colloid cyst

is to "think blood vessels." Nonvascular causes of thunderclap headache do exist, though. These include large colloid cysts which can intermittently block the third ventricle (producing transient hydrocephalus), and pituitary apoplexy.

If secondary causes of thunderclap headache are ruled out, several primary headache disorders that can sometimes present in this way should be considered. These include headaches provoked by activity (such as exertional headache, cough headache, and headache associated with sexual activity) as well as primary thunderclap headache. More controversial is so-called "crash migraine." This is an informal diagnostic term used by some headache experts to describe migraine attacks that build up quickly to peak intensity, rather than exhibiting the more gradual increase in pain intensity that is more common in migraine.

For the patient described in this vignette, all of these diagnoses must be considered. In particular, her previous history of migraine does not protect her against the many secondary causes of thunderclap headache. She requires urgent evaluation for dangerous causes of thunderclap headache, and the investigation should be as thorough as it would be in a patient with no prior history of headaches.

What workup should she have?

All patients presenting to the emergency department with thunderclap headache, including this patient, should have a noncontrast-enhanced CT of the head to evaluate for subarachnoid hemorrhage. It is well established that CT may be negative in 5% of cases of subarachnoid hemorrhage, however, so a follow-up LP in this situation is mandatory. False-negative findings on

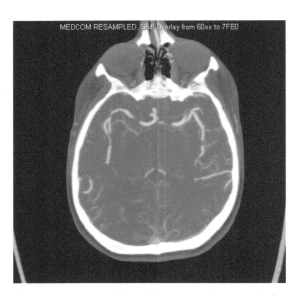

Figure 4.1 One image from a CT angiogram showing multifocal segmental areas of vascular narrowing that can be associated with reversible cerebral vasoconstrictive syndrome (RCVS).

LP can occur, however, since xanthochromia may not be seen until several hours after the initial development of headache. This means that visual inspection may not detect xanthochromia when LP has been performed very early after onset of headache. Spectrophotometry is helpful in these cases.

Even when subarachnoid hemorrhage has been ruled out by appropriate investigation, however, further diagnostic testing should be strongly considered. Reversible cerebral vasoconstrictive syndrome is increasingly recognized as a frequent cause of thunderclap headache. In RCVS there is segmental constriction of cerebral arteries, which produces a classic beaded appearance of the vessels. Typically this constriction begins in the distal vessels and spreads proximally. RCVS (as well as arterial dissection) can be recognized with MRI and MRA. Depending on the history, a magnetic resonance venogram may also be warranted. In the patient described in the vignette, the initial CT and LP were normal but a CT angiogram (Figure 4.1) demonstrated the characteristic beading appearance of RCVS.

Discussion

Thunderclap headache is an important presentation of headache in emergency settings. In our experience, most physicians are aware of the importance of obtaining a head CT in this setting, and most also would perform an LP if the CT is negative. In contrast, fewer physicians seem to be aware of RCVS or other potentially dangerous causes of thunderclap headache. Nonetheless, we believe that the standard of care in such cases is evolving rapidly and that it is prudent to perform additional testing when the CT and LP are normal in patients with thunderclap headache.

This level of diagnostic testing is justified because many of the conditions which cause secondary thunderclap headache are life-threatening. If RCVS is suspected it is useful to obtain a detailed history of recent substance use. Vasoconstrictive substances, both prescribed and illicit, are often associated with RCVS. Patients should be carefully questioned about the use of sympathomimetic agents such as decongestants or cocaine. Selective serotonin reuptake inhibitors and selective serotonin–norepinephrine reuptake inhibitors, as well as marijuana, are also suspected of being occasional causes of RCVS.

Treatment of thunderclap headache depends on the underlying cause. If RCVS is found or strongly suspected despite negative imaging, most clinicians would consider the use of a calcium channel antagonist such as verapamil or nimodipine. If secondary causes of thunderclap headache have been convincingly ruled out, treatment for a primary cause is usually in order. This may include the use of calcium channel antagonists or such things as indomethacin if exertional headache is suspected. Reassurance is also important; most cases of drug-induced or primary thunderclap headache resolve spontaneously, usually within a few months. Avoidance of vasoconstrictive medications during this period of time is important, however. Evidence is lacking, however, about whether avoidance of vasoconstrictive substances should be continued beyond this period of time.

Diagnosis

Reversible vasoconstrictive syndrome (RCVS) presenting as thunderclap headache.

Tip

Thunderclap headache is a clinical presentation rather than a diagnosis. Workup of thunderclap headache in the emergency department begins with a noncontrast head CT and LP; if these are negative an MR or CT angiogram should be strongly considered to assess for RCVS.

Incidental white matter lesions in a migraineur

Case

A 34-year-old woman reported intermittent headaches since age 14. About three-quarters of headaches were preceded by visual aura lasting roughly 45 minutes. On four occasions these visual symptoms had lasted six to eight hours. Upon hearing this history, the patient's primary care physician was concerned about the possibility of a stroke or other intracranial lesion and ordered an MRI scan of the head. The MRI report described "several small areas of abnormal increased signal seen in the white matter of the hemispheres bilaterally on the T2 and FLAIR (fluid attenuated inversion recovery) sequences. This can be seen in migraine but other demyelinating process cannot be entirely excluded. Clinical correlation is advised." Despite an explanation that isolated T2 hyperintensities are commonly found in people with migraine and are not worrisome, the patient did not seem reassured. She later called to request testing for Lyme disease and referral to a multiple sclerosis specialist.

What is known about white matter lesions in people with migraine?

White matter lesions on MRI brain scans are more commonly found in migraineurs than the general population. A Dutch population-based study showed that patients with migraine were more likely than controls to have deep white matter lesions. The increased risk of white matter lesions in migraineurs was also found in a meta-analysis of case–control studies. A number of studies have also suggested an increased risk of cerebellar infarcts in migraineurs.

In the Dutch study, the risk of white matter lesions was greater for patients with migraine with aura (compared to no aura) and in those with higher attack frequency (at least 12 attacks per year). After nine years of follow-up, the original lesions persisted but had not increased in size. However, women with migraine had an increased incidence of new white matter lesions, but the overall volume of lesions remained low. There was no evidence of such progression in men, and migraine was not associated with progression of other brain lesions. There also was no association between the presence of white matter lesions and cognitive processing or speed. This finding is consistent with evidence from a French study that showed no association between migraine and the risk of dementia or cognitive impairment.

Is any further workup or treatment required?

If the white matter lesions are small, few in number, and the patient has no symptoms other than migraine, as with the patient in this vignette, no further workup is recommended. If the lesions are extensive, large, or distributed in locations that are characteristic of specific demyelinating disease, additional investigation may be warranted. White matter lesions seen on MRI have a broad differential diagnosis. Etiologies to consider include multiple sclerosis, cerebral autosomal dominant arteriopathy with subcortical infarcts and leukoencephalopathy (CADASIL), mitochondrial disease, vasculitis, or infectious etiologies such as Lyme disease. Many of these disorders have characteristic appearances on imaging. Most patients with these disorders also have accompanying neurologic signs and symptoms in addition to headache which suggest a diagnosis other than migraine.

There is no specific treatment for white matter lesions. Obviously, treatment of the headache disorder that the patient initially presented with is usually advisable. It is unknown whether preventive treatment of migraine might decrease the risk of developing new white matter lesions. The use of triptans or ergots is not contraindicated in patients with white matter lesions, since the use of these medications has not been associated with their development. However, some studies showed that patients with white matter lesions had more cardiovascular risk factors than those without, for example smoking or hypertension. It remains possible that there are subgroups of migraineurs who are at elevated risk of not only white matter lesions but also ischemic brain lesions. Thus, it is prudent to search for and address modifiable cardiovascular risk factors in patients with migraine.

There is no evidence to support the use of antiplatelet or antithrombotic therapy such as low-dose aspirin in migraine patients with white matter lesions. In fact, a recent analysis of data from the Women's Health Study showed that women who had migraine with aura randomized to daily aspirin had an increased risk of myocardial infarction compared with those who did not receive aspirin. In view of this finding, we do not recommend aspirin therapy in patients with migraine who have white matter lesions and no other indication for aspirin therapy.

Discussion

Patients with migraine who have scattered small white matter lesions on MRI can be reassured that the lesions do not indicate a dangerous underlying condition. It can be difficult to reassure patients, however, if this finding is unexpected, and particularly when the radiologist's report mentions possible diagnoses such as multiple sclerosis. This is a situation where discussing possible test results with patients *before* a scan is ordered can help allay anxiety when results come back. When ordering an MRI scan of the brain, for example, we routinely tell patients that it is not uncommon to find "white bright spots" on the MRI. We tell them that the importance of these findings is not known for sure, but that we do not believe they are anything to worry about.

It is not clear why white matter lesions occur in migraineurs. Evidence is conflicting about whether the presence of a right-to-left cardiac shunt (such as patent foramen ovale) is associated with a greater burden of white matter lesions. Some theorize that the lesions are caused by transient localized hypoperfusion during migraine or migraine aura, possibly caused by oligemia of the deep penetrating vessels, or by neuronal hyperexcitability. An alternative hypothesis is that migraine and migraine aura are associated with increased permeability of small meningeal vessels, perhaps triggered by cortical spreading depression, the phenomenon generally accepted as the pathophysiologic process underlying migraine aura. This breakdown in the blood–brain barrier could theoretically allow neurotoxic substances into the surrounding white matter, which might act in unknown ways to cause white matter lesions.

Diagnosis

Migraine with aura.

Tip

Nonspecific white matter FLAIR hyperintensities are often seen on MRI in patients with migraine and if the pattern is not suggestive of another disorder, no further workup or treatment is required. Patients should be reassured that these lesions are common and are not associated with any adverse outcomes.

Familial occurrence of white matter lesions

Case

A 44-year-old woman was referred to the headache clinic for evaluation of an abnormal MRI brain scan. The patient reported a three-month history of near-daily headaches in the context of substantial work and family stress. Headaches were located behind both eyes and were mild or moderate in intensity and described as "squeezing, like a hat that's too tight." She felt cognitively "fuzzy" during headaches but had no nausea, vomiting, or sensitivity to light or sound. Headaches responded well to ibuprofen. The headaches were getting better and her preference was not to add additional treatment. She had been referred because her primary care doctor ordered an MRI scan of the head to assess her headaches. The scan (Figure 4.2) showed white matter abnormalities that were felt by the radiologist to be unusual for her age.

What is the differential diagnosis of this pattern of white matter abnormalities?

The list of conditions that can produce white matter abnormalities is very long. These lesions can be seen in demyelinating conditions; with inflammatory or neoplastic processes; as a result of trauma; or in association with congenital, metabolic, toxic, degenerative, or vascular disorders. This patient has no hypertension, is not a smoker, and does not have diabetes. Testing for Lyme disease and coagulopathies was negative. Her neurologic examination was normal with the exception of a blunted affect and some subtle cognitive abnormalities.

The patient reported that her 71-year-old mother had experienced troublesome headaches for many years, and had recently developed cognitive problems. Her mother had radiation therapy for a

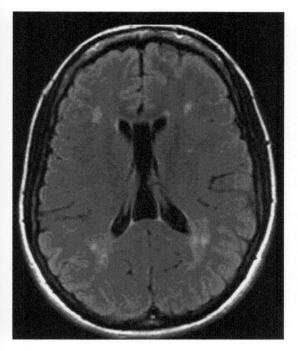

Figure 4.2 An MRI showing extensive white matter lesions in a 44-year-old woman.

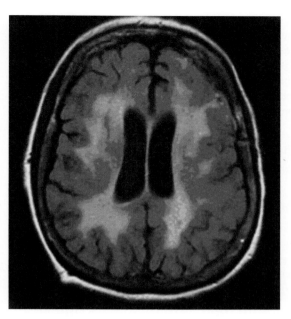

Figure 4.3 The MRI scan of the patient's mother, showing extensive white matter lesions of a size and distribution compatible with a diagnosis of CADASIL.

pituitary tumor over a decade ago. Two years ago she had developed confusion and the family had her evaluated for dementia. A meningioma was found and removed, but the cognitive problems persisted. The patient remarked that her mother "also had some other abnormalities on her MRI scan" but could not recall what they were.

What is the next step?

This patient's white matter lesions are extensive for her age. This in conjunction with her mild cognitive abnormalities and the report of headache and MRI abnormalities in her mother raise the possibility of a familial syndrome. The next step in this case was to obtain the mother's MRI scan for comparison. The list of genetic disorders that manifest as white matter abnormalities in conjunction with headache is quite short, and consists of mitochondrial abnormalities (such as mitochondrial encephalomyopathy, lactic acidosis, and stroke-like episodes [MELAS] and myoclonic epilepsy with ragged red fibers [MERFF]) or neurocutaneous disorders such as neurofibromatosis. These disorders can usually be easily distinguished from

CADASIL, however, by associated physical examination findings and laboratory testing. In this case, the mother's scan (Figure 4.3) shows extensive white matter lesions of a size and distribution compatible with a diagnosis of CADASIL.

Discussion

CADASIL is a genetically determined disorder caused by a *NOTCH3* mutation on chromosome 19. Initial symptoms can include migraine-like headaches or vague psychiatric symptoms. The disorder usually presents with brain dysfunction but it is actually a systemic disorder, due to abnormal accumulation of the NOTCH3 protein in vascular smooth muscle and the brain. A single-gene, autosomal recessive form of arteriopathy with similar clinical manifestations has recently been discovered and termed CARASIL (cerebral autosomal recessive arteriopathy with subcortical infarcts and leukoencephalopathy).

Molecular genetic testing can be done for CADASIL to identify the *NOTCH3* gene. Skin biopsy can also be diagnostic, since NOTCH3 protein accumulates at the cytoplasmic membrane of smooth muscle in peripheral as well as cerebral blood vessels.

The biopsy specimen, however, needs to be deep enough to include material from the border zone between the deep dermis and the upper subcutis. This patient was offered referral for genetic counseling and possible testing for CADASIL but declined the referral. She preferred to adopt a "watchful waiting" approach.

Diagnosis

Probable CADASIL.

Tip

Extensive white matter abnormalities in conjunction with a family history of headache and neurologic abnormalities should prompt consideration of a genetic syndrome.

A young man with headache following lumbar puncture

Case

A 28-year-old man who had an LP developed a headache within 12 hours of the procedure. It worsened within a few minutes when he stood upright and improved rapidly when he lay flat. It was associated with nausea and photophobia. The pain was severe. He was treated conservatively with bed rest, hydration, and caffeine for several days but the headache did not improve. On the basis of his clinical presentation, a diagnosis of post-dural puncture headache was made. He underwent a blood patch which provided some relief of headache for a day, but it then returned full force. His neurologic examination was benign. A gadolinium-enhanced MRI of the brain showed flattening of the pons and pachymeningeal enhancement. (Similar to changes depicted in Figure 4.5, although that is not the scan of this patient.)

Did this patient need neuroimaging or additional testing?

This patient had postural headache that occurred immediately following dural puncture. He had no additional features such as fever or focal neurologic findings that suggested an ominous cause of headache. The most likely diagnosis was post-dural puncture headache due to a persistent spinal fluid leak.

Diagnostic criteria for post-dural puncture headache do not require confirmation of the diagnosis with neuroimaging or other testing in the setting of a known dural puncture that is followed within five days by a postural headache. The criteria specify that the headache should worsen within 15 minutes of standing up, and improve within 15 minutes of lying down. One of the following must also be present: nausea, photophobia, hypacusia, tinnitus, or neck stiffness. Finally, the headache must improve spontaneously within a week or within 48 hours of effective treatment of the leak.

Thus, neuroimaging was not required to make the diagnosis in this case. It did, however, show characteristic abnormalities that supported a diagnosis of post-dural puncture headache, in this case brain sagging and diffuse pachymeningeal enhancement on an MRI with gadolinium. Similarly, a demonstration of low cerebrospinal fluid (CSF) pressure on LP is not required to make a diagnosis of post-dural puncture headache. If there is no history of a dural puncture, however, then confirmation of a diagnosis of low CSF pressure headache requires at least one of the following to be demonstrated: pachymeningeal enhancement on MRI, evidence of a CSF leak (with myelography or cisternography), or a CSF opening pressure of less than 6 mm Hg in the sitting position on LP.

Since the epidural blood patch was only temporarily successful, should this patient be treated with an epidural saline infusion or intravenous caffeine?

Epidural saline infusions, intravenous caffeine, and the use of abdominal binders are all treatments that have been reported helpful in cases of low CSF pressure headache. Before resorting to such measures, though, it is appropriate to repeat the epidural blood patch. A recent Cochrane review confirmed the benefits of epidural blood patches for treatment of post-dural puncture headache. Epidural blood patches should be done with at least 20 mL of autologous blood, which is typically injected one segment below the level of the dural puncture. The blood is thought to form a fibrin clot over the dural tear so that healing can occur. If a first blood patch does not succeed, a second one should be performed, and many experts would repeat this a third time if needed. A day or so of bed rest following the patch is often recommended although there is no strong evidence that this improves outcomes.

Pharmacologic therapy can be helpful when an epidural blood patch is ineffective. A recent Cochrane review concluded that caffeine is more effective than placebo for treating post-dural puncture headache. Theophylline, gabapentin, and hydrocortisone decreased pain severity scores compared with usual care or placebo. Evidence was uncertain for the effectiveness of sumatriptan or adrenocorticotropic hormone (ACTH). The role of intravenous fluids in treatment of post-dural puncture headache is also uncertain.

Discussion

The decreased volume of CSF that results from a spinal fluid leak causes headache through traction and tugging on pain-sensitive structures such as the large vessels of the brain. It also results in pachymeningeal enhancement on MRI because of compensatory engorgement of venous structures, which expand to fill the void caused by low levels of CSF. Almost a quarter of patients with low CSF pressure documented on LP, however, have normal imaging findings.

The use of smaller gauge pencil-point needles (rather than cutting needles) when performing an LP appears to reduce the incidence of post-dural puncture headache. Routine bed rest following LP does not appear to decrease the likelihood of post-dural puncture headache. Although blood patches are effective for treating post-dural puncture headache once it has occurred, evidence does not support using blood patches *prophylactically* to prevent the problem.

Diagnosis

Post-dural puncture headache.

Tip

Neuroimaging is not required to make a diagnosis of low CSF pressure headache in the setting of a known dural puncture followed by postural headache. If a first epidural blood patch is not successful, it should be repeated with a larger volume of blood up to three times.

A college student with malaise and a change in headache pattern

Case

A young male college student and athlete with a history of episodic migraine without aura sought evaluation for a recent change in headache pattern. He reported malaise and a three-day generalized, nondescript headache of moderate severity. He continued to attend class but was not concentrating well and was not able to exercise because it made his headache worse. On examination, he was afebrile but his neck was slightly stiff. Because he was very muscular, the physician thought this might be due to an inability to relax his neck muscles during the examination, which was otherwise normal. The physician considered performing an LP but recalled the patient he had seen earlier in the day who developed a post-dural puncture headache. She had been angry and reported that none of her prior headaches had been as bad as "the one you gave me." The physician advised the college student that his symptoms were likely to be from viral meningitis, were probably benign, and should respond to rest and analgesic medication.

When should a lumbar puncture be performed for the evaluation of headache?

The broad answer is that LP should be considered in the evaluation of any patient where the physician suspects a possible hemorrhage, infection, malignancy, or alteration in spinal fluid pressure as a possible cause of headache. When an LP is performed, it is routine to order laboratory testing of the fluid that includes a cell count on the first and last (usually the fourth) tubes of spinal fluid obtained, a spinal fluid protein level, and glucose determinations as well as infection-related testing. Additionally, the physician may order other special studies depending on the individual patient's situation. In our view, an opening pressure should be obtained routinely in all patients undergoing LP for the evaluation of headache, and the result should be recorded in the chart; a closing pressure can be obtained as well if warranted, which is usually in the setting of elevated intracranial pressure.

It can be challenging to decide when there is sufficient suspicion of one of these secondary headaches to warrant performing an LP. The possibilities of adverse effects of the LP, particularly post-dural puncture headaches, weigh heavily in this decision. The overall severity of the clinical situation and an assessment of how sick a patient is are both commonly taken into account. When the physician is still undecided, a clinical pearl that has been passed on from senior to younger physicians is that "the indication for an LP is whenever you think of it." In other words, experienced physicians have learned that it is important to maintain a high index of suspicion for dangerous illnesses that can only be diagnosed by LP.

The patient described in this vignette had a witnessed seizure at home later that night. He was taken to the emergency department where a CT of the head was negative but an MRI of the brain showed subtle bitemporal enhancement. His spinal fluid test results were consistent with a viral process. Antiviral therapy was started. Polymerase chain reaction (PCR) testing for herpes simplex virus (HSV) was later reported as positive. The patient was diagnosed with herpes simplex encephalitis and eventually recovered.

Was the hesitance to perform a lumbar puncture in this patient warranted?

Post-dural puncture headache is a complication of LP that occurs in up to 30% of procedures. The likelihood of this problem, and physician memories of unhappy patients who have experienced this complication, may make some physicians reluctant to perform the procedure, especially when secondary pathology is not highly suspected and the study is being considered simply to "rule out" other more serious conditions. On the other hand, in this particular case, the physician involved probably weighed the risk of post-dural puncture headache too highly based on his recent and easily recalled adverse experience with another patient. This is another example of availability bias, in which memorable events are easily recalled and erroneously thought to be more likely or common than is the case.

Discussion

Risk factors for the development of post-dural puncture are listed in Table 4.2. Some, such as the choice of needle used in the procedure, are modifiable, but others, such as patient sex, are not. Migraineurs may be at increased risk for post-dural puncture headache, so it is especially important that the pre-procedure informed consent discussion includes a review of post-dural puncture headache.

Table 4.2. Selected risk factors for headache following dural puncture

- Female sex
- Age between 31 and 50 years
- Prior history of post-dural puncture headache
- Use of a cutting needle (e.g. Quinke)
- Needle size
- Cutting needle bevel orientation perpendicular to the long axis of the spinal column during the procedure

It is unknown whether post-dural puncture headaches in migraineurs last longer or are more difficult to treat than in non-migraineurs, but our clinical experience suggests this might be the case. Fortunately, there is no evidence to suggest that the development of post-dural puncture headache will have a lasting negative effect on the patient's headache pattern. Thus, the decision to perform an LP in situations that warrant it should not depend on whether the patient has a history of migraine. The physician in this vignette was clearly hoping to avoid adding to this patient's existing burden of headache by avoiding a post-dural puncture headache. Unfortunately, his reluctance to perform an indicated diagnostic procedure led to a delay in diagnosis of a serious condition.

It is our impression that, for a variety of reasons, LP is an underused diagnostic procedure in a referral headache clinic and even emergency department settings. Careful attention to optimal procedural technique, as described in the next vignette, could improve both the clinician's and patient's experience with LP and decrease reluctance to perform it when indicated.

Diagnosis

Herpes simplex encephalitis.

Tip

Indicated diagnostic procedures such as LP should not be avoided in migraineurs because of a fear of complications.

Optimizing the performance of lumbar puncture

Case

A physician was covering the neurology consultation service of his local hospital one weekend. A

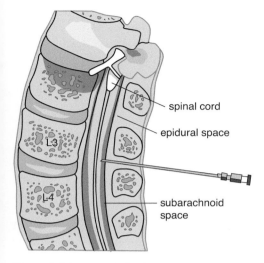

Figure 4.4 Anatomy of a lumbar puncture.

spinal cord

epidural space

L3

L4

subarachnoid space

first-year resident approached him and explained that she needed to perform an LP on a patient she had just admitted. She was not confident of her ability to do the procedure and asked if the physician could "walk her through" the technique.

How do you advise the resident?

LP is considered a routine medical procedure and most physicians gain experience performing LPs in their first post-graduate year. As with the resident in the vignette, though, most residents rely on advice and guidance from senior physicians to learn how to perform the procedure, which they then perfect through trial and error. The use of simulation-based training techniques has been shown to improve the performance of LP in clinical settings, but not all training programs provide simulator training. Figure 4.4 illustrates the anatomic structures and approach to doing an LP. There are many descriptions in the medical literature of the techniques for performing LPs. The following is a description of our preferred approach.

Procedure

1. Obtain informed consent; discuss with the patient the possibility of complications, including post-dural puncture headache, bleeding, or infection, and how those complications would be handled.

2. Explain the major steps of the procedure, how the patient will be positioned, and review aftercare recommendations.

3. Have the patient lie on an examining table or bed in the lateral decubitus position with knees curled up to the chin, or if seated ask them to lean over a solid surface on which they rest their elbows, since these positions spread the vertebrae and create maximum space between the interspinous processes.

4. Palpate for landmarks over the spinous processes at L4–5, L3–4, or L2–3 levels. If these cannot be palpated, locate the sacral promontory, which marks the interspace of L5–S1. Use this reference to locate L4–5 for the entry point.

5. Sterilize and drape the area after identifying landmarks. Use lidocaine 1% with or without epinephrine to anesthetize the skin and the deeper tissues under the insertion site.

6. Assemble needle and manometer. Attach the 3-way stopcock to manometer.

7. Insert LP needle through the skin and advance through the deeper tissues. A slight pop or give is felt when the dura is punctured. The angle of insertion should be slightly towards the navel, between the vertebrae. If you hit bone, partially withdraw the needle, reposition, and re-advance.

8. When CSF flows, attach the 3-way stopcock and manometer. Measure intracranial pressure, which should be 20 mm H_2O or less. Remember that any pressure reading performed when the patient is sitting will be unreliable.

9. If CSF does not flow, or you hit bone, withdraw needle partially, recheck landmarks, and re-advance.

10. Once the pressure has been recorded, remove the 3-way stopcock, and begin filling collection tubes 1–4 with 1–2 mL of CSF each:

    a. Tube 1: glucose, protein, protein electrophoresis, cell count
    b. Tube 2: Gram's stain, bacterial and viral cultures
    c. Tube 3: cell count and differential
    d. Tube 4: reserve tube for any special tests.

11. After tap, remove needle, and place a bandage over the puncture site.

a. Document the procedure in the patient's medical record.
b. Include in your note a brief history and physical examination of the patient, the reasons for performing the LP, and consent. Note in particular a brief examination of the cranial nerves, presence or absence of papilledema, or any other lateralizing neurologic finding. Also include a brief note of examination of the patient's spine with attention to any obvious spinal deformity.
c. Document position of patient during the procedure, opening pressure, and clarity/color of the CSF. Once results of the CSF analysis are available, they can be appended to your note.

Are there guidelines for the performance of lumbar puncture?

The American Academy of Neurology has published recommendations for the performance of LP. These suggest: (1) using the smallest needle size possible; (2) using noncutting atraumatic 22 gauge Sprotte spinal needles to reduce the frequency of post-dural puncture headache. If noncutting needles are used, the stylet should be replaced before the needle is withdrawn from the intradural space. (3) Keeping bevel orientation parallel to the long axis of the spinal canal if cutting needles are used. (4) Bed rest or fluid loading have not been shown to reduce the risk of post-dural puncture headache, so it is not necessary to limit activity after the procedure.

Misinterpreting the workup in low CSF pressure headache

Case

A 68-year-old male presented with a persistent headache of six months' duration. There was no past personal or family history of migraine. There was no history of trauma or instrumentation. Initially he had noticed a brief intermittent global headache triggered by coughing and at times associated with neck pain and tinnitus. The headache progressed to become daily with or without trigger but had cleared completely within five minutes when the patient lay down.

The headache was absent when he awakened in the morning but would recur within ten minutes after the patient got out of bed. A noncontrast head CT scan was normal. Low CSF pressure headache was considered as a diagnosis but excluded when a normal CSF opening pressure was found on LP and a normal CSF tracer study showed no apparent leak. The patient was diagnosed with cervical degenerative disease and cervicogenic headache. He unsuccessfully tried a variety of treatments, including nerve blocks and facet joint injections, and when seen in follow-up was no better.

Is cervicogenic headache the best diagnosis in this patient?

Certainly this story is more suggestive of a secondary headache than of migraine, and given the patient's age it was almost a certainty that testing would show some osteoarthritis of the neck. There is, however, very little specific history or diagnostic information in his case to suggest cervicogenic headache as a likely diagnosis. The term cervicogenic headache is used to describe a disorder of the cervical spine or adjacent structures that produces pain referred to the head or face. Apart from the finding of degenerative changes consistent with cervical spondylosis, there is little here to suggest cervical pathology as the cause of the patient's headache. Furthermore, cervical spondylosis and osteochondritis, since they are so commonly present asymptomatically, are explicitly mentioned in International Classification of Headache Disorders (ICHD)-3 beta as conditions that "may or may not be a cause of cervicogenic headache." In this patient, who has no physical findings of decreased cervical range of motion or worsening of headache with provocative neck maneuvers, cervicogenic headache does not seem a likely diagnosis. In addition, the patient did not improve with blockade of nerves supplying cervical structures, which makes the diagnosis even less likely.

What features of the history are of most value in establishing the correct diagnosis in this case?

Historical features of note in this case included the positional nature of the headaches, which began

Table 4.3. Conditions that can be missed on CT

- **Vascular diseases including:**
  - Aneurysms
  - Arteriovenous malformations (especially posterior fossa)
  - Subarachnoid hemorrhage
  - Arterial dissections
  - Acute infarcts
  - Venous thrombosis
  - Vasculitis
  - Subdural and epidural hematomas
- **Neoplastic diseases including:**
  - Posterior fossa neoplasms
  - Meningeal carcinomatosis
  - Small pituitary tumors
- **Infections:**
  - Paranasal sinusitis
  - Meningoencephalitis
  - Brain abscess
- **Other:**
  - Low CSF pressure

Table 4.4. Headache attributed to spontaneous intracranial hypotension: clinical and diagnostic characteristics

A headache, often but not always positional in nature and usually accompanied by stiffness of the neck or hearing abnormalities

CSF pressure of less than 60 mm H_2O (in the sitting position) or radiologic evidence of a CSF leak

Discussion

The clinical characteristics of headache due to spontaneous intracranial hypotension are listed in Table 4.4. The headache is usually diffuse or dull and often worsens within 15 minutes after standing. It commonly remits, sometimes slowly, after the patient lies flat for some time. Neck stiffness, tinnitus, diminished hearing acuity, photophobia or nausea may be reported. Diagnostically, we like to see that one or more of the following are present: MRI evidence of low pressure, radiographic evidence of a CSF leak, OR a CSF opening pressure of less than 60 mm H_2O in the sitting position. Although this is not the typical position for measurement of CSF pressure we find that a measurement obtained in the recumbent position may be normal in a low CSF pressure headache. In patients who are known to have had a procedure that might have punctured the dura or who have MRI evidence of a low CSF pressure headache, an LP to establish a low pressure is not needed prior to treatment.

Even when the history strongly implicates a low CSF pressure headache, it can be difficult or impossible to actually detect the leak. In fact some patients may not have an actual leak at all: patients who have multiple dural diverticulae in the lumbar region may sequester CSF in the diverticulae when they are upright, leading to low CSF pressure without an actual leak. This is sometimes termed a "compliance" headache.

Table 4.3 lists conditions in addition to low CSF pressure headaches that may be missed by CT but which are usually detected by MRI. CT may be suboptimal compared to MRI in the evaluation of a number of central nervous system conditions; a report of a normal head CT scan may be reassuring by indicating the absence of a large mass or bleed but does little to clarify some of the other conditions listed, including low CSF pressure headache, and should not be relied upon to confirm the diagnosis. In many neurologic conditions, including suspected low CSF

shortly after rising each day, and their rapid disappearance when the patient lay flat. This pattern is most consistent with a diagnosis of headache attributed to low CSF pressure. Practitioners often assume that there must be a history of a prior LP or other instrumentation in order to consider such a diagnosis, but there is ample evidence that spontaneous CSF leaks can develop and lead to low pressure or volume headache.

Although this diagnosis was considered, it was apparently discarded based on the normal CT report, the normal CSF opening pressure, and the normal tracer study. However, the clinical presentation is so characteristic of low CSF pressure headache that it is important to consider the possibility of false-negative or inaccurately interpreted test results. The CSF opening pressure may be normal in low CSF pressure headache when it is measured with the patient recumbent; taking a pressure reading with the patient in a sitting position will often show the pressure to be low. Tracer studies are notoriously likely to be negative in patients who have a slow leak. And finally, CT scanning is known to be inferior to MRI for demonstrating the pachymeningeal enhancement that is seen in many (but not all) patients with low CSF pressure headaches (Table 4.3). Taken as a whole, the best explanation of this patient's headache presentation remains headache due to low CSF pressure – despite his apparently normal test results.

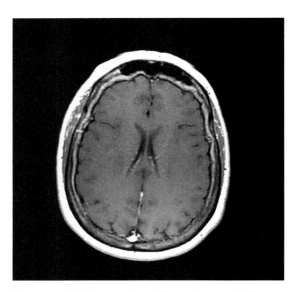

Figure 4.5 Gadolinium enhanced T1-weighted axial MRI showing pachymeningeal enhancement.

Table 4.5. MRI features of low pressure headache

- Diffuse pachymeningeal enhancement after gadolinium
- Cerebellar tonsillar descent
- Downward descent (sagging) of the brain/brainstem
- Crowding of the posterior fossa
- Pituitary enlargement
- Bilateral convexity subdural hygroma
- Paraspinal extra-arachnoid CSF collection

spinal MRI. Changes are enhanced with the use of gadolinium.

Diagnosis

Headache attributed to spontaneous intracranial hypotension.

Tip

Overreliance on the results of the wrong diagnostic study can obscure the clinical picture and lead to premature, and unwarranted, diagnostic conclusions and unsuccessful management. Selecting the correct study for the suspected condition is essential.

Further reading

Radiation risks from scanning

Brenner DJ, Hall EJ. Computed tomography – an increasing source of radiation exposure. *N Engl J Med.* 2007;357: 2277–84.

Mettler FA Jr., Huda W, Yoshizumi TT, Mahesh M. Effective doses in radiology and diagnostic nuclear medicine: a catalog. *Radiology.* 2008;248:254–63.

Does testing relieve anxiety?

Fitzpatrick R. Telling patients there is nothing wrong. *BMJ.* 1996;313:311–12.

Frishberg, BM. The utility of neuroimaging in the evaluation of headache patients with normal neurologic examinations. *Neurology.* 1994;44:1191–7.

Howard L, Wessely S, Leese M, *et al.* Are investigations anxiolytic or anxiogenic? A randomised controlled trial of neuroimaging to provide reassurance in chronic daily headache. *Neurol Neurosurg Psychiatry.* 2005;76:1558–64.

McDonald IG, Daly J, Jelinek VM, Panetta F, Gutman JM. Opening Pandora's box: the unpredictability of reassurance by a normal test result. *BMJ.* 1996;313: 329–32.

Petrie KJ, Muller JT, Schirmbeck F, *et al.* Effect of providing information about normal test results on patients'

pressure headache, the evaluation may be considered incomplete in the absence of MRI scanning, although even MRI can produce false negatives. In one study, the sensitivity of MRI with and without gadolinium was 83%. Thus, about a fifth of patients with low CSF pressure headaches will have normal MRI scans.

In this patient, an MRI scan was ordered (Figure 4.5) and showed clear evidence of pachymeningeal enhancement consistent with a low CSF pressure headache. He was treated with a 20 mL autologous epidural blood patch and experienced complete resolution of his headaches almost immediately after the procedure.

The characteristic MRI features of low CSF pressure headache (Table 4.5) are likely to be related to the suspected pathophysiology of the condition; in the setting of reduced CSF volume and support in an upright patient, contents of the skull may respond to gravitational force producing the sagging appearance with crowding of the posterior fossa and reduced size of the cisterns. Downward traction on meningeal structures has been associated with increased volume of the epidural space, leading to increased venous volume, producing the appearance of pachymeningeal enhancement, and to increased epidural fluid, leading to hygroma formation. Diagnostic changes likely related to pressure changes may also be apparent on

reassurance: randomized controlled trial. *BMJ.* 2007;334:
352–4.

van Ravesteijn H, van Dijk I, Darmon D, *et al.* The
reassuring value of diagnostic tests: a systematic review.
Patient Educ Couns. 2012;86:3–8.

Defensive medicine

Birbeck GL, Gifford DR, Song J, *et al.* Do malpractice
concerns, payment mechanisms, and attitudes influence
test-ordering decisions? *Neurology.* 2004;62(1):
119–21.

DeKay ML, Asch DA. Is the defensive use of diagnostic tests
good for patients, or bad? *Med Decis Making.* 1998;18(1):
19–28.

Thunderclap headache

Ducros A, Bousser M-G. Thunderclap headache. *BMJ.*
2013;346:e8557.

Schwedt, TJ. Thunderclap headaches: a focus on etiology
and diagnostic evaluation. *Headache.* 2013;53(3):563–
9.

White matter lesions in migraine

Agostoni E, Rigamonti A. Migraine and small vessel
diseases. *Neurol Sci.* 2012;33(Suppl 1):S51–4.

Debette S, Markus HS. The clinical importance of white
matter hyperintensities on brain magnetic resonance
imaging: systematic review and meta-analysis. *BMJ.*
2010;341:c3666.

Kruit MC, van Buchem MA, Hofman PA, *et al.* Migraine as
a risk factor for subclinical brain lesions. *JAMA.* 2004;
291(4):427–34.

Kruit MC, van Buchem MA, Launer LJ, Terwindt GM.
Migraine is associated with an increased risk of deep
white matter lesions, subclinical posterior circulation
infarcts and brain iron accumulation: the population-
based MRI CAMERA study. *Cephalalgia.* 2010;30(2):
129–36.

Kurth T, Diener H-C, Buring JE. Migraine and
cardiovascular disease in women and the role of aspirin:
subgroup analyses in the Women's Health Study.
Cephalalgia. 2011;31(10):1106–15.

Kurth T, Mohamed S, Maillard P, *et al.* Headache, migraine,
and structural brain lesions and function: population
based Epidemiology of Vascular Ageing-MRI study.
BMJ. 2011;342:c7357.

Palm-Meinders IH, Koppen H, Terwindt GM, *et al.*
Structural brain changes in migraine. *JAMA.*
2012;308(18):1889–96.

CADASIL

Federico A, Di Donato I, Bianchi S, *et al.* Hereditary
cerebral small vessel diseases: a review. *J Neurol Sci.*
2012;322(1–2):25–30.

Fukutake T. Cerebral autosomal recessive arteriopathy with
subcortical infarcts and leukoencephalopathy
(CARASIL): from discovery to gene identification.
J Stroke Cerebrovasc Dis. 2011;20(2):85–93.

Reimschisel T. Ethical perspectives in neurology. Accessed
August 29, 2012 at: http://www.aan.com/globals/axon/
assets/5585.pdf.

Post-dural puncture headache

Basurto Ona X, Martínez García L, Solà I, Bonfill Cosp X.
Drug therapy for treating post-dural puncture headache.
Cochrane Database Syst Rev. 2011;(8):CD007887.

Ghaleb A, Khorasani A, Mangar D. Post-dural puncture
headache. *Int J Gen Med.* 2012;5:45–51.

Schievink WI, Maya MM, Louy C, Moser FG, Tourje J.
Diagnostic criteria for spontaneous spinal CSF leaks and
intracranial hypotension. *AJNR Am J Neuroradiol.*
2008;29:853–6.

Sencakova D, Mokri B, McClelland RL. The efficacy of
epidural blood patch in spontaneous CSF leaks.
Neurology. 2001;57(10):1921–3.

Sudlow C, Warlow C. Posture and fluids for preventing
post-dural puncture headache. *Cochrane Database Syst
Rev.* 2002;(2):CD001790.

Vakharia SB, Thomas PS, Rosenbaum AE, Wasenko JJ,
Fellows DG. Magnetic resonance imaging of
cerebrospinal fluid leak and tamponade effect of blood
patch in post-dural puncture headache. *Anesth Analg.*
1997;84(3):585–90.

Lumbar puncture

Barsuk JH, Cohen ER, Caprio T, *et al.* Simulation-based
education with mastery learning improves residents'
lumbar puncture skills. *Neurology.* 2012;79(2):132–
7.

Ellenby MS, Tegtmeyer K, Lai S, Brano DAV. Lumbar
puncture. *N Engl J Med.* 2006;355:e1 (video).

Straus SE, Thorpe KE, Holroyd-Leduc J. How do I perform
a lumbar puncture and analyze the results to diagnose
bacterial meningitis? *JAMA.* 2006;296(16):2012–22.

Low CSF pressure headache

Agarwal P, Menon S, Shah R, Singhal BS. Spontaneous
intracranial hypotension: two cases including one
treated with epidural blood patch. *Ann Indian Acad
Neurol.* 2009;12(3):179–82.

Chung SJ, Kim JS, Lee MC. Syndrome of cerebral spinal fluid hypovolemia: clinical and imaging features and outcome. *Neurology*. 2000;55(9):1321–7.

Rando TA, Fishman RA. Spontaneous intracranial hypotension: report of two cases and review of the literature. *Neurology*. 1992;42(3 Pt 1):481–7.

Schievink WI. Spontaneous spinal cerebrospinal fluid leaks and intracranial hypotension. *JAMA*. 2006;295(19): 2286–96.

Watanabe A, Horikoshi T, Uchida M, *et al*. Diagnostic value of spinal MR imaging in spontaneous intracranial hypotension syndrome. *AJNR Am J Neuroradiol*. 2009; 30(1):147–51.

Chapter 5

Pitfalls in diagnostic testing: blood, urine, and other tests

In addition to imaging studies and lumbar puncture, a variety of other tests can be useful in the evaluation or treatment of patients with headache disorders. Blood and urine tests are the most commonly ordered additional tests in the headache clinic, but electrocardiograms, electroencephalograms, and other tests may also be used. Such tests are most helpful in assessing the possibility of secondary causes of headache but are only rarely *required* for such a diagnosis.

Of the hundreds of headache types described in the International Classification of Headache Disorders (ICHD), only four secondary forms of headache require blood or urine tests for a definitive diagnosis: urine testing is necessary to make a diagnosis of headache due to preeclampsia or eclampsia, while blood tests are required to make a definitive diagnosis of headache due to human immunodeficiency virus (HIV) infection or hypothyroidism. For a large number of other disorders, blood or urine testing is helpful in making a diagnosis but not absolutely required. A diagnosis of giant cell arteritis, for example, can be based solely on suggestive symptoms in conjunction with a positive temporal artery biopsy.

Laboratory testing is frequently needed to monitor headache treatment. Lithium and verapamil, the two most commonly used preventive treatments for cluster headache, require careful monitoring to minimize the chance of adverse events from treatment. Patients on chronic opioid therapy also require regular monitoring with blood or urine tests to ensure adherence to recommended treatment and minimize the likelihood of drug diversion or other aberrant drug-related behavior. For some drugs, monitoring of renal or liver function tests may be advisable.

The judicious use of laboratory and other forms of testing is an important part of the practice of headache medicine. Because abnormal results on testing can create anxiety and lead to further, potentially harmful, interventions, careful consideration should be given to the need for every test. Testing should be ordered after consideration of the patient's individual clinical situation, rather than ordered as part of a routine workup.

Hormone testing in women with menstrual headaches

Case

A 36-year-old woman sought treatment because of severe headaches associated with her menstrual cycle. Her description of headaches was consistent with a diagnosis of migraine and her neurologic examination was normal. The patient reported that although she had headaches at other times of the month, they were more likely to occur just before the onset of menstrual bleeding. She was treating headaches with over-the-counter ibuprofen with little success. A friend had suggested that her problems might be due to hormonal abnormalities. The patient had her estrogen levels checked by a naturopathic physician who told her they were "completely off" and recommended treatment with add-back bio-identical estrogen during the perimenstrual period. The patient had tried this for several months, but treatment was expensive and while she thought perhaps it had been helpful for her period-associated headaches, she still had an average of five or six other migraines a month.

What is the patient describing and how can that diagnosis be confirmed?

Migraine headaches that occur in predictable relation to the menstrual cycle are commonly referred to as "menstrual migraines." According to diagnostic criteria in the appendix of ICHD-3 beta, menstrual migraine attacks must occur during a five-day window of time beginning two days before and extending to three days after the onset of vaginal bleeding.

Furthermore, this must occur on average in two of every three cycles. The diagnostic criteria suggest that these attacks are without aura, and say that headaches occurring with aura are unlikely to be associated with menstruation.

The diagnostic criteria define "pure menstrual migraine" as a situation in which migraine attacks occur *only* during this five-day menstrual window and at no other time of the month. In contrast, "menstrually related migraine" is diagnosed when headaches occur predictably during this five-day window but also at other times of the month.

Confirmation of a diagnosis of menstrual migraine requires objective evidence of the timing of headaches in relation to the patient's menstrual cycle. In general, we recommend basing the diagnosis on at least three months of headache diary records. In our clinical experience, it is very important to take the time to do this, to identify correctly a menstrual trigger for headaches. Patient self-report of menstrual migraine is not reliable. One study showed that roughly 20% of women who self-reported a diagnosis of menstrual migraine did not actually meet criteria for a diagnosis of menstrual migraine when headache diaries were kept.

In this case, the patient's headache diary showed migraine attacks during the five-day menstrual window during all three months of recording. The patient also had attacks at other times of the month, so she met criteria for a diagnosis of menstrually related migraine.

Is it useful to check hormone levels in women who have menstrual migraine?

Good evidence suggests that estrogen withdrawal is the likely cause of menstrual attacks of migraine, although other hormonal changes at this time of the menstrual cycle may contribute to migraine susceptibility. Estradiol levels are high following ovulation. These high levels are sustained until the late luteal phase of the cycle, when they fall quickly. A similar fall in estrogen levels also occurs and can provoke headache in susceptible women during the placebo pill week of some oral contraceptive regimens, following childbirth, and with certain types of noncontinuous hormone replacement regimens.

Many patients with menstrually triggered migraine attacks wonder whether there is "something wrong" with their hormone levels. There is no evidence, however, that treatable hormonal abnormalities are the cause of menstrual migraine. Rather, women who have

inherited a migraine-prone nervous system are unusually sensitive to normal fluctuations in steroid hormone levels. There is no clinical reason to check serum levels of estrogen in women with menstrual migraine.

In this case, an emphasis on menstrual-associated headaches meant that the patient's many nonmenstrual headaches were ignored. The patient was begun on 10 mg of amitriptyline daily and asked to use eletriptan 40 mg for up to two headaches a week. At a follow-up visit she reported that her headache frequency was down to two headaches a month and that those headaches were effectively treated by eletriptan.

Discussion

Menstruation is a highly noticeable, culturally significant recurrent event. For these reasons it is what sociologists sometimes refer to as a "magnet explanation." In other words, events that occur in association with menstruation are highly likely to be attributed to it, sometimes mistakenly. This is an example of the cognitive error or bias known as "illusory correlation," in which coincidental events are falsely assumed to be causally related, often as a result of strongly held prior beliefs.

In women with frequent migraine attacks, headaches may occur in conjunction with menstruation simply by chance. It is important to verify even strongly held assumptions about the connection between headaches and hormonal events, ideally using a headache diary. Exclusive emphasis on hormonal causes of headaches may limit attention to other explanations for headache or may lead to misguided attempts at treatment. In the case described in the vignette, treatment aimed solely at hormonal causes of headache did nothing to help the patient with her many nonhormonal headaches. In contrast, all of her headaches were successfully managed using traditional nonhormonal migraine therapies.

Diagnosis

Menstrually related migraine.

Tip

Headache diaries, not blood or urine hormone levels, are most helpful in making a diagnosis of menstrually related migraine attacks, and are necessary to avoid falsely attributing headaches to a hormonal cause. A hormonal trigger for headaches does not mean that treatment must also be hormonal.

Monitoring verapamil treatment in cluster headache

Case

A 40-year-old man presented to the headache clinic for follow-up care. He reported daily 90-minute episodes of 10/10 right-sided retro-orbital pain with right-sided nasal congestion and ptosis. He had been seen in the clinic ten years earlier and diagnosed with episodic cluster headache. Treatment with verapamil was effective and he returned to the care of his personal physician who continued to prescribe verapamil.

The patient's cluster headache bouts typically occurred for just three months every year but he accumulated a stockpile of verapamil by filling prescriptions year-round. When his personal physician retired he used medication from this stockpile to manage his annual bout of cluster headaches. Through trial and error he found that a dose of 720 mg daily was more effective than the lower doses of medication recommended by the headache clinic and his personal physician.

At this appointment the patient said that his annual bout of cluster headaches had begun. His neurologic examination was normal, but on review of systems he complained of fatigue, constipation, and shortness of breath, noting that recently he had barely been able to get through his workday. He attributed these symptoms to cigarette smoking and planned to discuss them when he obtained an appointment with a new primary care physician. He was about to run out of verapamil and requested a refill.

Should this patient's verapamil prescription be refilled?

Verapamil is the drug of choice for prevention of cluster headaches, although the US Food and Drug Administration (FDA) has not approved it for that purpose. In our experience, the dose of verapamil required to suppress cluster headaches successfully is higher than the doses that are typically used to treat other conditions such as hypertension. Most experts begin with a dose of 240 mg a day, either given as a once-daily, sustained release preparation or as 80 mg three times daily. Many patients require an even higher dose

for control of headaches. One recommended titration strategy is to increase the drug by 80 mg a day every two weeks until headache control is gained or intolerable side effects occur.

These high doses increase the likelihood and severity of side effects, which can include constipation, peripheral edema, fatigue, and heart block. The patient in the vignette has achieved excellent control of his cluster headaches with verapamil. Although this patient could be experiencing an unrelated or smoking-related respiratory condition, the best option in this case before continuing verapamil would be to assess the patient for verapamil-related cardiac conduction delay, which may appear even after long periods of uneventful use.

How common are electrocardiographic abnormalities with verapamil treatment for cluster headache?

In one study, electrocardiographic abnormalities were detected in about a third of patients treated for cluster headaches with high doses of verapamil. Bradycardia (a heart rate of < 60 beats per minute) was the most common abnormality, followed by first-degree heart block (PR interval > 0.2 seconds). More severe degrees of heart block were rare. In this study, electrocardiographic changes were seen with mean verapamil doses of around 1000 mg daily and did not occur with doses lower than 800 mg a day. Although these abnormalities sometimes required cessation of verapamil, in many other cases they resolved with a decrease in dose. A reasonable monitoring strategy is to obtain an electrocardiogram before verapamil treatment is started, and after each dosage increase or with the appearance of symptoms that could have a cardiac cause.

The patient in the vignette had no history of heart disease and an electrocardiogram done two years ago had been normal. However, on examination at this visit his resting heart rate was 48 beats per minute. An electrocardiogram showed first-degree heart block with a PR interval > 0.2 seconds. The dose of verapamil was reduced to 80 mg three times daily. The patient's headaches did not recur and his symptoms of fatigue and shortness of breath resolved.

Discussion

Cluster headache is characterized by attacks of severe or very severe, strictly unilateral orbital, peri-orbital, or temporal pain that last from 15 minutes to 3 hours. During cluster periods or bouts, headaches may occur every other day up to several times a day. Attacks are associated with ipsilateral cranial autonomic features such as tearing, ptosis, miosis, or rhinorrhea. In episodic cluster headache, cluster bouts can last for weeks or months and often recur yearly at roughly the same time. Many patients have long periods of remission during which they are entirely free of headaches. In contrast, patients with chronic cluster headache do not experience remissions, or have remissions that are very short.

Injectable sumatriptan or inhalation of 100% oxygen are effective treatment for individual attacks of cluster headache, but their use on a daily or near-daily basis is impractical. Additionally, while waiting for them to take effect patients will experience a short period of incapacitating pain, which can severely disrupt daily life activities. Thus, essentially all patients with cluster headache should also receive preventive treatment, which is given daily during a cluster bout to decrease or eliminate cluster attacks.

Although verapamil is the first-line preventive treatment for cluster headache, other preventive treatments including lithium, melatonin, or the use of occipital nerve blocks can be tried. Successful use of verapamil may require titration to fairly high doses; a common reason for apparent failure of this treatment is the use of inadequate doses. In many instances doses over 360 mg daily are required up to and including the recommended maximum daily dose of 960 mg, doses that are far higher than those used in the management of cardiac conditions.

Once successful control of cluster headaches is achieved, many patients are reluctant to discontinue preventive treatment. Some patients with episodic cluster headache prefer to stay on preventive treatment such as verapamil year-round even if they have attacks for only three or four months a year. While this preference is understandable in view of the severity of cluster headache pain, we discourage this practice. Instead, we recommend that patients gradually lower the dose of preventive medication as they approach the expected time when their cluster bout should be ending. If headaches recur when the dose is lowered, a higher dose can be resumed for several more weeks, when another attempt should be made to taper the drug. In our experience, this is an often-overlooked aspect of managing cluster headaches.

Diagnosis

Episodic cluster headache and verapamil-induced cardiac conduction delay.

Tip

High doses of verapamil may be required for successful prevention of cluster headache. Regular electrocardiographic monitoring is needed to avoid the adverse effects of cardiac conduction delay.

Urine drug testing in patients taking opioids

Case

A 37-year-old woman returned to the headache clinic for a follow-up visit. The patient had severe post-traumatic head and face pain following a gunshot wound. The pain had not responded to treatment with gabapentin, amitriptyline, or numerous other medications for neuropathic pain. Because it was relieved by opioid medications, the patient had been started on sustained release morphine. Unfortunately, intermittent bouts of vomiting from pancreatitis made it difficult to use oral medications. At her last visit the oral morphine was discontinued and she was started on a fentanyl patch. The patient reported that her pain was well controlled on the fentanyl. Along with pancreatic enzymes and a multivitamin she was using carisoprodol intermittently for episodes of muscle spasm.

Because her usual physician was on maternity leave, the patient was seen by a resident who was rotating in the clinic. After consultation with a supervising physician, the resident refilled the patient's fentanyl prescription. He noticed that at her last visit a pain treatment urine drug screen had been obtained, so before the patient left he repeated this test. Later that day the resident reviewed the test results. He was startled to see that the urine drug test results did not mention the presence of fentanyl but instead reported that meprobamate, a tranquilizer, had been detected.

What are the possible explanations for these urine findings?

Fentanyl is not reliably detected by urine or blood drug testing, making it challenging to monitor the long-term use of this drug. Urine drug testing is still useful, though, in order to monitor the patient's possible use of other nonprescribed substances. In this case, the finding of meprobamate in the urine might be misinterpreted as a sign that the patient is taking a nonprescribed, possibily illicitly obtained, substance. However, carisoprodol is metabolized to meprobamate and thus the presence of meprobamate in this patient's urine sample is not unexpected. It is important to be aware of substances that can produce a false-positive urine drug test result. It is advisable to consult with the laboratory that you use to process the samples, to learn what tests they use, the limits of detection, and any other unique characteristics of the laboratory.

If this patient's urine sample had contained evidence of tetrahydrocannabinol (THC), an indication of marijuana use, the physician would have had more reason to be concerned. THC use is correlated with the use of other illicit substances and some studies suggest it is an indicator of high risk for abuse of opioids. An exception to this would be a patient who lives in a state where the use of "medical marijuana" is allowed. Such patients should have received the drug through approved channels, however, and should have informed the physician about its use prior to drug testing.

How else might this patient's use of fentanyl be monitored?

The purposes of monitoring in patients on chronic opioid therapy are two-fold: (1) to ensure the patient is benefitting from treatment; and (2) to detect problems with drug diversion or misuse. The benefits of treatment can be established through pain ratings that show meaningful reductions in pain intensity related to opioid treatment. Functional improvement is also important. Many physicians find it useful to monitor such things as return to work, reduced use of breakthrough pain medications, and fewer emergency department visits for poorly controlled pain. When urine or blood tests cannot reliably detect an opioid, as is the case in this vignette, other ways of monitoring compliance with long-term opioid therapy can be used. For example, the patient's skin can be inspected at each visit to ascertain that the expected patches are in place. Patients can also be asked to bring their unused patches along to appointments to show that these are in their possession and to ensure that the proper number of patches remains.

Patients may perceive these forms of monitoring as burdensome or intrusive. Before starting chronic opi-

oid therapy it is important to obtain informed consent from the patient for treatment and to outline in detail the rules of your practice about opioid treatment and monitoring. Most experts recommend the use of "treatment contracts" that outline the conditions under which the medication will be prescribed, the methods that will be used to monitor the treatment, and the circumstances under which lost prescriptions will be replaced or therapy discontinued. Sample treatment contracts can easily be located online. These treatment contracts do not have legal force but do stand as a clear record of the understanding you had with the patient about treatment. They are valuable if questions or disputes later arise about the patient's treatment.

Appropriate selection of patients for chronic opioid therapy may help reduce the risks of diversion or misuse, although there is no strong evidence about this. A number of tools can be used to identify patients who are at high risk of aberrant drug use, including the opioid risk tool, the Pain Medication Questionnaire, and others.

Discussion

The use of chronic opioid therapy in patients with non-malignant pain syndromes is controversial. Its long-term efficacy is uncertain, and the benefits and harms are often finely balanced. Risks of chronic opioid therapy include the development of addiction or dependence syndromes, opioid-induced hyperalgesia, and the potential for diversion or misuse of prescribed opioids. These problems have received a great deal of attention from the popular media, politicians, and regulators. For all of these reasons, patients on chronic opioid therapy must be closely monitored, with regular office visits and efforts to minimize the misuse or diversion of such drugs.

Urine or blood drug testing is nearly always an important part of a monitoring plan for patients on opioid maintenance therapy. In most cases, we recommend a baseline urine drug test before starting therapy, as well as regular random tests. The frequency of such testing depends on the patient's circumstances. In general, high-risk patients should be monitored more frequently, possibly at every visit. For long-term patients who appear to be stable and at low risk of diversion or misuse, we still recommend random testing once or twice a year. One study of headache patients receiving opioid maintenance therapy showed that unexpected urine drug test results suggesting aberrant drug-related behavior occurred in a sizeable proportion of apparently stable patients, sometimes even after long periods of trouble-free use.

Patients can be referred to independent laboratories for such testing, but many physicians obtain the urine samples in their own offices. These samples are not usually handled with the same strict "chain of custody" procedures applied in professional laboratories.

Diagnosis

Post-traumatic head and facial pain, treated with chronic opioid therapy.

Tip

Urine or blood drug testing does not reliably detect some opioids, such as fentanyl, but such tests are still valuable to detect use of other nonprescribed substances. Knowledge of cross-reactive substances that can produce false-positive urine drug tests is important to avoid inaccurately accusing patients of non-compliance with treatment standards.

Lithium levels in a patient with cluster headache

Case

A 45-year-old man presented to the headache clinic with a ten-year history of right retro-orbital attacks of 10/10 pain. These lasted 45 minutes to an hour and were associated with right-sided ptosis, rhinorrhea, and tearing of the right eye. During attacks the patient was restless and sometimes banged his head on the wall. Initially these attacks occurred infrequently and he was diagnosed with a possible sinus problem. He underwent sinus surgery with no improvement, and attacks began to increase in frequency. He was referred to a neurologist who diagnosed cluster headache and treated him with verapamil after he failed to respond to a course of oral steroid therapy. Over the last year and a half, the headache attacks had become daily despite continued treatment with verapamil, which had been increased to 320 mg/day. The patient was also using oral zolmitriptan and hydrocodone to treat individual attacks of headache, but reported they were not always effective.

The headache specialist obtained an electrocardiogram, which showed a PR interval of 0.2 seconds. She asked the patient to decrease his verapamil dose to 240 mg/day, and suggested that he add lithium carbonate, 300 mg twice a day, to his treatment regimen. She also recommended subcutaneous sumatriptan in place of oral zolmitriptan to treat individual attacks of headache. She asked the patient to return a week later to have his lithium level and an electrocardiogram checked. The electrocardiogram showed the PR interval had returned to normal, but the patient's lithium level was low at 0.3 mmol/L (normal range for this laboratory was 0.5–1.3 mmol/L). The doctor asked the patient to increase his lithium dose to 300 mg of lithium carbonate three times daily. When checked a month later, his lithium level was still low at 0.3 mmol/L and his headaches were no better. The doctor increased the lithium dose again, but a week later a third lithium level was 0.2 mmol/L.

What are the possible explanations for this patient's lithium level?

This patient's lithium level was low when he began taking lithium and remained essentially unchanged despite two increases in the prescribed dose of lithium. It is unlikely that these multiple test results were incorrect. Although lithium can interact with a number of medications, this patient's medication regimen was otherwise unchanged during the period when his lithium dosage had been increased. Thus, the most likely explanation for these consistently low levels was that the patient was nonadherent with the prescribed dose of lithium.

There are many reasons for nonadherence to drug therapy, which are discussed below. In this case, the patient's physician approached the matter in a non-judgmental way, since she knew that patients are often reluctant to admit they have not adhered to therapeutic recommendations. She told the patient that his lithium level had remained unchanged despite the recommended increases in dose; she then "normalized" the behavior of nonadherence by remarking that "many patients find it difficult to take their medicine regularly" and asking the patient if that was true for him. The patient appeared relieved and responded that his busy workday made it difficult to remember his morning dose of medication, and that he sometimes forgot to take his evening dose because of the demands of his three children when he returned home at night.

The patient and physician then strategized about ways in which he might remember to take his medication, and the patient decided to program an alarm on his cellphone. The doctor also reviewed the expected benefits of lithium and the fact that alternative treatments that might be used in its place had less evidence of benefit. Both she and the patient were pleased when at his next visit his headaches were greatly diminished and his lithium level had increased to 0.8 mmol/L.

How common is nonadherence to drug therapy in headache patients and why does it occur?

Nonadherence or poor compliance to recommended treatment is an important problem with all types of medical treatment, particularly with complex treatment regimens for chronic illnesses. There is no evidence that nonadherence is more common among headache patients than the general medical population. Failure to adhere to recommended treatment can take the form of overuse of prescribed or over-the-counter treatments, or underuse, which may consist of never filling a prescription at all, using less than the recommended dose, or premature cessation of treatment. One study of headache patients found that only slightly more than a third of patients were fully compliant with their prescribed treatment regimens.

There are many reasons for nonadherence to prescribed therapy. One study found that medication costs, patient uncertainty that the drug was indicated, or fears of side effects were the most common reasons for nonadherence.

Poor adherence is also related to the complexity of the treatment regimen. The more frequently a drug must be taken, for example, the less likely patients are to adhere to the regimen. When feasible, switching to once-daily treatments can improve the likelihood of adherence to drug regimens. Nonadherence to prescribed medications is probably an underappreciated reason for the apparent failure of headache treatment regimens. In the case described in this vignette, the patient happened to be taking one of the few headache drugs that require monitoring of serum drug levels. If blood tests had not been obtained, it is likely that his nonadherence would have gone undetected and

lithium would have been inaccurately regarded as ineffective for his cluster headache.

Discussion

The FDA has not approved any drugs for preventive treatment of cluster headache, but verapamil and lithium are widely used off-label. Verapamil is the preferred initial drug because it seems to have a quicker onset of action and fewer side effects. Lithium is used alone when verapamil is ineffective or not tolerated, or as an add-on to verapamil when combination therapy is needed. The scientific evidence supporting its use is modest, but clinically it is perceived to be quite effective, particularly in chronic cluster headache. A typical starting dose is 300 mg of lithium carbonate given twice a day, which can be increased in 300 mg increments based on treatment response and blood levels. Most patients who respond to the drug do so at doses between 600 and 1200 mg/day.

Nuisance side effects such as tremor, nausea, or diarrhea are relatively common, and at higher doses lithium toxicity can occur. This can produce kidney dysfunction, ataxia, or convulsions that may be fatal. Sodium depletion, which can occur with the use of some diuretics, may increase the likelihood of lithium toxicity. Nonsteroidal anti-inflammatory medications may increase lithium levels. Verapamil has been reported both to increase and decrease lithium levels.

Because lithium has a narrow therapeutic window, periodic monitoring of blood levels is necessary to avoid toxicity. Levels should be checked after any dosage increase, when symptoms related to toxicity occur, or when other medications that might affect lithium levels are started or stopped. Blood levels do not, however, correlate with response to the drug, so there is no "target" blood level. In patients on long-term lithium therapy most physicians also check yearly kidney function and thyroid function tests.

Diagnosis

Chronic cluster headache with nonadherence to lithium treatment.

Tip

Blood levels should be periodically monitored in patients taking lithium. Although principally intended to avoid toxicity, blood levels may also be used to assess adherence to the prescribed treatment regimen.

A young man with body aches, rash, and headache

Case

A 24-year-old man sought treatment in the emergency department for a chronic headache. He described the headache as dull and generalized. He also complained of body aches and sensitivity to light. He was afebrile and his physical examination was normal with the exception of a macular red rash over the torso and some cervical lymphadenopathy. The emergency department physician made a diagnosis of possible mononucleosis and sent the patient home with instructions to see his primary care physician if the symptoms did not remit.

A week later the patient saw his primary care doctor because of continued headache and body aches. The doctor asked the patient whether he had other reasons for seeking treatment and what he thought might be the cause of his problems. The patient confided that his new girlfriend had been an intravenous drug abuser; over the last few months they had had many unsafe sexual encounters and he worried that he might have "some kind of infection." The physician recognized that the patient was at high risk for a variety of sexually transmitted infections and ordered appropriate testing, including an HIV antibody test and an HIV RNA (viral load) test. The HIV antibody test was positive and the patient's viral load was > 100 000 copies/mL.

Can headache be a symptom of HIV infection?

This case is a reminder that a half to two-thirds of people with newly acquired HIV infection will experience a constellation of signs and symptoms as they seroconvert, usually about two to eight weeks following infection. Headache may be a prominent symptom of this influenza-like event, which is often termed "acute retroviral syndrome" and lasts an average of about a month. In one series of 218 patients with acute HIV infection, headache was reported by 51%. Only fever (77%), lethargy (66%), and skin rash (56%) were more common. Other neurologic symptoms of photophobia and meningismus (stiff neck) were reported by 12% and 9% of patients, respectively, making headache by far the most common neurologic symptom of acute

HIV infection. In our experience, such patients do not usually come to the headache clinic but are more likely to present in an emergency department or urgent care setting, given the abrupt nature and relatively short duration of symptoms. The reason for headache or other symptoms is not fully understood, but may involve release of cytokines.

A more chronic form of headache has been described in people with stable HIV infection. Once superimposed infections related to immunosuppression have been eliminated as a cause of headache, a diagnosis of headache attributed to human immunodeficiency syndrome/acquired immunodeficiency syndrome (HIV/AIDS) can be considered. This diagnosis is contained in the appendix of ICHD-3 beta rather than the main body of the classification because the validity of the diagnostic criteria has not been firmly established. This is largely due to the fact that it can be very challenging to distinguish the low-grade headache likely to be attributable to HIV from other forms of primary headache commonly reported by HIV patients. Additionally, some antiretroviral drugs can produce headache.

Nonetheless, most experts believe that low-grade headache is a common feature of HIV infection. It is typically a dull, bilateral headache. This diagnosis should only be made after blood testing confirms infection with HIV and/or immunodeficiency, in conjunction with demonstration of disease-related pathophysiology "likely to cause headache." Blood or oral fluid samples can be tested with rapid tests but any positive results require confirmation using immunoassay procedures. Because antibody tests may be negative early in the infectious process, an HIV RNA (viral load) test should also be ordered in settings where infection may have been recent.

What are some other possible causes of headache in people with HIV infection?

A high index of suspicion for secondary causes of headache is appropriate in HIV-positive patients, particularly when immunosuppression is severe. A large number of opportunistic infections such as *Cryptococcus* or toxoplasmosis can produce headache, and patients with HIV also have an increased risk of central nervous system neoplasms.

The degree of immunosuppression is positively correlated with the likelihood of these secondary causes of headache, and can be useful in deciding whether or not an HIV-positive patient with headache needs a brain scan. One study found that important abnormalities on CT scans of the brain were far more likely in patients whose CD4 counts were below 200 cells/μL, and recommended this as a threshold below which imaging should be considered.

Discussion

A high degree of suspicion should be maintained for the possibility of acute HIV infection in people with headache and risk factors for sexually transmitted diseases. Individuals with acute HIV infection may have very high viral loads and be particularly infectious to others. Following the period of symptoms during seroconversion, infected people may experience a long interval during which they have relatively few signs or symptoms, and diagnosis may be delayed. Thus the correct recognition of the acute retroviral syndrome may allow early diagnosis of a potentially fatal illness and the opportunity to minimize the risk of transmission to others. Unfortunately, because the symptoms of acute retroviral syndrome are variable and nonspecific, this opportunity is often missed.

In the case described in the vignette, the emergency department physician missed an opportunity to identify the patient's HIV infection, but fortunately the patient again sought treatment. His primary care physician correctly recognized that the patient had risk factors for HIV infection through his exposure to a former intravenous drug abuser. The prevalence of HIV is high in intravenous drug users, and their sexual partners are at risk of infection with this and other blood-borne infections such as hepatitis. A recent study suggests that a short course of antiretroviral treatment early in HIV infection may delay disease progression, with important benefits for individual patients and public health, making it even more important to detect infection as early as possible.

Diagnosis

Headache related to acute retroviral syndrome (HIV seroconversion).

Tip

Acute retroviral syndrome should be considered in patients presenting with headache and influenza-like

illness who have risk factors for sexually transmitted diseases. To maximize the chance of detecting recent infection, both an HIV antibody test and an HIV RNA (viral load) test should be ordered.

A young woman with headache and multiple laboratory abnormalities

Case

A 19-year-old woman was seen in the headache clinic on referral from her primary care physician. She had developed headaches a few months earlier. These occurred on average twice a month and were very severe. She described them as pounding and usually located over her right temple. These headaches could last up to two days at a time and were associated with severe nausea and vomiting and sensitivity to noise. She was unable to function during the headaches and retreated to her darkened bedroom, although between headaches she was active and well.

The patient's primary care physician thought that migraine was the most likely diagnosis. However, the patient's parents were very concerned and insisted on a "complete workup" to rule out dangerous causes of headache. A CT scan of the brain was normal. A large number of blood tests had also been ordered, and several of these had been abnormal. Her antinuclear antibody (ANA) test was positive at 1:80 so the patient had been seen by a rheumatology consultant, who after extensive further testing did not find evidence that the patient had systemic lupus erythematosus (SLE) or any other rheumatic disease. Her thyroid-stimulating hormone (TSH) level was also slightly elevated, and the patient had been seen by an endocrinologist who, after further testing, did not find any evidence of thyroid dysfunction, but did note a small 1 cm thyroid nodule, which proved to be benign on fine-needle aspiration.

Was it a mistake to order all of these tests?

In a word, yes. Laboratory testing should be limited to patients who have a reasonable pre-test probability of the disease the test is meant to detect. The physician in this case meant well, but both he and the patient's parents failed to appreciate one of the common pitfalls of diagnostic testing, which is that testing should be ordered based on the clinical context. In trying to make sense of this concept, it is helpful to understand the concepts of sensitivity, specificity, and positive and negative predictive values. Together, these are the *operating characteristics* of a test. *Sensitivity* is the proportion of patients with a disease who have a positive test result. *Specificity* is the proportion of patients without a disease who have a negative test result. The predictive value of a test is the likelihood that a patient does or does not have a disease given a particular test result. *Positive predictive value* is the likelihood that a patient with a positive test result really has the disease in question, and *negative predictive value* is the likelihood that a patient with a negative test result really is disease-free.

The sensitivity and specificity of a test do not vary from patient to patient, but the positive and negative predictive values of a test can differ dramatically depending on the prevalence of the disease in the population that is being tested. In the patient in the vignette, the likelihood that she had lupus was low – for the purposes of demonstration, let's assume it was on the order of 1%. In other words, assume that in 100 otherwise healthy young women like our patient who have intermittent severe headaches, one truly has SLE. If an ANA test for SLE has a sensitivity of 100% and a specificity of 90%, the positive predictive value of the test is only 9%. In other words, there was still a 91% chance the patient did not have SLE even with a positive test. (If you are interested in the details of this calculation, positive predictive value is calculated by dividing the true-positive rate by the true-positive plus false-positive rate; in other words, 100%/[100% + 10%], which equals roughly 9%.) The bottom line is that when the prior probability of disease is low, the positive predictive value of a test is poor. Additionally, when a large number of tests are ordered, some are likely to be abnormal on the basis of chance alone.

Discussion

Laboratory and other tests are most helpful when ordered based on the clinical context of an individual patient's situation. They should be ordered selectively and interpreted very cautiously. It is difficult to defend the practice of routinely ordering a large panel of tests for all patients with a particular problem without consideration of the individual clinical situation.

The incidence (new onset of disease) of migraine is very high in young women, and this patient's headaches met criteria for that disorder. She was otherwise healthy and her physical and neurologic examinations were normal. Thus, the likelihood of a sinister cause of headache was very low. She had no other signs or symptoms that might suggest thyroid abnormalities or an autoimmune disorder or any of the other diseases for which she was tested. Specifically, she had not experienced recent fatigue, constipation, skin rash, or any other systemic indicators of underlying disease. The extensive testing that was ordered was not done because of any suspicion that a particular disease was present, but rather to appease the patient's parents and ease their anxiety about a possible dangerous cause of headache.

Although blood tests are not invasive and are commonly perceived as harmless, a good case can be made that indiscriminate testing harmed the patient in this vignette. Not only was attention to her presenting problem – migraine – delayed by additional fruitless investigation, she was exposed to radiation from a CT scan of the head and underwent invasive aspiration needle biopsy for an incidental thyroid nodule. This sort of additional investigation triggered by an abnormal finding is often referred to as the "medical cascade." Additional invasive diagnostic procedures always carry a risk of harm, and certainly the wait for results creates anxiety. These harms and the costs of additional testing may be low for an individual patient, but if such unnecessary testing occurs on a widespread scale the iatrogenic harms and costs can be substantial on a population level. Ordering a large number of tests in the absence of specific indications for testing does not represent high value medical care.

Patients (and sometimes physicians) commonly overestimate the value of laboratory or other forms of testing and have unrealistic ideas about the accuracy of many tests. No test is perfect: not all positive or abnormal test results indicate disease – instead, some are false positives. Similarly, not all negative or normal test results mean that a patient does not have the disease in question – these are false negatives. In situations where the likelihood of disease is low, as in the patient in this vignette, positive results on a test are more likely to be false positives than true indicators of disease. In other words, their *positive predictive value* (the likelihood that a patient with a positive test actually has the disease in question) is low.

Diagnosis

Migraine and iatrogenic harm from unnecessary testing.

Tip

A shotgun approach to testing in patients with headache is inadvisable. In settings where the prior probability of a particular disorder is low, most abnormal test results will be false positives, evaluation of which can lead to unnecessary anxiety and possible harm from unneeded additional testing or interventions – the so-called "medical cascade."

Further reading

Menstrual migraine

Loder E, Rizzoli P, Golub J. Hormonal management of migraine associated with menses and the menopause: a clinical review. *Headache*. 2007;47(2):329–40.

Marcus DA, Bernstein CD, Sullivan EA, Rudy TE. A prospective comparison between ICHD-II and probability menstrual migraine diagnostic criteria. *Headache*. 2010;50:539–50.

Somerville BW. The role of estradiol withdrawal in the etiology of menstrual migraine. *Neurology*. 1972; 22(4):355–65.

Verapamil treatment of cluster headache

Cohen AS, Matharu MS, Goadsby PJ. Electrocardiographic abnormalities in patients with cluster headache on verapamil therapy. *Neurology*. 2007;69:668–75.

Leone M, D'Amico D, Frediani F, *et al.* Verapamil in the prophylaxis of episodic cluster headache: a double-blind study versus placebo. *Neurology*. 2000;54:1382–5.

Nesbitt AD, Goadsby PJ. Clinical review: cluster headache. *BMJ*. 2012;344:e2407.

Chronic opioid therapy

Manchikanti L, Abdi S, Atluri S, *et al.* American Society of Interventional Pain Physicians (ASIPP) guidelines for responsible opioid prescribing in chronic non-cancer pain, Parts 1 and 2. *Pain Physician*. 2012;15:S1–100.

Owen GT, Burton AW, Schade CM, Passik S. Urine drug testing: current recommendations and best practices. *Pain Physician*. 2012;15:ES119–33.

Lithium for cluster headache and nonadherence to medication

Hedenrud T, Jonsson P, Linde M. Beliefs about medicines and adherence among Swedish migraineurs. *Ann Pharmacother*. 2007;42:39–45.

May A, Leone M, Afra J, *et al.* EFNS guidelines on the treatment of cluster headache and other trigeminal-autonomic cephalalgias. *Eur J Neurol*. 2006;13:1066–77.

Rains JC, Penzien DB, Lipchik GL. Behavioral facilitation of medical treatment for headache – Part II: Theoretical models and behavioral strategies for improving adherence. *Headache*. 2006;46:1395–403.

Tfeldt-Hansen PC, Jensen RH. Management of cluster headache. *CNS Drugs*. 2012;26(7):571–80.

Acute retroviral syndrome

Cohen HS, Gay CL, Busch MP, Hecht FM. The detection of acute HIV infection. *J Infect Dis*. 2010;202(Suppl 2): S270–7.

Graham CB, Wippold FJ, Pilgram TK, Fisher EJ, Smoker WRK. Screening CT of the brain determined by CD4 count in HIV-positive patients presenting with headache. *AJNR Am J Neuroradiol*. 2000;21:451–4.

The SPARTAC Trial Investigators. Short-course antiretroviral therapy in primary HIV infection. *N Engl J Med*. 2013;368:207–17.

Vanhems P, Allard R, Cooper DA, *et al.* Acute human immunodeficiency virus type 1 disease as a mononucleosis-like illness: is the diagnosis too restrictive? *Clin Infect Dis*. 1997;24:965–70.

Vanhems P, Dassa C, Lambert J, *et al.* Comprehensive classification of symptoms and signs reported among 218 patients with acute HIV-1 infection. *J Acquir Immune Defic Syndr*. 1999;21:99–106.

Iatrogenic harms of unnecessary testing

Gough J, Scott-Coombes D, Palazzo FF. Thyroid incidentaloma: an evidence-based assessment of management strategy. *World J Surg*. 2008;32(7): 1264–8.

Loder E, Cardona L. Evaluation for secondary causes of headache: the role of blood and urine testing. *Headache*. 2011;51:338–45.

Qaseem A, Alguire P, Dallas P, *et al.* Appropriate use of screening and diagnostic tests to foster high-value, cost-conscious care. *Ann Intern Med*. 2012;156(2): 147–9.

Ulvestad E, Kanestrøm A, Madland TM, *et al.* Evaluation of diagnostic tests for antinuclear antibodies in rheumatological practice. *Scand J Immunol*. 2000;52:309–15.

Chapter 6

When historical or examination findings are missed or misinterpreted

There are no biomarkers for benign headache disorders such as migraine, and laboratory or imaging studies serve mainly to exclude other causes of headache. Thorough patient evaluation, especially a careful history and physical examination, is therefore essential for the accurate diagnosis of headache problems. Headache diagnosis has important treatment implications, since management that is effective for one form of headache may be ineffective for another. Overlooked or misinterpreted historical or examination findings can result in missed diagnoses and lost opportunities for appropriate therapy. One common example is a patient with cluster headache who has been misdiagnosed with migraine and treated ineffectively with anti-migraine drugs for years.

Most seasoned headache experts recognize that the patient history is usually more informative than the physical examination. In fact, the physical examination is expected to be normal in most patients with primary headache disorders. Despite this, additional findings such as occipito-nuchal tenderness, abnormal neck posture, or temporomandibular joint dysfunction can identify problems that might be contributing to a primary headache disorder. Documentation of these findings also can be helpful to patients for insurance reasons or disability determination. The fact that physical or neurologic abnormalities are uncommonly encountered in headache patients may lull doctors into a false sense of security. Thorough examination of all patients with headache is important since, as cases in this chapter illustrate, subtle findings can change a diagnosis and influence treatment.

Considerable skill is sometimes required to obtain a thorough history of headache problems, especially in cases of long-standing headache with many failed treatment attempts. We find it helpful to begin with the open-ended question "Tell me about your headaches." This allows the patient uninterrupted time to tell their story. The resulting narrative is often therapeutic for the patient and instructive for the physician. Many patients will spontaneously describe features such as photophobia or vomiting that are required for headache diagnosis; the physician can query missing information later.

It is important to note that although most patients should be allowed to tell their story in an unfettered way, some patients may require different degrees of active guidance from the provider. This can help retain a focus on the most salient details, the result being a narrative crafted from a balance of conversational flow and what could be termed "supportive" redirection on the part of the provider: for example, "Let's put your visit to the emergency department aside for now and go back to what you were saying about your headache."

With only some practice and without any special or expensive technology, the provider can, after an effective history and physical examination, expect to arrive at a correct headache diagnosis much of the time. When the process breaks down or shortcuts are taken, various complications can occur, as illustrated by the following cases.

A young man with visual changes and a sore head

Case

A 28-year-old man with a prior history of hypertension was seen in the emergency department with a complaint of sudden visual changes. The patient described a "flashing" in his peripheral vision that started in one eye and spread to both over a period of about ten minutes. This gradually evolved into what he described as a "flashing floater" along the edges of his vision bilaterally. This was followed by blurred vision in the originally affected eye.

The visual symptoms, which had lasted a total of 20 minutes, gradually disappeared while the patient

Table 6.1. Features suggestive of retinal detachment

Acute visual loss (this is an ophthalmologic emergency)
Recent onset of visual "floaters"
Sudden onset of flashes of light
Darkening of vision or development of a curtain or shadow across vision

Table 6.2. Selected features that distinguish the visual aura of migraine from ischemic events

Visual aura of migraine	Ischemic events
Visual phenomena begin in the periphery and develop gradually	Sudden onset of visual loss
Both positive and negative visual phenomena are present	Negative visual symptoms predominate
Reversible, with duration of event no longer than an hour	Short duration (typically no more than 15 minutes)
If other aura symptoms are present, they occur in sequence	If other neurologic symptoms are present, they occur simultaneously with visual phenomena
Similar events on multiple occasions	No prior history of similar events
Symptoms are followed by headache (usually within 15 minutes)	Headache is not a common associated feature

was on the way to the emergency department. There was no associated headache. The emergency department physicians were concerned about the possibility of a transient ischemic attack and he underwent an evaluation that included a carotid ultrasound, a CT scan of his head, and consultation by an ophthalmology resident. The results of these investigations were normal and he was discharged home with instructions to take 81 mg of aspirin daily and follow up in the outpatient neurology clinic.

He was seen in the clinic several days later where a neurologist elicited a history of several similar episodes of visual disturbance when the patient was in his teens. Those were described as periods of "fluttery" peripheral vision lasting 5–25 minutes and followed by a period of mild head "soreness." These episodes had occurred sporadically over a period of several years and then disappeared. The patient had sought ophthalmologic examination at the time but no abnormalities were found.

What is the differential diagnosis of these visual symptoms?

Isolated visual symptoms can be related to intraocular pathology, transient ischemic attacks, migraine aura, retinal detachment, or seizures. Visual phenomena are often described as "positive" or "negative." Positive visual phenomena include false visual images or distortions of normal vision, such as sparkling lights, lines, or geometric shapes, spots of color, or shimmering vision. Negative visual phenomena, on the other hand, include visual deficits such as dark or blind spots.

The differential diagnosis for visual symptoms that resolve spontaneously includes seizures, migraine aura, and transient ischemic attacks. Symptoms that persist beyond an hour or two require urgent investigation for intraocular pathology such as retinal detachment; features characteristic of this diagnosis are listed in Table 6.1. It can be difficult to distinguish tran-

sient ischemic attacks from more benign causes of visual symptoms such as migraine aura, but several historical features, which are listed in Table 6.2, can help.

The patient described in the case experienced a mixture of positive and negative visual features that developed gradually and were followed by headache. These are all more characteristic of visual aura than of transient ischemic attack. Patients often find it difficult to describe visual aura. Obtaining a previous history of such attacks can be very helpful. We make a special point of inquiring about such attacks at a younger age, since in our experience patients may not spontaneously report them.

What bedside test may have helped clarify the diagnosis?

Almost all patients who have any type of migraine aura also have visual aura. Thus, in order to recognize patients with aura, it is only necessary to establish the presence of visual aura. This can be done using the Visual Aura Rating Scale (VARS), which is a validated tool developed for this purpose. The point system used by the VARS is described in Table 6.3. The VARS is simple to administer at the bedside or in the office. Points are assigned for the presence of any of five characteristics of visual aura: duration from 5 to 60 minutes, gradual onset, visual scotoma, zig-zag lines, or unilateral location of the visual phenomena. The patient

Table 6.3. The Visual Aura Rating Scale for the diagnosis of migraine with aura

Feature	Points
Duration 5–60 minutes	3 points
Develops gradually ≥ 5 minutes	2 points
Presence of associated scotoma (blind spot)	2 points
Zig-zag lines (fortification spectra)	2 points
Unilateral location	1 point

A VARS score of 5 or more diagnosed migraine with aura with a sensitivity of 96% (95% confidence interval [CI] 92–99%) and a specificity of 98% (95% CI 95–100%).

Reproduced with permission from: Eriksen MK, Thomsen LL, Olesen J. The Visual Aura Rating Scale (VARS) for migraine aura diagnosis. *Cephalalgia*. 2005;25(10):801–10.

Table 6.4. Clinical characteristics of aura

One of the following features should be present:
1. Fully reversible (usually homonymous) visual symptoms including positive features (e.g. flickering lights, spots, or lines) and/or negative features (e.g. loss of vision)
2. Fully reversible (usually unilateral) sensory symptoms including positive features (e.g. pins and needles) and/or negative features (e.g. numbness)
3. Fully reversible dysphasic speech disturbance

described in this case would have scored five of ten possible points. The use of the VARS or elicitation of the history of similar episodes when he was younger might have spared him an unnecessary workup for transient ischemic attack, and unnecessary treatment with aspirin. In the past, some physicians prescribed low-dose aspirin therapy for patients with aura, but there is no evidence that this is beneficial, and some recent evidence suggests it may be harmful. Thus, we do not recommend the use of low-dose aspirin therapy in patients with migraine aura.

Discussion

Aura occurs in about a third of patients with migraine. Visual aura is by far the most common type of aura, occurring in 99% of subjects with aura. This is followed by sensory aura (31%) and aura involving language symptoms such as aphasia (18%). Motor aura is rare, and this special form of aura is separately recognized as hemiplegic migraine. Some forms of hemiplegic migraine are autosomal dominant single gene disorders; these have provided an important opportunity to study the genetics of migraine.

Migraine aura is thought to be due to the phenomenon of cortical spreading depression, which is an orderly wave of depolarization that spreads anteriorly across the cerebral cortex. This is followed by a prolonged period during which neurons struggle to repolarize (hence the term "depression") and is followed by a small reduction in regional cerebral blood flow. The wave of neuronal depolarization spreads at a rate of 2–5 mm per minute, which correlates closely with

the evolution of visual or sensory symptoms during an aura.

Aura symptoms usually develop gradually over five or more minutes, and different aura symptoms, when present, usually develop in succession, each lasting between 5 and 60 minutes. Associated loss of vision or blurred vision may be present, but blurred vision alone is not sufficient to make a diagnosis of visual aura. Table 6.4 lists the typical features of aura.

Aura may occur without a subsequent headache or can be followed by a mild, non-migrainous headache. With age, patients may lose characteristic migraine headache features or may not experience headache at all after an aura. The diagnosis of visual aura without headache thus occurs more frequently in older patients.

Diagnosis

Typical aura with headache.

Tip

Failure to elicit historical features consistent with migraine aura can lead to an erroneous diagnosis of cerebral ischemia in patients with aura.

A young woman with a headache that was "worse than ever"

Case

A 30-year-old obese female presented to a headache clinic with records from her initial evaluation at another clinic for the same symptoms. These records indicated that she had initially reported several months of a "worse than ever" daily headache sometimes associated with "black spots" in her vision, nausea, vomiting, and photo and phonophobia. She was taking a combination estrogen–progestin contraceptive pill, and was a smoker. Her examination was normal. The physician, hearing that she was having "the worst headache ever," was concerned about a secondary headache. He sent her for an emergent MRI followed by an unsuccessful attempt at lumbar puncture. A second lumbar puncture was attempted under fluoroscopy and was finally successful. This was followed by an MRV. The results of these tests were normal.

Was the physician's level of concern appropriate?

The phrase "worst headache ever" was understandably worrying to this patient's doctor, who undoubtedly was concerned about secondary causes of headache such as cerebral venous thrombosis or stroke. However, when viewed in the context of the patient's history this situation is not so alarming. In the headache clinic, the patient was asked to provide a chronologic history that included childhood headache symptoms and the evolution of her headaches from onset to their current pattern. This revealed a strong family history of migraine, and a personal history of years of episodic migraine headache with a gradual transformation to a chronic situation.

This pattern is very typical of the evolution of episodic to chronic migraine, caught around the time of transformation of the headache pattern. Furthermore, the patient's sex and obesity are factors associated with an increased risk of transformation from episodic to chronic migraine. When this patient's headache history is considered as a whole, the extensive diagnostic workup that was undertaken seems superfluous, costly, and unnecessarily invasive.

Two evaluations of the same historical information produced divergent outcomes. What went wrong?

The initial examiner failed to take into account the context into which the current headache situation fits. This is another example of the cognitive error of premature closure. The doctor settled on a likely diagnosis of a dangerous secondary headache based on some details but minus other useful information. This does not mean that his concern was completely

unfounded: certainly the patient's nicotine addiction deserves attention.

The picture that emerged of this patient's headaches appeared very different when considered in the overall context of her headaches. She reported childhood carsickness and subsequent onset of headaches with migrainous features in her 20s. These headaches slowly progressed in frequency and severity over many years. The change in her headache pattern in the preceding four months before the current evaluation was probably the point at which the patient recognized that her headaches were becoming chronic and more disabling. Because the initial headache history did not elicit this story of gradual progression, unnecessary diagnostic testing and treatment ensued. Unnecessary diagnostic investigation is often uncomfortable for the patient, provokes anxiety, and creates the potential for iatrogenesis.

Discussion

In most cases the patient history is the most important part of headache evaluation and sets the stage for decision-making about testing and treatment. Conventional teaching is that the patient history is a stepwise process that begins with the history of the present illness, proceeds through a review of what brought the patient in for evaluation at that moment (the chief complaint), and then the details of the current problem.

In the evaluation of headache, however, it is often wise to begin with an open-ended question such as "tell me about your headaches" and then fill in details using a time-based or chronologic approach. This begins with questions about family history and childhood headache symptoms, followed by detailed longitudinal questioning about migraine-related symptoms during the teenage years and then in each decade beyond the teens, with appropriate attention devoted to headache changes associated with such events as menarche, pregnancy, marriage, or job changes. The headache history can then be considered in the context of the overall history of headaches, which provides a more complete picture and is likely to produce a more accurate diagnosis.

Diagnosis

Migraine without aura, with transformation to chronic migraine.

Tip

Failure to consider a patient's current headache problem in the context of the overall headache history can lead to unnecessary testing and treatment.

Intractable headache and psychiatric illness in a young woman

Case

A 24-year-old female had been followed in adult neurology since age 16, and before that in a pediatric neurology clinic, for debilitating and limiting headache associated with multiple psychiatric comorbidities. Over the span of eight years, five neurologists had evaluated her for her headaches. She was also receiving treatment from a psychiatrist and psychologist for anxiety, major depression, and suicidal gestures. She had been hospitalized twice for management of psychiatric problems, and had periodically been unable to attend school for weeks at a time. Both her headaches and her psychiatric problems had not improved despite multiple trials of treatment.

When seen at her most recent visit, the patient told her neurologist that she had read a magazine article about the possible connection between headaches and abuse. She told the doctor that she had been sexually abused as a child by a relative. She said she had just mentioned this to her therapist and was beginning to explore the issue. A recent psychiatry chart note confirmed that the abuse history had "been revealed for the first time." Review of the patient's record showed no documentation of any previous questions or discussions about physical, emotional, or sexual abuse or trauma, with the exception of a note in the psychiatry intake form that stated: "Not evaluated at this time."

Should the patient's doctors have suspected a prior history of abuse or trauma?

This patient's doctors probably should have been more alert to the possibility that this patient had experienced prior maltreatment, since a history of abuse is very common in patients with refractory headache disorders. Traumatic experiences in childhood are linked with an elevated risk of a large number of childhood and adult medical problems, including headache. Trauma can result not only from the personal experience of violence or abuse, but also from witnessing

Table 6.5. Types of adverse or traumatic experiences

Physical abuse or neglect

Sexual abuse

Intimate partner violence

Emotional abuse or neglect

Alcohol or drug abuser in the home

No parents in the home or single parent

Chronically physically or mentally ill person in the home

Witnessing violence in the home or social environment

such events. Table 6.5 lists some common forms of adverse or traumatic experiences. The prevalence of childhood sexual or physical abuse or neglect is high in the general population and is not confined to a particular ethnic or socioeconomic group. For example, some sources estimate that as many as one in four girls and one in six boys experience sexual abuse in childhood. Abuse is not confined to children, however. Intimate partner violence or other traumatic events frequently occur in adulthood, and those with a childhood history of adverse experiences may be at high risk for later revictimization.

The prevalence of abuse or trauma is even higher in patients with chronic headache disorders than in the general population. A large multicenter study performed in specialty headache clinics found that roughly a quarter of patients with migraine acknowledged a history of physical or sexual abuse or neglect, and over a third reported a history of emotional abuse or neglect. There was substantial overlap of the different forms of maltreatment, and almost half of those who experienced abuse in childhood reported experiencing abuse in adulthood.

In our experience, it is prudent to maintain a high index of suspicion about abuse or trauma in patients with difficult-to-treat headaches. This patient had intractable, debilitating headaches from a young age, associated with severe, difficult to treat psychiatric disease.

It is difficult to prove a causal relationship between maltreatment and headache occurrence or intractability, but several lines of evidence suggest this connection. For example, several studies have demonstrated a dose–response relationship between the number of adverse childhood experiences and the prevalence and risk of frequent headaches in both sexes. Some evidence suggests that childhood trauma can produce permanent changes in the hypothalamic–pituitary axis, while other work implicates the development of poor coping strategies, somatization, or dissociation.

How and when should questions about abuse or trauma be asked?

Good quality evidence supports an association between maltreatment and chronic headache, but there is no consensus about whether all patients should be questioned about a history of abuse. At present recommendations for screening are limited to particular subgroups. For example, the United States Preventive Services Task Force (USPSTF) has reviewed available evidence and recommends that "clinicians screen women of childbearing age for intimate partner violence, such as domestic violence, and provide or refer women who screen positive to intervention services…The USPSTF concludes that the current evidence is insufficient to assess the balance of benefits and harms of screening all elderly or vulnerable adults (physically or mentally dysfunctional) for abuse and neglect."

This patient was prompted to tell her caregivers about a previous history of childhood sexual abuse after reading about its possible connection with chronic headaches. Her providers were distressed to find that this history had remained undocumented for so long. Few patients are likely to be as forthcoming as this patient was. Our belief is that it makes sense to ask about abuse routinely in patients seeking treatment for headache problems, especially those whose problems have resisted treatment or occur in the context of other psychiatric disorders. Psychiatrists often include a history of abuse in their patient evaluations, but as this case illustrates, this cannot be assumed.

There are several ways in which information about maltreatment can be obtained. If patients are asked to fill out written surveys or questionnaires prior to being seen, the question can be asked in writing. Validated instruments such as the Childhood Trauma Questionnaire can be used. In our practice we include a written question about a history of trauma or abuse in the information we ask patients to complete before being seen. However, since patients may be reluctant to disclose this information on a form we also follow up with a routine question during our initial meeting with the patient.

We usually ask these questions when inquiring about other aspects of the social history, first asking patients about their living situation, and then moving on to whether they feel safe in their current living situation, finally asking whether they have ever been in a situation that was unsafe or abusive. As with other sensitive information, it is helpful to frame the questions carefully. We try to "normalize" the disclosure of such information by telling patients that many people with chronic headache have experienced prior sexual or physical abuse or trauma. We then let them know that we routinely ask all patients about abuse, and finish with more specific questions.

How should doctors respond when patients disclose abuse or trauma?

Most physicians are subject to mandatory reporting requirements if abuse is suspected in vulnerable patients such as minor children or the elderly, and some states have additional reporting requirements. These vary and physicians are encouraged to stay up to date with local regulations. In the case of competent adult patients without immediate injuries, the physician usually is legally obligated to respect the privacy of information disclosed in the doctor–patient relationship. The clinician's role in these cases is limited to helping the patient make decisions and ensuring they have access to information about available help and resources.

We tell adult patients who disclose abuse or trauma that we are glad they told us about the maltreatment. It is also important to tell the patient that "you do not deserve to be treated like this." The next step is to evaluate the immediate safety of patients who are currently involved in abusive situations, and to give the patient information about resources such as abuse hotlines, legal resources, and healthcare resources. We keep a variety of information pamphlets on hand for this purpose.

In the case of patients who are involved in abusive relationships, many clinicians are tempted to advise the patient to leave the relationship or ask them why they put up with such treatment. Although well intentioned, such questions or advice may imply that you hold the patient responsible for the abusive situation. In some cases, such advice if acted upon may put the patient or any involved children in danger from the abuser. It is important to respect the patient's choices about whether or when to end a relationship. We tell patients experiencing abuse that we are very concerned about their welfare, recommend that they contact local counseling resources, and urge them to make follow-up appointments so that we can monitor the situation.

Discussion

Good quality evidence supports a link between various forms of childhood abuse (sexual, physical, or emotional) and later life pain syndromes, including migraine. One study found that a past history of emotional abuse was almost four times more common in patients, mostly female, with migraine. Migraine patients with a past history of such "adverse childhood experiences" may be more likely to experience not only chronic migraine in later years but also depression and anxiety. They may also be less compliant with treatment or medical appointments, particularly if the situation at home remains chaotic.

Because this is a relatively new area of research, there are no clear implications for patient management when a history of abuse is uncovered. We find, however, that patients who have experienced intimate partner or sexual violence may have difficulty with treatments that remind them of the circumstances of any abuse. For example, a female patient who has been sexually abused by an older male may become anxious during physical therapy or relaxation sessions with an older male therapist.

It is not clear that the outcome of this patient's care would have been different if her abuse history had been known. It does, however, seem evident that it is an integral part of her medical and psychosocial history. Knowledge of this part of the patient's history might have helped her caregivers to understand the patient's headaches in the context of her life experiences. It is important not to underestimate the effect that traumatic life experiences can have on a patient's headache problems.

Diagnosis

Chronic migraine in a patient with a history of childhood sexual abuse.

Tip

Do not forget to ask all headache patients, especially those with treatment-refractory headaches, about a history of sexual, physical, or emotional abuse or trauma. These high-yield historical questions can clarify a complex situation.

A man with headache, neurologic symptoms, and spinal fluid pleocytosis

Case

A 33-year-old male was seen in the emergency department with headache and neurologic symptoms. There was a past history of occasional episodic migraine but the patient had not been troubled by migraines for several years. He was otherwise healthy and taking no medications. The patient had developed a constant mild frontal headache three days prior to evaluation. On the fourth day, he had noted migratory right-sided numbness and paresthesias in the arm, leg, and face. Shortly thereafter he was unable to speak for a short time, and following that he developed a "worst ever" headache with associated nausea and vomiting. This prompted urgent evaluation including a plain CT scan of the head followed by lumbar puncture, MRA, and MRV. Test results were normal except for the finding of elevated white blood cells (150 cells/μL) in the CSF, lymphocyte predominant. He was afebrile. He was advised that the diagnosis was viral meningitis.

One week later he noted a return of the numbness followed by a one-hour episode of confusion and a moderately severe headache. He returned to the emergency department where evaluation was again normal apart from elevated white cells in the CSF (450 cells/μL) and a mildly elevated CSF protein at 113 mg/dL. The diagnosis at that point was possible viral encephalitis. He was admitted to the hospital and placed on seizure prophylaxis and antiviral agents.

Was a diagnosis of encephalitis appropriate in this case?

At the initial presentation, viral meningitis was a reasonable diagnosis, although the patient did not report a full range of typical symptoms such as fever, stiff neck, or other viral features (malaise, muscle aches, etc.). Additionally, the patient had reported the most severe headache of his life and there was no history of prior headache or migraine. In this setting, a secondary headache of some kind was a leading diagnostic possibility. During his second presentation the patient's symptoms included confusion, which indicates a process affecting either the brainstem or both halves of the cortex. On the other hand, no localizing neurologic findings were noted and imaging findings remained normal. Although the patient appeared less

Table 6.6. Clinical characteristics of headache with neurologic deficits and CSF lymphocytosis (HaNDL)

- Episodes of moderate headache occurring with or quickly followed by transient neurologic deficits
- Episodes of headache and focal neurologic deficits recur over a period of less than 3 months
- Lumbar puncture findings show cerebrospinal fluid pleocytosis with lymphocytic predominance (> 15 cells/μL)
- CSF culture and neuroimaging findings are normal

ill than might be expected with encephalitis, an early or incomplete encephalitic process was plausible and management for this potentially severe condition was reasonable.

The patient stayed in the hospital for several days. He remained afebrile and looked well at the time of discharge. However, he returned again to the emergency department three days later with a similar presentation: headache, confusion, and paresthesias, though now these were all milder than at the time of the initial presentation. He was afebrile, looked well, and had a normal examination at this last emergency department visit. He underwent a diagnostic workup similar to his previous episodes and was again admitted to the hospital.

What is the best diagnosis at this point?

The diagnostic possibilities in this case are becoming clearer as a history emerges of repeated benign episodes of headache and CSF abnormalities. This patient presented with new-onset headache without migrainous features, with mild reversible focal neurologic deficits, and CSF lymphocytosis. Furthermore, such episodes recurred. This is the classic description of headache with neurologic deficits and CSF lymphocytosis (HaNDL), which was first described in 1981. Features of the syndrome that are helpful for diagnostic purposes include a finding of CSF lymphocytosis along with negative cultures (Table 6.6).

Clinical mimics of this syndrome include migraine aura, transient ischemic attacks or stroke, as well as viral meningitis or encephalitis. In this case, there were no migraine features to the headache and the episodes were not stereotyped, as would be expected in migraine aura. Although about a third of patients with HaNDL have a history of migraine, the clinical significance of this is uncertain because the prevalence of migraine is so high in the general population.

In hindsight, what historical and examination features might have suggested this patient's condition was benign?

Although abrupt headaches in combination with focal neurologic deficits may indicate a serious disorder, they can also be due to benign, self-limited problems. In this patient there were no signs of ischemia on imaging and it would be unusual for repeated transient ischemic attacks to occur in an otherwise healthy young man. Although CSF lymphocytosis was documented, there were no other signs of infection. The patient continued to feel and act better than would be expected if he had an ongoing encephalitic or ischemic process. Additionally, he was completely well between episodes and his spinal fluid cultures were negative, lowering the likelihood of any ongoing infectious process.

Although physicians worry about missing potentially severe but treatable conditions, they also have a duty to protect patients from unnecessary testing, iatrogenesis, and undue anxiety. In this case, more restraint in testing and treatment was probably warranted when, despite the worrisome diagnoses under consideration, the patient continued to look and do well.

Discussion

HaNDL is a rare but well-described syndrome that may be confused with meningoencephalitis or other serious conditions. It is benign and usually resolves on its own. There are several case reports of patients with HaNDL who were suspected of having acute stroke and treated with systemic thrombolysis. Failure to recognize the characteristic historical and examination features of this illness can thus have serious consequences. In this case the patient was unnecessarily treated with antiepileptic and antiviral therapies.

HaNDL was initially thought to represent a form of migraine, but current thinking centers on the possibility of a post-viral syndrome. The reversible focal deficits have been attributed to transient vasoconstriction. Some authors report that steroid treatment can be helpful, although there are no large-scale studies to support this view. Catheter angiography may worsen symptoms and should be avoided if this condition is suspected.

Diagnosis

Headache with neurologic deficits and CSF lymphocytosis (HaNDL).

Tip

Prompt recognition of benign historical and examination findings can save patients from invasive and dangerous treatments or multiple hospitalizations.

An elderly woman with giant cell arteritis and persistent headache on steroids

Case

A 73-year-old female presented for evaluation of a mild to moderately severe headache of three months' duration. She described an achy global headache associated with mild photophobia, ear pain and nausea. She did not have distended temporal arteries or any head soreness. There were no constitutional or jaw claudication symptoms. As part of her evaluation, an erythrocyte sedimentation rate (ESR) and C-reactive protein (CRP) were obtained. Both were moderately elevated, and a subsequent temporal artery biopsy reportedly showed giant cell arteritis.

Her headache initially improved on initial doses of prednisone but later returned during the prednisone taper. The physician attributed this worsened headache to ongoing arteritis and recommended an increase in the patient's corticosteroid dose. At the patient's next visit she reported that this increased dose had not improved her symptoms. The physician asked her to give a more complete description of the headache. She reported that the headache was absent on waking each day, but would begin after becoming upright for 10–15 minutes and progress throughout the day to a severity of 6 on a 0–10 pain scale. The headache was dull and bilateral. Her MRI was reviewed and, although it had originally been read as normal, showed subtle findings consistent with low CSF volume. Her symptoms improved with use of an abdominal binder when she was upright and a regimen of daily caffeine tablets. She was eventually sent for an epidural blood patch and her headache cleared completely.

Was giant cell arteritis the best initial explanation of the headache pattern?

Headache associated with giant cell arteritis has been described as generalized and throbbing, intermittent or constant; but it can also be nonspecific, as it was in this case. Temporal artery tenderness and enlargement may be found on physical examination. In this case, a temporal artery biopsy was positive and the patient initially improved with corticosteroid treatment. When her headache recurred, the physician assumed the symptoms were due to the original diagnosis but failed to consider other possible explanations for the continued headache. This is an example of "anchoring bias," in which new historical information is interpreted in the light of an established diagnosis, without consideration of other explanations. In hindsight, although this patient certainly did have giant cell arteritis, it is unclear how much of the initial headache report was explained by the arteritis. It is plausible that the symptoms of low CSF volume prompted her initial evaluation. The possibility that this patient had two causes of headache was not considered until relatively late in her course.

When should a diagnosis be reconsidered?

In our experience, headaches attributable to giant cell arteritis typically improve promptly with corticosteroid treatment, although there are occasional patients where headaches linger. Worsening of headache is sometimes attributable to incomplete treatment of the arteritis and an elevation in steroid dose is a reasonable first step. However, failure to respond as expected to treatment (in this case to an elevation of the corticosteroid dose) should raise concern about alternative or additional diagnostic possibilities.

As was done by the physician in this case, it is helpful in such situations to put aside assumptions and re-evaluate the headache history from the beginning. It can also be useful to discuss the case with a colleague, since presenting a case to someone forces a reconsideration of the entire clinical picture.

Discussion

The physician in this case initially did not recognize that the historical evolution of the patient's headache deviated from the clinical course expected with her initial diagnosis. Upon revisiting the history, however, he elicited important information about postural features of headache. This eventually led to the diagnosis of an additional cause of headache: low CSF pressure, presumably from a spontaneous leak.

It is important to be vigilant for giant cell arteritis in older patients, since it is a medical emergency. The clinical picture of giant cell arteritis can be highly variable, and early treatment with corticosteroids may prevent permanent visual loss. Thus, a low threshold for biopsy and treatment is appropriate. It is useful to remember, however, that corticosteroid treatment may produce temporary improvement in a wide variety of headache types, so response to steroid treatment is not diagnostic.

Diagnosis

Giant cell arteritis; low CSF pressure headache.

Tip

Patients can have more than one cause of headache. When patients do not respond as expected to treatment, the history should be carefully reviewed for overlooked clues.

A man with unilateral headache and subtle eye findings

Case

A 62-year-old man was seen for evaluation of a headache that had started about three weeks ago. He had a prior history of occasional bilateral, mild headaches that lasted a few hours at most, but this headache was located behind the right eye and was continuous since onset. The patient reported that the headache began after he had been target shooting for several hours. This required him to close his left eye frequently and hold his neck in a particular posture. The evening of target practice and for two days after, the patient had experienced blurry vision. His vision then normalized, but he developed a continuous dull right retro-orbital headache that radiated to the angle of his jaw on the right. He had photophobia and wore sunglasses, but denied any associated features such as nausea or vomiting. He mentioned that he felt as if he had some grit or sand in his right eye. Based on the unilateral location of the headache, the physician made a

diagnosis of hemicrania continua and recommended treatment with indomethacin.

The physician performed a brief examination but the patient declined to remove his sunglasses for a funduscopic inspection. As the patient was about to leave, however, the patient's wife asked the doctor why her husband was "squinting" and noted "It's been like that since the headache started." Upon further examination, the patient was noted to have right-sided ptosis and miosis, with warmer skin on the right side of his forehead. Further examination revealed a suggestion of a slight left-sided central facial palsy and mild left upper extremity weakness.

What is the differential diagnosis, and what tests should be performed next?

Autonomic features are frequent accompaniments of many types of headache, most notably the trigeminal autonomic cephalgias and hemicrania continua. They can also be seen in migraine. Thus, the differential diagnosis of side-locked headache in association with ipsilateral autonomic features includes benign headaches such as cluster headache, hemicrania continua, or even migraine, but also dangerous conditions such as giant cell arteritis, carotid dissection, or cervical facet disease.

Neuroimaging should be considered in all patients with side-locked headaches, even when they appear to meet criteria for a benign headache disorder. MRI of the cervical spine and MRA of the extracranial carotid circulation are indicated when there are abnormal examination findings, as there were in this case. In older patients an ESR and CRP should also be considered, since giant cell arteritis can present as a unilateral headache.

This patient had a normal ESR and CRP, but MRA showed dissection of the extracranial part of the right internal carotid artery with significant stenosis. The patient was treated with aspirin.

What is the cause of the physical examination findings in this patient?

The combination of ptosis and miosis is characteristic of Horner's syndrome. A lesion of sympathetic fibers that innervate the face and eye causes this problem. Other findings in Horner's syndrome may include anhidrosis (decreased sweating) on the side of the lesion. Flushing and conjunctival injection are less frequent. First-order neurons from the posterior hypothalamus travel to the upper cervical and lower thoracic segments of the spinal cord, where they synapse with second-order preganglionic neurons. These travel over the apex of the lung, pass around the subclavian artery, and finally end in the superior cervical ganglion. Here they synapse with third-order postganglionic neurons, some of which travel with the internal carotid artery through the cavernous sinus to innervate the pupil and muscles of the eyelid, others of which travel with the external carotid artery to the facial sweat glands.

Suspicion should be high that patients with new-onset Horner's syndrome and headache may have a dangerous secondary explanation for their problems. This is true even when, as in this case, the headaches appear to meet criteria for a benign form of headache. A Horner's syndrome may occur from a lesion anywhere along the sympathetic pathway. If needed, special pupillary testing can establish whether lesions are pre- or postganglionic. One frequent cause that also presents with head or neck pain is carotid dissection. As described above, the sympathetic fibers lie just outside the carotid artery and a dissection may cause stretching of the fibers sufficient to disrupt functioning. For this reason, a patient who presents with headache and a Horner's syndrome, or neck pain and a Horner's syndrome, should be evaluated with carotid imaging. This could be accomplished with duplex sonography, a CTA of the neck, or an MRA with fat suppression sequences.

What accounts for the diagnostic "near miss" in this case and how can mistakes like this be avoided?

The physician in this case did not perform a careful physical examination, perhaps because she fell prey to the cognitive error of "premature closure." No additional diagnoses were considered once a verdict that "fits the facts" had been found. The physical examination findings in this patient were subtle, and his sunglasses probably masked the eye abnormalities. He refused funduscopic examination, but that is not unusual in patients with primary headache disorders who are sensitive to light. In addition, the patient's history was highly suggestive of a particular form of benign headache, including the "classic" feature of a

foreign body sensation in the eye. The physician in this case probably reasoned that she was unlikely to find anything on physical examination and so skipped this step.

When autonomic features occur in close association with discrete episodes of headache pain, and especially if lacrimation or rhinorrhea also occur, the cause is most likely to be benign activation of the autonomic nervous system by a headache. It is easy to understand how the physician in this case made a diagnosis of hemicrania continua, especially since the feeling of "grit" in the eye is a common complaint in that disorder. More careful examination, however, prompted by the wife's parting question about "squinting," revealed subtle neurologic signs that raised suspicion of a more sinister explanation for the patient's problem.

Physicians may perform brief physical exams for many reasons: a shortage of time or a belief that the diagnosis is clear based upon a characteristic history. They may reason that therefore the physical examination is an afterthought, or wish to spare the patient discomfort. In this case, several of these factors were likely at play. This case is a reminder of the importance of a thorough physical exam even if it means putting the patient through temporary discomfort, such as exposing a photophobic patient to a brief ophthalmologic exam.

Discussion

Headache is present in roughly two-thirds of patients with carotid dissection, and is usually ipsilateral to the dissection. Horner's syndrome is also common. A history of previous minor head or neck trauma, as in this case, is also common. Dissection is thought to occur when small tears in the intimal layer of the artery allow arterial blood (which is under high pressure) to penetrate into the medial layers of the arterial wall. The resulting hematoma can produce partial or complete occlusion of the artery, and emboli arising in this area may also result in ischemia.

Cardiac risk factors such as hypertension or hypercholesterolemia may raise the risk of dissection, as do connective tissue disorders. Chiropractic manipulation of the neck has also been associated with dissection of cranial arteries, and this is one reason we do not recommend it for the treatment of headache. Dissection is usually treated with either anticoagulation or antiplatelet agents. A recent nonrandomized study did not show clear benefit for either approach so in view of the potential risks of full anticoagulation, many physicians opt for treatment with aspirin or other antiplatelet regimens.

Diagnosis

Carotid dissection with Horner's syndrome.

Tip

A careful ophthalmologic examination is important in all patients who present with headache. A cursory examination can miss subtle but important findings.

An older woman with focal headache

Case

A 68-year-old woman was seen in the urgent care department of the hospital because she had awakened earlier that day with a headache. The pain was burning, throbbing, and located over the left temple and forehead. She rated it 8 on a pain scale of 0–10. The headache was not associated with additional symptoms such as nausea, vomiting, photo or phonophobia. She had a remote history of episodic migraine without aura but had not experienced any migraine headaches for the last 12 years. Her physical examination was normal with the exception of elevated blood pressure of 178/96 mm Hg. Her neurologic examination was also normal, with no bruits or tender or indurated temporal blood vessels.

What is the differential diagnosis?

There is a long list of diagnostic possibilities that should be considered in an older patient with the subacute onset of a new type of headache. This patient has a history of migraine but her current headache has few migrainous features. It would be unusual for severe migraine to recur abruptly at this age.

Some sort of vascular problem is at the top of the list of differential diagnoses in this case. While sudden, severe elevations in blood pressure can provoke headache, this patient's modest degree of hypertension is an unlikely explanation for her headache. Could this be a cerebral hemorrhage or infarct? This patient is alert and has no focal neurologic deficits, making this possibility less likely. Giant cell arteritis is a possibility, but this patient does not have additional systemic signs or symptoms suggestive of that disorder. A mass lesion of some sort or a slowly expanding subdural hematoma is also a possibility, but again there are no focal symptoms to support these diagnoses. An inflammatory process also seems unlikely.

What laboratory or other investigation should this patient have?

A careful workup to exclude the dangerous diagnoses discussed above is appropriate in this situation. The patient in this case underwent a full battery of blood tests, including an ESR and CRP. A computed tomographic scan of the head with and without contrast showed no abnormalities, and a lumbar puncture showed clear fluid with a normal pressure. The patient was diagnosed with recurrent migraine. She was given a prescription for acetaminophen with codeine and advised to see her primary care physician in a few days if the symptoms did not improve.

The pain continued over the next day and was only partially relieved by acetaminophen with codeine. On the afternoon of the second day, the patient began to experience itching as well as pain and noticed the development of a vesicular rash over her left forehead. She saw her primary care physician who diagnosed herpes zoster (shingles).

How should this patient's herpes zoster be treated?

Soothing topical lotions and analgesics are appropriate symptomatic treatments for the rash of herpes zoster. Eye involvement occurs in 10–25% of patients with zoster, when zoster affects the ophthalmic division of the trigeminal nerve. This patient should be referred for ophthalmologic evaluation since zoster affecting the eye can pose a threat to vision. Ophthalmologists may prescribe antiviral eye drops, or ointments may be helpful.

Because the pain of zoster can be intense, many patients require the use of opioid analgesics. Most doctors also treat patients with systemic antiviral agents such as acyclovir or famciclovir. These may reduce the duration of the attack and speed healing, but the drugs are likely to be most effective when started as soon as possible after symptoms begin, so time is of the essence.

Timely use of antiviral agents may decrease the chance that patients will develop persistent postherpetic pain, and additional treatment with corticosteroids may help some patient subgroups. Many doctors thus use both antiviral agents and steroids to treat herpes zoster. Postherpetic neuralgia occurs in 10–18% of patients with zoster, and is frustrating to treat. The usual treatment is amitriptyline, but results are often disappointing and anticholinergic side effects may limit its use in elderly patients. Carbamazepine and gabapentin are also used.

Discussion

Herpes zoster results from spontaneous reactivation of the varicella zoster (chickenpox) virus, which remains latent in the sensory ganglia after the initial chickenpox infection. It is a common viral infection, with an incidence of about 4 per 1000 people per year. The elderly and immunocompromised individuals are at highest risk. Zoster is easy to diagnose when the characteristic vesicular rash is present but, as illustrated by this case, pain may precede the appearance of the rash by several days. In those patients, the severe localized pain can easily be mistaken for other illnesses such as migraine.

A zoster vaccine has recently become available and is recommended for use in those over the age of 60. It is intended to prevent zoster, and is not a treatment for existing cases of shingles or postherpetic neuralgia. One clinical trial suggested that vaccination of 1000 patients of age 60 or older would prevent one case of postherpetic neuralgia over the subsequent three years. Unfortunately, vaccination is least effective in patients who need it most: the very elderly and those who are immunocompromised. Nonetheless, we strongly recommend to all of our patients over the age of 60 that they consider vaccination. There is no evidence that pre-existing headache disorders such as migraine increase the risk of developing zoster or its complications, but we think it is worth minimizing the chance that patients with an existing headache disorder will also have to cope with postherpetic neuralgia.

Diagnosis

Herpes zoster.

Tip

The diagnosis of herpes zoster is easily missed in patients who present with pain and no rash. The possibility of herpes zoster infection should be considered in elderly or immunocompromised patients with the subacute onset of severe unilateral head pain.

A 27-year-old woman with weakness and headache

Case

A 27-year-old woman presented to the headache clinic for a new patient visit after moving to the area for work. She had developed migraines at the age of six but was otherwise healthy. Headaches had varied in frequency over the years and were now occurring two or three times a month. The headaches were typical of migraine and a previous brain MRI had been normal.

The patient reported that all of her headaches were preceded by right-sided numbness and weakness. She could tell when a headache was likely because she began to drop things and experienced some difficulty walking. The patient had multiple family members with migraine, but no one else had experienced preceding symptoms like hers. These symptoms typically lasted about an hour and cleared as the headache began.

Her previous neurologist had diagnosed hemiplegic migraine and told her that she should stop using sumatriptan, which she had taken since she was 18 and which had worked well for her severe headaches. Instead, he prescribed a butalbital-containing combination analgesic but the patient reported it was not very effective.

Her new neurologist asked the patient to call for an urgent appointment the next time she experienced an episode of weakness. On examination during such an episode, the patient had dense numbness of the right hand, arm, foot, and calf. Her motor strength, however, was 5/5 throughout. Because of this, her diagnosis was revised to that of migraine with typical sensory aura rather than hemiplegic migraine. She resumed the use of sumatriptan, which was again effective.

What were the diagnostic possibilities based on the history?

This patient had a long history of headaches that met criteria for migraine and responded well to migraine-specific therapy with triptans. She also experienced stereotyped focal neurologic deficits prior to her headache episodes that from her description sounded like transient right hemiparesis. The list of diagnostic possibilities in this case includes migraine with aura; familial or sporadic hemiplegic migraine; a seizure disorder; vascular disorders such as arteritis or transient ischemic attacks; mitochondrial myopathy, encephalopathy, lactic acidosis, and stroke-like symptoms (MELAS); and cerebral autosomal dominant arteriopathy with subcortical infarcts and leukoencephalopathy (CADASIL).

Many of these diagnoses can be immediately excluded based on the patient's history. She had no cognitive impairment or complex motor behavior associated with her episodes, so a seizure disorder was unlikely. MELAS or CADASIL were likewise improbable based on a normal brain MRI that showed no evidence of prior infarcts or other abnormalities. Likewise, vascular disorders are an unlikely explanation for headaches in a healthy young woman who has experienced no permanent problems despite multiple similar attacks over two decades.

About a third of patients with migraine experience focal neurologic deficits before a headache. Typical aura symptoms can include visual, sensory, or speech phenomena. Patients who experience true motor weakness in association with migraine are classified separately as having hemiplegic migraine. This is usually an inherited autosomal dominant disorder and a number of single-gene mutations have been identified that are associated with hemiplegic migraine. Non-familial cases also occur and are attributed to spontaneous mutations. The patient's history is suggestive of transient hemiplegia in association with headaches, so the differential diagnosis in this case is between migraine with typical aura and hemiplegic migraine.

What historical and physical examination findings were at odds with the diagnosis of hemiplegic migraine?

It can be challenging to discriminate between typical migraine aura and hemiplegic migraine. These disorders share many features of migraine including severe headache and neurologic accompaniments to those headaches. One common pitfall is accepting at face value a patient's report of motor weakness. Patients can have difficulty distinguishing between sensory and motor symptoms. Numbness can make it difficult to grasp or hold objects, and the resulting clumsiness may be interpreted as due to weakness. In this case, the patient's new physician correctly recognized that it was important to examine the patient during an episode to assess for objective signs of true motor weakness.

Other features of this patient's presentation were not wholly compatible with a diagnosis of hemiplegic migraine. She did have a family history of migraine, but no one else in the family had similar neurologic accompaniments to headache. This makes a history of hemiplegic migraine less likely since in most cases there is a strong family history compatible with autosomal dominant transmission of the disorder. Speech disturbances are also common in hemiplegic migraine, but this patient had no speech component to her aura. Additionally, this patient's aura symptoms preceded her headache and faded as the headache began. Most patients with hemiplegic migraine experience aura symptoms throughout the headache and occasionally beyond.

How does the management of migraine with typical aura differ from that of hemiplegic migraine?

Vasoconstrictive medications such as triptans that are routinely used for the treatment of patients with migraine without aura and migraine with typical aura are contraindicated in patients who have familial hemiplegic migraine. This contraindication is based on fears that triptans or ergots might be more likely to cause vasoconstrictive complications in patients who have complex forms of aura such as hemiplegic migraine. There is no firm scientific foundation for these worries, but formal package labeling contraindicates the use of these agents. Because of this, most physicians are understandably reluctant to allow their use in patients who carry a diagnosis of hemiplegic migraine.

Most patients with hemiplegic migraine have relatively infrequent attacks. Depending upon the subtype, these are sometimes triggered by head injury, emotional stress, or hormonal fluctuations. In most cases of hemiplegic migraine the neurologic deficits are reversible, but there are cases in which neurologic deficits have progressed over time or become permanent. Because attacks are usually infrequent, most patients do not require preventive medications. There is a clinical impression, but no firm evidence, that calcium channel antagonists or acetazolamide may be more desirable preventive agents for hemiplegic migraine than for migraine with typical aura. Many physicians believe it is prudent to avoid beta-blockers in patients with hemiplegic migraine.

Discussion

Hemiplegic migraine is a diagnosis of exclusion that can have serious implications for patients. In this case the patient was prevented from using highly effective treatment for her migraine based on a mistaken diagnosis of hemiplegic migraine. This could have been avoided if the physician who made the diagnosis had made efforts to verify the patient's report of weakness.

Diagnosis

Migraine with typical (sensory) aura.

Tip

Patients can easily confuse numbness and weakness. Patient reports of motor weakness in association with headache should be verified by examination during an episode.

Further reading

Typical aura with headache

Hansen JM, Lipton, RB, Dodick, DW, *et al.* Migraine headache is present in the aura phase: a prospective study. *Neurology.* 2012;79:2044–9.

Russell MB, Olesen J. A nosographic analysis of the migraine aura in a general population. *Brain.* 1996;119:355–61.

Transformed migraine

Scher AI, Stewart WF, Buse D, Krantz DS, Lipton RB. Major life changes before and after the onset of chronic daily headache: a population-based study. *Cephalalgia.* 2008;28(8):868–76.

Scher AI, Stewart WF, Ricci JA, Lipton RB. Factors associated with the onset and remission of chronic daily headache in a population-based study. *Pain.* 2003;106(1–2):81–9.

Headache and maltreatment

Nelson HD, Bougatsos C, Blazina I. Screening women for intimate partner violence: a systematic review to update the U.S. Preventive Services Task Force recommendation. *Ann Intern Med.* 2012;156(11): 796–808, W-279, W-280, W-281, W-282.

Norman RE, Byambaa M, De R, *et al.* The long-term health consequences of child physical abuse, emotional abuse, and neglect: a systematic review and meta-analysis. *PLoS Med.* 2012;9(11):e1001349.

Tietjen GE, Brandes JL, Peterlin BL, *et al.* Childhood maltreatment and migraine. *Headache.* 2010;50(1): 20–51.

Tietjen GE, Khubchandani J, Herial NA, Shah K. Adverse childhood experiences are associated with migraine and vascular biomarkers. *Headache.* 2012;52:920–9.

Teitjen GE, Peterlin BL. Childhood abuse and migraine: epidemiology, sex differences, and potential mechanisms. *Headache.* 2011;51:869–9.

HaNDL

Bartleson JD, Swanson JW, Whisnant JP. A migrainous syndrome with cerebrospinal fluid pleocytosis. *Neurology.* 1981;31:1257–62.

Berg MJ, Williams JS. The transient syndrome of headache with neurologic deficits and CSF lymphocytosis. *Neurology.* 1995;45:1648–54.

Krause T, Nolte CH. The syndrome of transient headache and neurological deficits with cerebrospinal fluid lymphocytosis (HaNDL) as an acute ischemic stroke mimic leading to systemic thrombolysis: a case report. *Clin Neurol Neurosurg.* 2012;114(6):689–90.

Nakashima K. Syndrome of transient headache and neurological deficits with cerebrospinal fluid lymphocytosis: HaNDL. *Intern Med.* 2005;44(7):690–1.

Low CSF pressure headache

Mokri B. Spontaneous low cerebrospinal pressure/volume headaches. *Curr Neurol Neurosci Rep.* 2004;4(2):117–24.

Tseng YL, Chang YY, Lan MY, Wu HS, Liu JS. Spontaneous intracranial hypotension in a patient with reversible pachymeningeal enhancement and brain descent. *Chang Gung Med J.* 2003;26(4):293–8.

Carotid artery dissection

Kennedy F, Lanfranconi S, Hicks C, *et al.*; CADISS Investigators. Antiplatelets vs anticoagulation for dissection: CADISS nonrandomized arm and meta-analysis. *Neurology.* 2012;79(7):686–9.

Parwar BL, Fawzi AA, Arnold AC, Schwartz SD. Horner's syndrome and dissection of the internal carotid artery after chiropractic manipulation of the neck. *Am J Ophthalmol.* 2001;131(4):523–4.

Patel RR, Adam R, Maldjian C, *et al.* Cervical carotid artery dissection: current review of diagnosis and treatment. *Cardiol Rev.* 2012;20(3):145–52.

Herpes zoster

Harpaz R, Ortega-Sanchez IR, Seward JF; Advisory Committee on Immunization Practices (ACIP) Centers for Disease Control and Prevention (CDC). Prevention of herpes zoster: recommendations of the Advisory Committee on Immunization Practices (ACIP). *MMWR Recomm Rep*. 2008;57(RR-5):1–30.

Sanford M, Keating GM. Zoster vaccine (Zostavax): a review of its use in preventing herpes zoster and postherpetic neuralgia in older adults. *Drugs Aging*. 2010;27(2):159–76.

Hemiplegic migraine

Lafrenière RG, Rouleau GA. Identification of novel genes involved in migraine. *Headache*. 2012;52:107–10.

Russell MB, Ducros A. Sporadic and familial hemiplegic migraine: pathophysiological mechanisms, clinical characteristics, diagnosis, and management. *Lancet Neurol*. 2011;10(5):457–70.

Errors in management of acute headache

Nearly every patient who experiences headache will use some form of therapy to treat his or her acute headaches. Also known as abortive or symptomatic therapies, these treatments are intended to relieve the pain of headache, as well as accompanying symptoms such as nausea. Acute therapies can range from non-pharmacologic treatments such as topical ice or heat, to nonspecific over-the-counter and prescription analgesics, to treatments specific to the headache type. Triptan therapy for treatment of migraine falls into this last category.

In addition to the particular pitfalls illustrated by the cases in this chapter, a few general principles should be kept in mind. Treatments for acute episodes of headache are generally more effective when taken early in the headache, before central sensitization develops. One study showed that triptans were less effective once cutaneous allodynia (a marker for central sensitization) had developed. Unfortunately, many patients wait until a full-blown headache has developed before taking a triptan, so education about the importance of treating early can by itself improve response rates.

When a single treatment for headache is not effective, a combination of treatments may be more effective. For example, some patients respond well to a combination of triptans and nonsteroidal anti-inflammatory drugs (NSAIDs) but not to either medication given alone. Likewise, patients who develop nausea early in the course of their migraines will likely have a better response to oral triptan therapy if they are also treated with an antiemetic. The phenothiazine antiemetics (such as promethazine and prochlorperazine) probably have some intrinsic anti-migraine effects as a result of their anti-dopaminergic effects.

Lastly, it is worth mentioning the debate about whether stepped or stratified care is a better approach to treatment of acute headaches. In stepped care,

patients treat headaches first with a nonspecific agent such as an NSAID, and then go on to a specific therapy (usually a triptan) only if the NSAID is not effective. In stratified care, patients use nonspecific agents as first-line therapy for less severe and specific therapies as first line for more severe headaches; in other words, the treatment is tailored to the patient's individual circumstances. A randomized trial comparing stepped care with stratified care in the treatment of acute migraine showed that stratified care was more effective and associated with higher patient satisfaction. For this reason, we strongly recommend that patients with troublesome migraine should be treated with stratified care approaches rather than required to fail therapies that are usually ineffective before being allowed to use highly effective therapy.

A migraineur who does not respond to triptan treatment

Case

A 30-year-old woman was referred for consultation because of recurrent headaches for several years. She was in good health and her neurologic examination was normal. Her headaches met diagnostic criteria for migraine without aura and occurred on average twice a month. She had successfully treated headaches with 550 mg of naproxen sodium until two years ago when she underwent gastric bypass surgery for obesity. Post-operatively, the surgeon told her that she should not use naproxen or other nonsteroidal anti-inflammatory drugs. To replace naproxen she was given a prescription for 1 mg naratriptan tablets. These were not effective, so her physician prescribed 2.5 mg of zolmitriptan, which also did not help.

Eventually the patient was given a prescription for oxycodone. This partially relieved her headache pain but produced nausea and made it impossible for her to function at her job as a nurse. The patient tried several migraine preventive drugs that were not tolerable or effective. She does not want to take medicine every day for something that happens only twice a month.

Why should NSAIDs be avoided after bariatric surgery?

Gastric ulceration is a well-known side effect of NSAIDs. Bariatric surgery does not necessarily increase the risk of gastric ulceration. Rather, ulcerations that do occur can be more difficult to detect after bariatric surgery and may produce more serious complications. Thus most bariatric surgeons recommend that patients avoid this class of drugs following surgery.

The most common type of gastric bypass surgery in the United States is the Roux-en-Y gastric bypass, which sections off a portion of the stomach into a small pouch to limit food intake. The small intestine is repositioned and connected to the pouch at the top of the stomach, where its narrow opening slows stomach emptying. After this procedure the stomach cannot easily be visualized with gastroscopy, making it difficult to detect ulcers if they are suspected. Nonsteroidal anti-inflammatory drugs also may increase the risk of anastomotic leakage. Finally, because the active portion of the stomach is very small, any ulceration that does occur covers a larger proportion of the total surface of the stomach.

A common misconception among patients and some physicians is that avoiding oral ingestion of non-steroidal anti-inflammatory medications will circumvent this problem. Nonsteroidal anti-inflammatory drugs can be administered intranasally, parenterally, or as rectal suppositories, but these formulations do not reduce the risk of stomach ulceration. The risk of gastric ulceration is related to systemic inhibition of prostaglandins and not to direct irritation of the gastric mucosa, so non-oral administration of NSAIDs does not reduce the risk.

What are the possible explanations for this patient's failure to respond to triptans?

Triptans are very effective but do not work for everyone. One possibility is that this patient is truly refractory to triptans. On the other hand, it is possible that she has been treated with subtherapeutic doses or for-

mulations of triptans or that treatment has not been properly timed. In our experience, these are the most common explanations for an apparent lack of response to triptan treatment.

Clinical trials suggest that the maximum response rate to triptans is approximately 70%, although in clinical practice they seem to be slightly less effective, with response in about 60% of treated attacks. The likelihood of a good response to a triptan seems to depend on the dose and formulation of the drug, and the timing of treatment. A recent meta-analysis of sumatriptan trials showed the 100 mg dose was effective for a larger percentage of patients than the 50 mg dose, which in turn was more effective than the 25 mg dose. This dose–response relationship has been demonstrated for other triptans. The patient in this vignette was treated with the lowest commercially available doses of naratriptan and zolmitriptan. It is possible that higher doses of these drugs (e.g. 2.5 mg of naratriptan or 5 mg of zolmitriptan) would have been effective.

Most patients prefer oral migraine treatments but parenteral drugs have higher bioavailability. The therapeutic gain for subcutaneous sumatriptan, for example, is higher than for any of the oral triptans. Intranasal formulations of sumatriptan and zolmitriptan are available, but these are not more effective than oral triptans. Only a small amount of these intranasal triptans is absorbed through the nasal mucosa; rather, most of the liquid drips down the back of the throat, is swallowed, and absorbed through the gastrointestinal tract in the same way as orally administered drugs. Likewise, the orally disintegrating formulations of rizatriptan and zolmitriptan are not well absorbed sublingually but dissolve and are swallowed. The patient in this case was treated with oral triptans, and it is possible that parenteral sumatriptan would have been more effective.

Finally, the timing of drug administration may spell the difference between successful triptan treatment of a migraine attack and apparent drug failure. Some research suggests that triptan treatment is less likely to be effective when delayed until headache intensity is severe or the attack is well established. This lack of benefit may be due to the development of central sensitization. We do not know at what point in her headaches this patient treated her attacks, but it is possible that early treatment when the headaches were mild would have been more effective.

Table 7.1. Selected strategies for optimizing triptan treatment of acute headache

Use adequate doses
Try a different triptan
Try combination therapy
– Triptans with NSAIDs
– Triptans with antiemetics
Treat early
Use alternative formulations (nasal spray, injection, orally dissolving tablet)

Discussion

Most patients with migraine or cluster headache respond to a triptan if the right dose and formulation are used. Treatment is most effective when adequate doses of the drug are used early in a headache. Thus, our position is that "no patient has failed a triptan until they have failed a full dose of an injectable triptan given early in a headache." In practice, this means a 6 mg dose of subcutaneous sumatriptan administered as soon as the headache begins. In our experience, the subcutaneous formulation of sumatriptan is remarkably underused and is often effective in patients who have apparently "failed" triptan therapy. It is administered using an auto-injector that can hold cartridges of 6 or 4 mg of sumatriptan. The dose can be repeated at any point after two hours if needed. The maximum daily dose is 12 mg, which translates to two 6 mg or three 4 mg injections in a 24-hour period.

If triptans alone are not effective, or are only partially effective, we commonly recommend that patients use them in combination with an NSAID. (Obviously, however, that is not an option for the patient in the vignette.) Naproxen sodium is available in a fixed-dose tablet formulation with sumatriptan, but this combination pill is expensive. Unless patients prefer the convenience of a single tablet, we prefer to provide this combination of treatments using separate pills. This also allows for customization of the dose of both triptan and the NSAID. For patients who have prominent nausea, we may even add a third anti-nausea drug to this regimen, such as 10 mg of metoclopramide or a promethazine rectal suppository, a regimen we refer to as "triple therapy." Strategies for improving treatment results of acute headache using triptans are summarized in Table 7.1. Many of these are generalizable to other forms of treatment for acute migraine as well.

Diagnosis

Migraine without aura.

Tip

It is a mistake to conclude that patients do not respond to triptans without ensuring that they have used an adequate dose and formulation early in a headache.

A young woman with chest pressure from sumatriptan

Case

A 19-year-old woman with episodic migraine without aura was seen in the emergency department (ED) with a headache and nausea. The headache was similar to her previous attacks but had not responded to her usual treatment of 1000 mg of aspirin and 10 mg of metoclopramide. Her neurologic examination was normal. She had no other major medical problems or illnesses and was taking no regular medications. She was given a subcutaneous injection of 6 mg of sumatriptan. Her headache disappeared and nausea improved, but she experienced chest pressure and neck tightness lasting 15 minutes. She had no associated symptoms. She had an electrocardiogram that was normal and was referred for outpatient cardiovascular evaluation.

Were the electrocardiogram and cardiovascular investigation indicated?

No. This young patient at low risk of cardiovascular disease experienced short-lived chest pressure in close temporal relation to an injection of sumatriptan. Nonserious side effects such as flushing, paresthesias, and transient neck or chest tightness are well-recognized triptan side effects. They occur often enough that they are referred to as "triptan sensations." They usually begin within a few minutes to half an hour of drug administration and can last up to an hour, although in our experience they are typically of relatively short duration. For unclear reasons, triptan sensations seem to be most common in younger women such as the patient in the vignette.

Triptan sensations may frighten patients and doctors because of their similarity to more serious cardiac symptoms. Although cardiovascular events, some serious, have been reported with triptan use, they are not common. Most have occurred in patients with many risk factors for coronary artery disease. Research suggests that the clinically used doses of triptans do

Table 7.2. Triptan characteristics.

Generic name	Brand name	Formulations	Dosing	Comments
Almotriptan	Axert	Tablet	12.5 mg	
Eletriptan	Relpax	Tablet	20/40 mg	
Frovatriptan	Frova	Tablet	2.5 mg	Longest half-life
Naratriptan	Amerge	Tablet	1/2.5 mg	Second longest half-life
Rizatriptan	Maxalt	Tablet Orally disintegrating tablet	5/10 mg 5/10 mg	Decrease dose when used with propranolol
Sumatriptan	Imitrex	Tablet Nasal spray Subcutaneous injection	25/50/100 mg 5/20 mg 4/6 mg	Also available in a fixed-dose combination tablet containing sumatriptan and naproxen
Zolmitriptan	Zomig	Tablet Nasal spray Orally disintegrating tablet	2.5/5 mg 5 mg 2.5/5 mg	

not cause coronary artery constriction sufficient to provoke myocardial ischemia. Furthermore, studies of patients who have chest or neck pain with triptan administration have not shown electrocardiographic or other evidence of reductions in myocardial perfusion. Based on this evidence, we do not believe that cardiovascular evaluation is warranted in young patients like the one in this vignette who have transient triptan sensations.

Should this patient be advised to avoid triptans?

There is no safety reason for this patient to avoid the use of triptans in the future. Sumatriptan was effective for a severe headache that had not responded to nonsteroidal anti-inflammatory treatment. She is likely to have similar bad headaches in the future. It is important not to foreclose the use of an effective treatment unnecessarily. We find that many of our patients believe the benefits of sumatriptan outweigh short-lived side effects such as chest pain, especially once they are reassured these side effects are not serious. Furthermore, most patients who are prone to triptan sensations do not experience them every time they take a triptan, and those who do often come to view them as a sign that "the drug is working."

Triptan sensations may be more common in patients who receive parenteral rather than oral triptans, so one strategy for this patient might be to use an oral formulation of sumatriptan. In one study about half of patients treated with subcutaneous sumatriptan reported such side effects compared with roughly a quarter who were treated with the oral drug. If the problem recurred with the use of oral sumatriptan, and was troubling to the patient, it would still be worthwhile to try a different oral triptan. Although triptan sensations can occur with any triptan, for individual patients the adverse effect profile of the different triptans may vary.

Since there are relatively few classes of drugs that can be used to treat individual migraine attacks, it is important to maximize the chances of success when a triptan is first prescribed. We find it useful to warn patients about the possibility of transient triptan sensations *before* they try the drug for the first time. This reduces the likelihood that they will be frightened if such symptoms occur and then refuse to use the drug again – thus foreclosing use of a highly effective treatment option. For patients who are very anxious about the possibility of triptan side effects, we sometimes suggest that they try the drug for the first time when they do *not* have a headache. This allows them to experience the effects of the drug without the added anxiety produced by a bad headache, and makes it possible to separate the side effects of the drug, if any, from the symptoms of a headache.

Discussion

Triptans have been in widespread clinical use since their introduction in the early 1990s, and have a good record of safety and tolerability. Table 7.2 lists the characteristics of the seven triptans that are available in the United States. All are US Food and Drug Administration (FDA) approved for treatment of acute migraine and sumatriptan injections are FDA approved for treatment of acute cluster headache. Triptans are appropriate treatment for patients whose attacks do not reliably respond to simple analgesics, which was the case for this patient. They provide good relief of pain and headache-related symptoms such as nausea.

For most patients, triptans have a more favorable side effect profile than other choices for treatment of acute migraine. Unlike opioids and barbiturate-containing medications, triptans do not generally produce sedation or cognitive impairment, nor are they associated with the development of abuse and dependence syndromes. Unlike NSAIDs, triptans do not impose a risk of gastrointestinal bleeding. Overuse of triptans may produce medication overuse headache, but evidence suggests that it is simpler to treat medication overuse headache that results from triptans than that resulting from overuse of opioids or barbiturates.

These are important long-term considerations. Unlike minor, transient side effects such as triptan sensations, these more serious adverse events must be taken into account when deciding what treatment to use for individual migraine attacks. Although treatment for individual headaches is used intermittently, migraine is a chronic condition for which such treatment will be used repeatedly over many years. Thus, adverse effects that are inconsequential when treatment is used for a single attack can be very important with long-term regular use. Conversely, side effects such as triptan sensations which are more unpleasant within the context of an individual headache may nonetheless not be as important in the larger perspective of treatment decisions.

Diagnosis

Migraine without aura and transient "triptan sensations" with sumatriptan.

Tip

Transient triptan sensations such as chest pressure, paresthesias, or flushing are common, nonserious side effects of triptans. When they occur in patients at low risk for cardiovascular disease they do not warrant cardiac investigation or require avoidance of triptans.

Worries about serotonin syndrome

Case

A 45-year-old female presented for evaluation of headache that had begun when she was in her late teens. Attacks were frequently related to her menstrual cycle. During each of two pregnancies, she had been free of headache. Since her second delivery, however, she had noted headaches with every menstrual period that were moderate to severe in intensity, lasted for two days each, and limited her activities. Each headache began with a prodrome of cervical muscle spasm after which she developed unilateral throbbing frontal and retro-orbital pain, increasing with physical activity and associated with photo and phonophobia and rare nausea. NSAIDs and oral sumatriptan were of incomplete benefit. She had previously been advised to try sumatriptan by injection but was reluctant since she recalled being told that it was contraindicated because she was also taking a low dose of sertraline. Her primary care physician had prescribed the sertraline for situational depression after a recent divorce.

The headache specialist told the patient that in his opinion the risk of using a triptan in combination with a selective serotonin reuptake inhibitor (SSRI) was low. He recommended early use of the sumatriptan injection in the hopes of reducing her typical level of disabling symptoms. The pharmacist, however, refused to fill the prescription without contacting the physician, citing the potential for a severe interaction between the sumatriptan and the sertraline. The patient was told that this was a "class one interaction." The patient, convinced that her prior worries had been warranted and now suspicious of the medical advice she had received, left the pharmacy without the prescription and cancelled her return visit to the headache clinic.

Were the physician's treatment recommendations appropriate?

A 2006 FDA warning advised caution in the use of triptans with other serotonergic drugs because of worries about serotonin syndrome. Experts have called the evidence used as the basis for this warning into question. For one thing, the concomitant use of SSRIs and triptans is very common, yet an epidemic of serotonin syndrome has not emerged. One study suggested that as many as 65 million patients in a one-year period in the United States were using an SSRI along with a triptan with no documented cases of serotonin syndrome identified among them. An American Headache Society Position Paper published in 2010 stated that "The currently available evidence does not support limiting the use of triptans with SSRIs or selective serotonin–norepinephrine reuptake inhibitors (SNRIs), or the use of triptan monotherapy, due to concerns for serotonin syndrome (Level U). However, given the seriousness of serotonin syndrome, caution is certainly warranted and clinicians should be vigilant to serotonin toxicity symptoms and signs to insure prompt treatment."

Many physicians and patients believe that menstrual migraine is often more severe and resistant to treatment than migraines occurring at other times of the month. Early and aggressive management can therefore be appropriate and necessary. In patients who do not respond to oral therapy, such as this one, treatment can include recommendations for an injectable triptan. As in this case, the goal is to reduce disability and improve the ability to function during this monthly event.

Is there anything that the provider could have done differently to avoid the patient leaving care?

Possibly. The provider could have warned the patient to expect advice of an interaction from the pharmacy and discussed the basis of his advice with her. The pharmacist, if concerned, could have discussed the matter with the physician to understand more fully the reasons for use of the agents before approaching the patient; a more balanced discussion may have resulted.

Discussion

Many headache specialists, feeling confident about the low risk of serotonin syndrome with concomitant use of SSRIs/SNRIs and triptans, and with limited time to spend with patients, may omit discussion of this matter. However, patients who search for information about these drugs online will encounter multiple sites which describe a "major interaction" that is "rare but serious and potentially fatal" and typically warn that concomitant use should be avoided.

Decision support software embedded in many electronic medical records will often show a warning when such agents are prescribed together, and presumably pharmacy software also produces similar warnings. Accumulated evidence is quite compelling, however, that the risk of serotonin syndrome with concomitant use of triptans and selective serotonin reuptake inhibitors is very low. Even after years of experience with triptans, however, pharmacists continue to contact our office frequently to discuss the possibility of serotonin syndrome. Unfortunately, as in the case

Table 7.3. Selected symptoms of serotonin syndrome

Tachycardia
Hypertension
Hyperthermia
Clonus (inducible or spontaneous)
Ocular clonus (slow horizontal eye movements)
Tremor
Hyperreflexia
Agitation or restlessness
Hypertonicity (muscle rigidity)
Autonomic signs: diaphoresis, dilated pupils, flushing, increased bowel activity

above, these "stops" can lead to disruption of care for the patient and contribute to distrust of the medical establishment.

The serotonin syndrome results from enhanced serotonergic activity in the brain usually as the result of use of medications which can increase serotonergic activity, either alone or in combination. This results in a constellation of symptoms and signs listed in Table 7.3 that include restlessness, confusion, autonomic instability, muscular irritability, tremor or myoclonus, and even coma.

Diagnosis

Menstrually related migraine.

Tip

Good quality evidence suggests that the risk of serotonin syndrome is low when triptans are prescribed in combination with other serotonergic drugs. It is prudent to discuss the balance of benefits and harms with patients prior to prescribing this combination of treatments, however, in order to avoid misunderstandings later.

A patient with sulfa allergy and migraine

Case

A young woman with episodic, infrequent migraine with aura not controlled with over-the-counter medications presented asking for better treatment of her individual attacks of headache. She was given a prescription for sumatriptan to manage her occasional

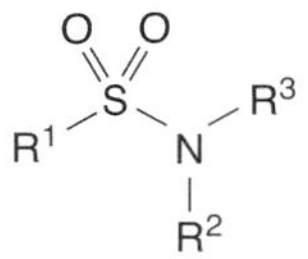

Figure 7.1 A sulfonamide group.

attacks, and appropriate use and side effects of the drug were discussed. The next day, the pharmacy called the office to notify the provider that the patient had a documented allergy to sulfa. Because the sumatriptan molecule contains a sulfa group (depicted in Figure 7.1), the pharmacist wanted to know if the patient should be switched to a different triptan.

Should the patient be switched to a different medication?

Of the seven commercially available triptans, naratriptan, eletriptan, and almotriptan all contain sulfonamide groups. These sulfa moieties are folded within the molecule and are not exposed, however. They do not appear to produce cross-reactivity in patients who are allergic to sulfonamide antibacterial drugs. The package insert for sumatriptan notes that hypersensitivity reactions to sumatriptan are rare but may be more likely in patients with hypersensitivity to multiple medications. In our experience, most patients with a history of sulfa allergy can use sulfonamide-containing non-antibacterial medications without risk and it would be reasonable to advise the patient in this case to fill her prescription. If her previous sulfa reaction was anaphylactic in nature, however, we would err on the side of caution and consider prescription of a triptan such as rizatriptan which does not contain a sulfa moiety. Otherwise, the patient could be advised not to be alone the first time she takes the medication.

Discussion

A number of studies have examined the question of cross-reactivity in patients who are allergic to sulfonamide-containing antibiotics, to which allergy is relatively common (3%), and other medications that contain sulfa moieties. The mechanism of the allergy to the antibacterial drugs is not completely understood and all types of hypersensitivity reaction have been described. Many studies, however, have failed to show clear cross-reactivity with other sulfonamide-containing medications and suggest that structural differences between the sulfonamide-containing antibi-

otics and non-antibiotics may explain the lack of association.

More technically, the sulphonamide-containing antibiotics are sulfonylarylamines, in which the sulfonamide moiety is attached to a benzene ring, and have an amine at the N4 position. The triptans are simple sulfonamides, in which the sulfonamide moiety is not connected to a ring structure. Incidentally the intermediate group, which includes carbonic anhydrase inhibitors, has the sulfonamide moiety attached to the ring structure but without the N4 amine.

It does appear that patients allergic to sulfonamide antibiotics may in general have a greater risk of allergy to other medications, thus creating a general increased risk of hypersensitivity but not a specific risk in relation to the sulfonamide derivatives. Given the described structural differences, and the lack of clinical reports of cross-reactivity between sulfa antibiotics and triptans, the risk of sumatriptan use in a patient with sulfa allergy is likely to be low.

In this case, the patient was reassured and went on to use sumatriptan without incident.

Diagnosis

Episodic migraine; sulfa allergy.

Tip

Although sumatriptan contains a sulfa moiety, it is not attached to a benzene ring. Cross-sensitivity in patients allergic to sulfonamide antibiotics is thus not likely to occur.

Adverse effects associated with regular long-term NSAID use

Case

A 45-year-old woman presented with headaches that had begun when she was in graduate school and which had gradually increased in frequency. They were now present more days than not. They were bifrontal, vise-like in quality, moderate in severity, and associated with low-grade phonophobia but not photophobia or nausea. The headaches were not worse with exercise and there was no aura. These headaches generally responded well to ibuprofen 400–800 mg, depending on severity, and she had been taking ibuprofen at least four days per week for as long as she could remember, sometimes requiring multiple doses a day. She had previously been diagnosed with tension-type headache and advised to continue ibuprofen, which she was told was the best treatment for tension-type headache. A friend of hers recently experienced liver damage as a result of excessive use of acetaminophen. This had caused her to wonder about whether it was safe to continue taking ibuprofen.

How would you advise this patient, and is any further evaluation indicated?

This patient has been taking NSAIDs for many years, and is therefore at risk for some of the health consequences of chronic NSAID use. Gastritis is the most common adverse effect associated with NSAIDs, and all patients taking NSAIDs should be queried about symptoms of heartburn or other signs of gastro-esophogeal reflux disease. Patients who are on chronic NSAIDs should probably also have renal function checked periodically. Lastly, NSAID use may increase the risk of cardiovascular events in patients with heart disease, and risk factors for heart disease should be evaluated periodically.

Upon further questioning, this patient reported progressively worsening heartburn over the last several years. She did not connect it with ibuprofen use as she had been using ibuprofen for many years and the heartburn had only developed recently. She had not been to a doctor in many years because she was healthy aside from her headaches, and she had not had lab work in the last five years. A creatinine level was obtained at her presenting visit and was 1.4 mg/dL.

What treatment options are available for this patient's headaches, and what could have been done to prevent her kidney problems?

This patient has experienced two possible complications of chronic NSAID use, namely gastritis and mild chronic renal failure. Because of these adverse events, she should be advised to discontinue the use of NSAIDs. In addition to these adverse events, the possibility that her chronic headaches are due to medication overuse should also be considered. If that is the case, her headaches may ultimately improve once she has discontinued the daily use of analgesic medications (although they may worsen temporarily as a result of drug withdrawal). If headaches do not improve fol-

lowing NSAID withdrawal, the patient would benefit from preventive therapy to reduce the frequency of headaches and the need for treatment of individual headaches.

Ideally, this patient's chronic headaches would have been recognized as a problem many years ago, and she might have been offered preventive therapy for them, perhaps when she initially presented to her physician's office and had been diagnosed with chronic tension-type headaches. Although NSAIDs are first-line therapy for treatment of many acute headache disorders, they are less appropriate in patients who have chronic headaches. Their use should be carefully monitored in patients with frequent headaches because daily or near-daily use can lead to medication overuse headaches and other complications. If patients are maintained on long-term NSAID treatment, regular monitoring for development of gastric or renal side effects is usually in order.

Discussion

NSAIDs are commonly used to treat many types of headache. Ibuprofen and naproxen are often used for tension-type headache or migraine, while indomethacin is a first-line therapy for the relatively uncommon syndromes of hemicrania continua, paroxysmal hemicranias, and exertional headaches. NSAIDs are also one of the most common over-the-counter treatments for headaches, particularly among patients with milder headache or those who have not sought medical treatment. Despite their nonprescription status, NSAIDs are associated with substantial risks, particularly when used long term or frequently. Important risks include gastrointestinal events, including gastritis, peptic ulcer disease, and gastrointestinal bleeding, and an increased risk of cardiovascular events. These two risks are listed in a black box warning on the prescription form of ibuprofen, and both of these risks may increase with prolonged duration of use. Indomethacin seems particularly prone to produce gastroduodenal toxicity.

Another potential adverse effect from long-term NSAID use is renal papillary necrosis, which can lead to renal failure. It is suspected that this is related to prostaglandin inhibition by NSAIDs; prostaglandins are responsible for pre-renal vasodilation and thus help maintain renal blood flow. Patients with pre-existing renal insufficiency, the elderly, and those taking diuretics or angiotensin-converting enzyme (ACE) inhibitors seem to be at the highest risk of renal complications with NSAIDs. Many patients return to baseline renal function after discontinuation of NSAIDs, but this may be more likely if the renal dysfunction is discovered early. In this case, it appeared that the patient's renal function had been compromised for some time, because her creatinine remained elevated despite discontinuation of NSAIDs.

Diagnosis

NSAID-induced gastritis and mild chronic renal failure; chronic tension-type headache.

Tip

Chronic use of NSAIDs can be associated with gastritis, renal failure, and cardiovascular events. Risks increase with duration of use and appropriate monitoring for safety is necessary.

Agitation after intravenous treatment for acute headache

Case

A 37-year-old woman with migraine was brought to the ED by her boyfriend. She had been suffering from a typical migraine headache that had begun the previous morning. It had not responded to several doses of her usual treatment of 6 mg subcutaneous sumatriptan and oral metoclopramide. For prevention of migraines, she also took venlafaxine 75 mg daily, topiramate 50 mg twice daily and lisinopril 10 mg daily. She had no neurologic findings on examination and further testing was not felt necessary. An intravenous line was placed and she was hydrated with normal saline and given 30 mg of intravenous ketorolac and 10 mg of intravenous prochlorperazine.

About an hour after receiving this treatment, the patient became restless and agitated. When asked how she was feeling she reported that she felt "terrible…I just can't explain it. I feel so bad and I can't lie still." Assuming that the patient was restless because of pain, an additional dose of 5 mg of intravenous prochlorperazine was administered. Ten minutes later the patient experienced a prolonged tightening of her right sternocleidomastoid muscle. Her chin was drawn down towards the right shoulder and she developed slurred speech. This slowly resolved but was followed

within 15 minutes by a similar episode involving the right side.

Given the clinical description provided, what is the likely cause of this patient's symptoms? Was the additional prochlorperazine a good idea?

This patient's agitation and uncontrolled muscular movements were typical of extra-pyramidal side effects that can occur with neuroleptic medications. Two types of extra-pyramidal side effects are relevant to migraine treatment: neuroleptic-induced acute dystonia results in abnormal muscle contractions with spasm or twisting of the head and abnormal movements of the trunk or limbs. Episodes of dystonia usually last 20–30 minutes and often produce pain. One well-described form of dystonia is the oculogyric crisis, in which the eyes deviate together to one side. Neuroleptic-induced akathisia is characterized by severe motor restlessness and agitation. This can be more difficult to recognize than dystonia. Patients may pace the room or rock from side to side if in bed. Dystonia and akathisia may occur separately or together; typically dystonic symptoms precede those of akathisia, although that was not so in this case.

The correct diagnosis of extra-pyramidal side effects in patients receiving neuroleptics for the treatment of migraine is a challenge. The differential diagnosis also includes neuroleptic malignant syndrome, serotonin syndrome, tricyclic antidepressant overdose, or cocaine intoxication, so a careful review of all possibilities is in order. An important management pitfall is that the agitation and discomfort associated with extra-pyramidal symptoms are easily mistaken for anxiety or for residual pain, as occurred in the case presented. Patients may then be given additional neuroleptic medication in the mistaken belief that pain is the problem. In hindsight, the additional 5 mg of prochlorperazine was a mistake.

How should this patient's symptoms be treated? Can neuroleptic-induced extra-pyramidal symptoms be prevented?

The traditional approach to treating neuroleptic-induced extra-pyramidal symptoms involves discontinuation of the offending neuroleptic drug. In addition, anticholinergic agents such as diphenhydramine or benztropine, or benzodiazepines, are often administered in the belief that they will cause more rapid resolution of symptoms. Anticholinergic agents are believed to work because extra-pyramidal reactions involve an imbalance between central dopaminergic and cholinergic systems. The acute blockade of dopaminergic systems by the neuroleptic drug is theorized to result in an excess of cholinergic activity. The dose of diphenhydramine is typically in the range of 0.5–1.0 mg/kg and for benztropine it is 0.010–0.015 mg/kg, both administered intramuscularly.

Good quality evidence suggests that anticholinergic medications are effective in treating neuroleptic-induced dystonia. Evidence is conflicting, however, about whether diphenhydramine or benzodiazepines should be used to treat akathisia. In our view, both drugs probably work but the evidence is stronger and more consistent for benzodiazepines. A study comparing diphenhydramine and midazolam for the treatment of acute akathisia due to metoclopramide found that midazolam was more effective than diphenhydramine, although sedation was a prominent side effect. A recent Cochrane Collaboration review also supports the view that benzodiazepines are effective for treatment of acute akathisia.

Given the discomfort associated with neuroleptic-induced extra-pyramidal side effects, it is reasonable to wonder whether these symptoms can be prevented. A randomized double-blind controlled trial compared midazolam 1.5 mg IV, diphenhydramine 20 mg IV, or placebo on the occurrence of akathisia related to metoclopramide used for the ED treatment of nausea or headache. Midazolam was effective in preventing akathisia but diphenhydramine was no more effective than placebo. Thus, benzodiazepines appear to be superior to diphenhydramine for both acute treatment and prevention of neuroleptic-induced extra-pyramidal symptoms. Another study suggested that a slower infusion rate of metoclopramide (15 minutes versus 2 minutes) lowered the incidence of akathisia without reducing the effectiveness of the drug for nausea.

Discussion

Neuroleptic medications such as prochlorperazine, metoclopramide, and chlorpromazine successfully relieve pain and nausea associated with acute attacks of migraine. They are the drugs of choice for severe headaches that have not responded to specific anti-

migraine therapy or where such therapy is contraindicated. Intravenous treatment with prochlorperazine 10 mg or metoclopramide 20 mg, given with diphenhydramine 25 mg, is more effective than placebo for acute migraine, and three-quarters of patients receiving these treatments say they would want them for their next headache. In fact, one study suggested that the combination of prochlorperazine and diphenhydramine was more effective than sumatriptan for migraine in the emergency setting.

Neuroleptic-induced extra-pyramidal symptoms are, however, important potential side effects that must be kept in mind when using these drugs. These effects are more common with prolonged administration but can also complicate short-term therapy. In fact, they can appear within minutes of treatment initiation. Their reported prevalence varies, but a reasonable estimate is that they may occur in about 20% of individuals who receive intravenous neuroleptic medications for migraine treatment.

Diagnosis may be difficult because of the variety of symptoms that can occur and their similarity to symptoms displayed with anxiety or pain. Extra-pyramidal symptoms are severely distressing for patients. Patients who have experienced inadequately treated dystonia or akathisia commonly refuse to use these drugs in the future, with the result that an important therapeutic option is lost.

Diagnosis

Neuroleptic-induced dystonia and akathisia.

Tip

Neuroleptic medications are useful for severe headaches, but clinicians should be careful not to misinterpret the extra-pyramidal side effects of dystonia or akathisia as being due to anxiety or pain and mistakenly treat the patient with additional neuroleptics.

A woman with intractable headache and vomiting

Case

While on call, a physician received a message to contact a patient. This 36-year-old woman had a long history of occasional migraine headaches that usually responded well to 10 mg of oral rizatriptan. The previous day she had developed a typical headache, but she was getting over a bout of norovirus and could not keep rizatriptan down. Her headache had lasted almost two days and she wanted to know if she should go to the ED.

When should someone with a bad headache go to the emergency department?

Even patients with a well-established history of primary headaches such as migraine can have other causes of headache. An ED visit is appropriate when there are "red flag" signs or symptoms that suggest a dangerous cause of headache. These include a headache that is unusually severe or sudden in onset – the so-called "thunderclap" headache – or headaches associated with fever or confusion. In this case, the patient reported that her headache was a typical one for her – what was unusual was that nausea prevented her from taking her usual oral medication. When questioned further she denied high fever, confusion, or any other alarm symptoms. She preferred to avoid a trip to the ED if possible. She was there several years ago under similar circumstances and ended up having a CT scan of her head and a lumbar puncture, complicated by a severe post-lumbar puncture headache that did not resolve until she had a blood patch.

What strategy might be helpful in treating this headache, and prevent similar situations in the future?

Migraine is a chronic illness. Even patients whose headaches typically respond to oral treatment are likely to have occasional headaches that do not. Sometimes the headache begins while they are sleeping and has progressed to the point of vomiting when they awaken. Perhaps treatment has been delayed if a headache developed when they were without medication. Or perhaps, as in this case, circumstances made it impossible to use customary treatment. Whatever the reason, a number of useful backup or "rescue" treatments may still be effective even when a patient's first-line treatment has failed. Often these will prevent the need for an ED visit.

As a general rule, rescue treatments should be non-oral. Non-oral treatments take effect quickly and will still be effective in patients who are vomiting. Table 7.4 lists common rescue treatments. They

Table 7.4. Commonly used rescue therapies

Triptans:
- Sumatriptan SC 4–6 mg

NSAIDs:
- Indomethacin 50 mg PO or PR (PR may be more effective)
- Ketorolac nasal spray/PO 15–30 mg

Sedating phenothiazines:
- Promethazine 25 mg PO
- Prochlorperazine 5–10 mg PO or 25 mg PR (PR may be more effective)

Ergot derivatives:
- Dihydroergotamine nasal spray 0.5 mg, 1 spray each nostril q15 min ×2

Steroids:
- Prednisone, dexamethaxone, or methylprednisolone

Used with caution due to concern of overuse or addiction syndromes:
- Butalbital-containing medications
- Narcotics

PO, by mouth; PR, per rectum; SC, subcutaneous

include injectable medications such as sumatriptan, which comes in an auto-injector that can be self-administered, nasal sprays, and rectal suppositories. In the latter category, we find promethazine suppositories to be particularly useful. They will usually stop vomiting and put a patient to sleep until a headache runs its course.

Discussion

Poorly controlled pain is an acceptable reason to go to the ED, but many patients with headache dislike seeking ED care. They report feeling labeled as "drug seekers" by medical staff, and dislike the long waiting times. Most also dread the fluorescent lights and loud, busy environment of the ED. Then, too, there is the danger of excessive diagnostic testing or investigation as ED staff seek to "rule out" dangerous causes of headache such as subarachnoid hemorrhage. Finally, patients who visit the ED with a bad headache are at risk of receiving nonspecific treatments such as narcotics, which may create expectations of future narcotic treatment that are difficult to reverse. In our experience, it is difficult to predict with certainty when or whether patients with well-controlled migraine might need to visit the ED for an out-of-control headache. We find it prudent to provide a backup "plan B" rescue treatment for every patient, even those who think they might not need it. Our advice is to "fill the prescription and keep it in your medicine cabinet. You may never need it, but if you do you will be glad it is there."

Diagnosis

Migraine in the setting of recent gastrointestinal illness.

Tip

Most headache patients benefit from having a "rescue" plan for backup treatment when their first-line strategies fail. In most cases this backup treatment should be non-oral so that it will be effective even if the patient is vomiting.

A never-ending migraine

Case

A 29-year-old woman presented to the ED with a severe headache. This was her second visit to the ED in four days for the same problem. She had a long history of intermittent migraine without aura that usually responded well to oral almotriptan. A week prior to this visit she had developed a typical headache, but her usual treatment was not effective, perhaps because she was vomiting and could not keep the medicine down. After three days of severe headache and persistent vomiting, she presented to the ED.

Her neurologic examination was normal, and a CT scan of the head and lumbar puncture were also normal. She was treated with subcutaneous sumatriptan and intravenous hydration, and the headache resolved. She returned home, but the headache and vomiting recurred. The headache was bilateral, throbbing, associated with phono and photophobia, and worse with movement. She rated her pain 10 on a 0–10 scale. Her neurologic examination was normal.

What is this patient's diagnosis and how should it be treated?

Migraine episodes that continue for at least three days are termed *status migrainosus*. Temporary improvement with medication or interruption during sleep is disregarded in determining the duration of an attack. Status migrainosus is considered a complication of migraine. Recurrence of migraine depends on many things, including the patient's age, sex, the initial severity of the headache, and the choice and timing of treat-

Table 7.5. Selected treatments for status migrainosus

Drug and dose	Comments
Dihydroergotamine (DHE) 0.5–1 mg IV as a single dose/ 1 mg IV q8 hours ×3 days: this is often referred to as the "DHE protocol" or "Raskinizing" a patient (since Dr. Neil Raskin first devised this protocol)	Pretreatment with an antiemetic such as metoclopramide is advisable. Patients may need to be admitted or treated in an outpatient infusion center in order to receive the full DHE protocol
Droperidol 2.5 mg IV every 30 minutes until three doses or patient is completely or almost headache-free	Patients should be warned of possible side effects of sedation and akathisia. Use is limited because of the potential for prolongation of the QT interval
Metoclopramide 10 mg IV	Monitor for dystonic reactions
Prochlorperazine 5–10 mg IV	Monitor for hypotension, sedation, and dystonic reactions

ments. In status migrainosus, the ongoing episodes are typical of a patient's previous migraine attacks, differing only in duration. Sometimes, as in this case, an attack may be long-lasting because vomiting interferes with the ability to treat the headache, but even patients who use parenteral therapies will sometimes have particularly stubborn attacks of migraine.

There are no large studies of treatments for status migrainosus. Status migrainosus is usually treated with parenteral medication in order to maximize bioavailability of the drug. Intravenous hydration is also helpful to counteract the volume depletion that may arise after several days of poor appetite or vomiting. Drugs with longer durations of action are preferred to treat this long-lasting form of migraine. (Of note, the patient in this vignette received subcutaneous sumatriptan, which has a half-life of only a few hours.) Table 7.5 lists some treatment regimens commonly recommended for the treatment of status migrainosus in the acute setting. Dihydroergotamine (DHE) is especially useful and the "DHE protocol" of repetitive parenteral administration of DHE-45 is an especially valuable strategy. Droperidol has also been employed with substantial clinical success, but its use is limited by the potential for prolongation of the QT interval.

How could migraine recurrence and return to the ED have been prevented?

About half of patients who receive ED treatment for migraine will experience headache recurrence within the next few days. Some, as the patient in this vignette, will return to the ED because of relapse. Several meta-analyses have evaluated clinical trials studying the use of steroids, mostly dexamethasone, as a treatment that will reduce headache recurrence. The way in which steroids might reduce the risk of headache recurrence is not clear, but may relate to suppression of neurogenic inflammation. There appear to be few adverse events associated with single doses of dexamethasone.

Discussion

Even patients whose migraines are well controlled will occasionally have headaches that do not respond well to treatment and which last beyond 72 hours. A single dose of dexamethasone is well tolerated and is moderately effective in preventing migraine relapse. One meta-analysis estimated a number needed to treat of 9. Because steroids take some time to become effective, they are not usually used as stand-alone treatment in the ED. In fact, there is little evidence to suggest that steroids are an effective symptomatic treatment. Rather, they are used in addition to standard abortive therapy for the attack.

Steroids are typically given intravenously under these circumstances, although one study suggested that oral treatment might also be effective. Doses in clinical trials have ranged from 10 to 24 mg IV, but higher doses ($\geq$ 15 mg of dexamethasone) appear to be most effective. For this reason, and because there are few adverse events associated with a one-time dose of dexamethasone, we recommend that a dose of at least 15 mg should be used. The importance of dose is underscored by a recent study that used just 10 mg of IV dexamethasone to treat status migrainosus in the ED, and did not find an effect compared with placebo.

Diagnosis

Status migrainosus.

Tip

The addition of a high dose ($\geq$ 15 mg IV) of dexamethasone to customary ED migraine treatment prevents headache recurrence with a number needed to treat of 9.

A man with cluster headache and limited sumatriptan access

Case

A 36-year-old man was referred for consultation because of headaches that awoke him from sleep nearly every night. The headaches were located behind the right eye and were described as sharp and stabbing. They lasted about an hour and were rated 10 on a 0–10 pain scale. With the pain, he had mild nausea and a stuffy nose on the side of the headache. The headaches occurred daily for the last month. He had a similar bout of headaches last fall that resolved after three months. His primary care physician diagnosed cluster headache, gave him a prescription for the sumatriptan auto-injector (4 mg), and arranged for him to have oxygen to use at home. The patient reported that sumatriptan was effective for the headaches but his insurance would only pay for only four boxes (eight doses) a month. He could not afford to pay for it out of pocket. He had tried the oxygen but said that it "doesn't do much and those nasal prongs hurt my nose."

The patient had not been started on preventive treatment to reduce the number of attacks he was experiencing. Since he had a history of bipolar disorder with previous episodes of mania requiring hospitalization, steroids were avoided but treatment with 240 mg of sustained release verapamil daily was started.

Was this patient receiving optimal treatment for individual attacks of headache?

Subcutaneous sumatriptan is approved by the FDA for treatment of cluster headache attacks. It can be self-administered with a reusable auto-injector. Individual cartridges containing the medication are inserted into the auto-injector and discarded after use. When the drug was first introduced the auto-injector cartridges were only available in a 6 mg "one size fits all" dose. Since the daily dose limit for sumatriptan is 12 mg a day, that meant patients could use just two injections in a 24-hour period. For patients with cluster headache, who can have more than two attacks in a 24-hour period, two injections a day are sometimes not sufficient to treat all headaches. Additionally, the 6 mg dose produced unpleasant side effects in some patients.

For these reasons, cartridges that contain only 4 mg of the drug have been introduced. This lower dose of subcutaneous sumatriptan is useful in a number of clinical settings, although some patients still need the full 6 mg dose. In this patient's case, however, the 4 mg dose reportedly worked well, so his sumatriptan treatment does appear to be optimized. It should be noted that parenteral sumatriptan can also be administered using a "needle-less" system that propels the drug through the skin using a blast of air. This system can only deliver a 6 mg dose, however, and in our experience is more expensive than the original auto-injector.

The patient's description of "nasal prongs" when asked about his oxygen treatment, however, suggested that oxygen is not being used correctly. Incorrect oxygen administration – too low a flow rate, use of nasal prongs instead of a face mask, or both – is probably the cause of apparent lack of benefit in this patient's case. When administered by face mask at a high rate of flow, oxygen therapy is highly effective for treatment of individual attacks of cluster headache. This patient should be encouraged to repeat a trial of 100% oxygen at 12 liters/minute administered via face mask for 15 minutes at the onset of headaches.

How does oxygen work to abort an attack of cluster headache?

The way in which oxygen works to stop an attack of cluster headache is not known. A number of theories have been advanced, including the possibility that oxygen inhibits firing of trigeminal afferent neurons, affects the parasympathetic pathway, or decreases cerebral blood flow through vasoconstrictive mechanisms. Some experts have postulated that there is a hypersensitivity to oxygen in cluster headache.

Discussion

The first clear description of cluster headache was provided by the English physician Wilfred Harris. He accurately described many features of the disorder, including the characteristic Horner's syndrome. The first systematic study of oxygen for cluster headache was done by Dr. Lee Kudrow, himself a cluster headache sufferer. He was reportedly prompted to investigate oxygen because of an account of its benefits by an optometrist with cluster headache who used it to abort his own attacks. Kudrow's study compared self-administered 100% oxygen (administered

Table 7.6. Selected studies of oxygen for treatment of individual attacks of cluster headache

Citation	Flow rate and method of administration	Results
Kudrow L. Response of cluster headache attacks to oxygen inhalation. *Headache.* 1981;21:1–4.	6 liters/minute via face mask for 15 minutes	Oxygen aborted more than 7/10 attacks in 82% of patients
Anthony M. Treatment of attacks of cluster headache with oxygen inhalation. *Clin Exp Neurol.* 1981;18:195.	8 liters/minute via face mask for 15 minutes	100% oxygen was effective in relieving pain in all 12 patients studied
Fogan L. Treatment of cluster headache. A double-blind comparison of oxygen v. air inhalation. *Arch Neurol.* 1985;42:362–3.	6 liters/minute via face mask for 15 minutes	56% of patients had relief of headache in over 80% of attacks
Cohen AS, Burns B, Goadsby PJ. High-flow oxygen for treatment of cluster headache. *JAMA.* 2009;302:2451–7.	12 liters/minute via face mask for 15 minutes	78% of patients had complete or substantial pain relief at 15 minutes

using a mask at a flow rate of 7 liters/minute for 15 minutes) with sublingual ergotamine. Oxygen aborted more than seven out of ten attacks in 82% of the patients. Ergotamine worked in 70% of patients but the response time for oxygen was faster, on average 6 minutes. Two small subsequent studies also reported good results using flow rates of 6 and 8 liters/minute. A larger, carefully done study used 100% oxygen at a rate of 12 liters/minute for 15 minutes. At 15 minutes after treatment 78% of patients were pain-free or had substantial pain relief, compared with only 20% who received high flow air placebo. These studies are summarized in Table 7.6. To summarize, high flow 100% oxygen administered at 12 liters/minute for 15 minutes at onset of an attack with a nonrebreather face mask should be prescribed.

Diagnosis

Episodic cluster headache.

Tip

Oxygen is an effective, evidence-based therapy for acute attacks of cluster headache, but high flow administration through a nonrebreather mask is important to avoid treatment failure.

A woman with migraine planning to attempt pregnancy

Case

A 30-year-old woman with a history of episodic migraine with aura presented for a routine follow-up visit to the headache clinic. At that visit, she told the physician that she was having headaches about three times a month and sumatriptan was reliably effective within an hour or so. She sometimes took metoclopramide for nausea. She was planning to try to conceive in the next six months, but wanted to know what options for treatment would be available. Her migraines were debilitating before she was started on sumatriptan, and she was concerned about missing work if she was unable to take the drug when she had headaches.

What options are available for treating her migraines during pregnancy?

Management of headache during pregnancy ideally starts even before pregnancy is attempted, when non-pharmacologic techniques such as biofeedback can be started. Lifestyle modifications such as regular meals, adequate hydration, regular sleep, and stress management can also be very helpful in decreasing the frequency of headache. If pharmacologic treatment is required, acetaminophen is first-line symptomatic therapy and several antiemetics are commonly used in pregnancy. Metoclopramide and ondansetron have an FDA safety in pregnancy rating of B (more on FDA ratings below). If these treatments are ineffective, other commonly used options include butalbital-containing medications and opiates, though these are both FDA Category C. Steroids such as prednisone or dexamethasone can also be used. Occipital nerve blocks are a low-risk procedural intervention. Conservative treatments are usually initiated first, and treatments with greater risk are added only if necessary.

Can she take sumatriptan?

Although controlled trials have not been performed, the limited available information regarding safety of sumatriptan in pregnancy is reassuring. In the population-based Norwegian Mother and Child Cohort Study, 1535 women had taken triptans during pregnancy. There was no significant association

Table 7.7. FDA use-in-pregnancy safety categories

Category A: Controlled human studies show no risk

Category B: No evidence of risk in humans but there are no controlled human studies

Category C: Risk to humans has not been ruled out

Category D: Positive evidence of risk in humans

Category X: Contraindicated in pregnancy

between triptan use in the first trimester and major congenital malformations or other adverse pregnancy outcomes. Triptan use in the second or third trimester was associated with a slightly increased risk of atonic uterus and blood loss during labor. A registry for sumatriptan and naratriptan sponsored by the manufacturer included 599 women, most of whom had taken sumatriptan. Although this was a small sample size, the number of birth defects in this group was comparable to that in the general population. Because of these studies, some headache specialists feel comfortable prescribing sumatriptan to patients whose headaches are not controlled by the therapies discussed above. While this clinical scenario arises rarely in our practice, we do keep this on the list of options for pregnant patients with otherwise intractable headaches.

Discussion

The FDA categorizes safety of medications during pregnancy into Categories A, B, C, D, and X (Table 7.7). Category A indicates the best evidence of safety, and is limited to drugs for which there are controlled human studies showing no risk. Category X indicates that a medication is contraindicated in pregnancy due to a clear risk of serious harm to the fetus. There are alternative systems for evaluating the safety of the medication during pregnancy, including the TERIS risk rating and narrative reports from proprietary databases such as REPROTox. The frequent disagreement and inconsistencies among these systems illustrates how difficult it can be to make determinations based on the limited data available.

Table 7.8 lists the FDA use-in-pregnancy ratings for commonly used symptomatic treatments of migraine in pregnancy. Acetaminophen is perhaps the most commonly used due to its B rating, but all of the antiemetics also have a long track record of safety. In fact, all of the antiemetics except ondansetron have received a TERIS rating indicating that after

Table 7.8. FDA use-in-pregnancy ratings of commonly used symptomatic therapies for migraine

Analgesics	
Acetaminophen	B
Aspirin and NSAIDs	C (D in the third trimester)
Butalbital	C
Caffeine	C
Codeine	C
Hydrocodone/acetaminophen (APAP)	C
Meperidine	C
Oxycodone	C
All triptans	C
Antiemetics	
Metoclopramide	B
Ondansetron	B
Promethazine	C
Prochlorperazine	C
Chlorpromazine	C

exposure during gestation, teratogenic risk is unlikely on the basis of evidence rated at least fair to good. As described above, there is so far no evidence suggesting teratogenicity associated with the use of sumatriptan. Ergots should be avoided because they decrease uterine blood flow. NSAIDs are also typically avoided during the first trimester, due to increased risk of spontaneous abortion, and third trimetester, due to risk of premature closure of the ductus arteriosus and renal abnormalities.

Despite the availability of symptomatic medications generally regarded as safe during pregnancy, nonpharmacologic therapy is the mainstay of acute headache treatment during pregnancy. Thermal biofeedback, relaxation training, and physical therapy are all effective. It may be helpful to start training in these therapies prior to attempting pregnancy, so that they are available when needed particularly during the first trimester. In addition, the importance of hydration should not be underestimated. Sometimes, IV fluids and resting in a dark quiet room are all that is needed to help a pregnant migraineur feel significantly better.

In developing a treatment plan, physicians should realize that the use of pharmacologic therapy to manage migraines during pregnancy is best based on balancing the harms and benefits for an individual patient. The FDA package inserts for most medications state that use of the medication in pregnancy is not recommended unless "benefit outweighs risk." Medications are not tested on pregnant women during clinical trials, so clear data about medication safety during

pregnancy are often lacking and rely on postmarketing registries or observational data. In patients whose migraines are severe, lead to frequent protracted vomiting and dehydration, or cause significant emotional distress, the benefits of using pharmacologic therapy may be felt to outweigh the potential risks. This conversation should be documented in the chart.

The natural history of migraine during pregnancy is discussed in greater detail in Chapter 8. Although migraine typically improves during pregnancy, it does not always do so and often does not improve until after the first trimester. For this reason, all patients planning to attempt pregnancy should have a treatment plan for any headaches that do occur.

Diagnosis

Episodic migraine without aura, planned pregnancy.

Tip

Many migraine treatments are contraindicated in pregnancy, but several medications with a long track record of safety are available. Patients should be reassured that treatments are available if headaches persist past the first trimester.

Treatment of headache during lactation

Case

The patient in the previous case had her baby and returned for follow-up. Her migraines had improved during the second half of the pregnancy, but they had recurred postpartum. She was having them about three days a week, and they seemed to be the same headaches that she had before she was pregnant. She thought the increased frequency might be related to disrupted sleep and the stress of returning to work. For treatment of acute headaches she was still using acetaminophen, which she had taken during during pregnancy, but this was not consistently effective.

How is medication safety during lactation determined?

The American Academy of Pediatrics (AAP) Committee on Drugs has provided a non-exhaustive list of medications, grouped into the following categories: usually compatible with breast-feeding; effects are unknown but may be of concern; require temporary cessation of breast-feeding; associated with significant effects on some infants and should be given with caution; contraindicated. This list was last updated in 2001. Another commonly used resource is Hale's *Medications and Mothers' Milk*, which is updated every two years. These ratings are based on large-scale clinical observations or controlled trials. Safety is rated L1–L5, with L1 indicating the safest drugs and L5 indicating those which are contraindicated during lactation.

What medications can be recommended to treat this patient's headaches while she is breast-feeding?

Good options for symptomatic therapy during lactation include acetaminophen, NSAIDs, and sumatriptan. Eletriptan is not listed in the AAP rating system, but has a Hale rating of L2. Steroids, including dexamethasone and prednisone, are usually compatible with breast-feeding. None of the antiemetics have been rated using the AAP rubric. Importantly, aspirin and ergots should be avoided.

In this case, the patient was started on propranolol for preventative therapy and had reduction of headaches to once per week. Minor headaches were treated with ibuprofen and the more severe headaches occurring about twice per month were treated with sumatriptan. The excretion of maternally ingested drugs into breast milk is determined by a number of factors, including their lipophilicity. The amount of maternally ingested sumatriptan that is excreted into breast milk is negligible; that fact in conjunction with the short half-life of the drug means that it is a good choice for treatment of acute migraine in women who are breast-feeding. Some women choose to pump and discard breast milk for a period of time after ingesting medications, but that is not medically necessary when sumatriptan is used.

Discussion

The postpartum period is a time when many women with migraine experience increased headache frequency. In this case, the patient identified two common triggers for increased frequency of migraine: disrupted sleep and increased psychologic stress. There is conflicting information about the effect of lactation itself on migraine frequency, with one study suggesting that breast-feeding did not change the frequency

Table 7.9. Medication safety during lactation

Medications usually compatible with breast-feeding (Hale rating is in parentheses where available)	Medications associated with significant effects/give with caution during lactation	Medications for which safety during lactation is unknown/may be of concern
Propranolol (L2)	Aspirin	Amitriptyline (L2)
Magnesium	Atenolol	Nortriptyline
Riboflavin	Ergotamine	SSRIs
Valproate (L2)	Lithium	
Verapamil (L2)		
Steroids		
Acetaminophen		
Ibuprofen (L1)		
Ketorolac		
Indomethacin		
Naproxen (L3)		
Simple opioids		
Sumatriptan (L3)		

of headaches postpartum, and another study showing that breast-feeding had a protective effect. At the very least, it is safe to say that migraine is not a contraindication to breast-feeding.

Because the mechanism of transmission of a medication to the infant during lactation is different from the mechanism of transmission to a fetus during pregnancy, the medication safety ratings of drugs may differ depending upon whether they are used during pregnancy or during breast-feeding. Valproate, for example, has a class X safety rating during pregnancy (positive evidence of risk in human or animal studies) but is listed as "usually compatible" with breast-feeding in the AAP rating system and has a Hale's L2 rating.

Likewise, some medications perceived to be safe during pregnancy are contraindicated during lactation, although this is less common. One important example of this is nadolol, which is probably safe when used in pregnancy, but is lipophilic and thus concentrated in breast milk. Case reports exist of several infants who experienced heart block when breast-fed by a mother taking this drug.

Several factors determine medication safety during lactation, including the amount excreted into breast milk, the concentration of drug in the mother, and the amount of milk ingested by the infant. Table 7.9 lists a selection of medications often used during lactation, along with their safety ratings. In general, there are fewer contraindications to migraine treatments during breast-feeding then during pregnancy.

If women remain concerned about exposing an infant to a specific medication, there are strategies to reduce further the infant's potential exposure. For example, the mother can take the medication just after she has breast-fed her infant or just before the infant is likely to have an extended sleep period. If the mother is willing to express milk, she can pump and discard the breast milk after taking the medication in question, the so-called "pump and dump" method.

Diagnosis

Episodic migraine without aura in a breast-feeding woman.

Tip

The safety profile of the same drug may differ depending upon whether it is used when a woman is pregnant or when she is breast-feeding. A number of medications can be safely used to treat headaches when women are breast-feeding, so there is no need for a woman to avoid lactation in order to treat headaches.

Further reading

Optimizing triptan use

Burstein R, Collins B, Jakubowski M. Defeating migraine pain with triptans: a race against the development of cutaneous allodynia. *Ann Neurol.* 2004;55:19–26.

Dodick DW. Triptan nonresponder studies: implications for clinical practice. Headache. 2005;45:156–62.

Tfelt-Hansen P. Maximum effect of triptans in migraine? A comment. *Cephalalgia.* 2008;28:767–8.

Triptan sensations

Dodick D, Lipton RB, Martin V, *et al.* Consensus statement: cardiovascular safety profile of triptans (5-HT agonists) in the acute treatment of migraine. *Headache.* 2004; 44(5):414–25.

Papademetriou V. Cardiovascular risk assessment and triptans. *Headache.* 2004;44(Suppl 1):S31–9.

Visser WH, Jaspers NM, de Vriend RH, Ferrari MD. Chest symptoms after sumatriptan: a two-year clinical practice review in 735 consecutive migraine patients. *Cephalalgia.* 1996;16(8):554–9.

Triptans, SSRIs, and serotonin syndrome

Evans RW, Tepper SJ, Shapiro RE, Sun-Edelstein C, Tietjen GE. The FDA alert on serotonin syndrome with use of

triptans combined with selective serotonin reuptake inhibitors or selective serotonin-norepinephrine reuptake inhibitors: American Headache Society position paper. *Headache.* 2010;50(6):1089–99.

Shapiro RE, Tepper SJ. The serotonin syndrome, triptans, and the potential for drug-drug interactions. *Headache.* 2007;47(2):266–9.

Sulfa allergies and triptan use

Platt D, Griggs RC. Use of acetazolamide in sulfonamide-allergic patients with neurologic channelopathies. *Arch Neurol.* 2012;69(4):527–9.

Strom BL, Schinnar R, Apter AJ, *et al.* Absence of cross-reactivity between sulfonamide antibiotics and sulfonamide nonantibiotics. *N Engl J Med.* 2003;349(17): 1628–35.

NSAID side effects

García Rodríguez LA, Barreales Tolosa L. Risk of upper gastrointestinal complications among users of traditional NSAIDs and COXIBs in the general population. *Gastroenterology.* 2007;132(2):498–506.

Harirforoosh S, Jamali F. Renal adverse effects of nonsteroidal anti-inflammatory drugs. *Expert Opin Drug Saf.* 2009;8(6):669–81.

Jacobsen RB, Phillips BB. Reducing clinically significant gastrointestinal toxicity associated with nonsteroidal antiinflammatory drugs. *Ann Pharmacother.* 2004;38(9): 1469–81.

Extra-pyramidal side effects with neuroleptics

Erdur B, Tura P, Aydin B, *et al.* A trial of midazolam vs diphenhydramine in prophylaxis of metoclopramide-induced akathisia. *Am J Emerg Med.* 2012;30(1): 84–91.

Kelley NE, Tepper DE. Rescue therapy for acute migraine, part 2: neuroleptics, antihistamines, and others. *Headache.* 2012;52(2):292–306.

Lima AR, Soares-Weiser K, Bacaltchuk J, Barnes TR. Benzodiazepines for neuroleptic-induced acute akathisia. *Cochrane Database Syst Rev.* 2002;(1): CD001950.

Parlak I, Erdur B, Parlak M, *et al.* Midazolam vs. diphenhydramine for the treatment of metoclopramide-induced akathisia: a randomized controlled trial. *Acad Emerg Med.* 2007;14(8):715–21.

Tura P, Erdur B, Aydin B, Turkcuer I, Parlak I. Slow infusion metoclopramide does not affect the improvement rate of nausea while reducing akathisia and sedation incidence. *Emerg Med J.* 2012;29(2):108–12.

Rescue treatments for migraine

Kelley NE, Tepper DE. Rescue therapy for acute migraine, part 1: triptans, dihydroergotamine, and magnesium. *Headache*. 2012;52(1):114–28.

Kelley NE, Tepper DE. Rescue therapy for acute migraine, part 2: neuroleptics, antihistamines, and others. *Headache*. 2012;52(2):292–306.

Kelley NE, Tepper DE. Rescue therapy for acute migraine, part 3: opioids, NSAIDs, steroids, and post-discharge medications. *Headache*. 2012;52(3):467–82.

Whyte C, Tepper SJ, Evans RW. Expert opinion: Rescue me: rescue medication for migraine. *Headache*. 2010;50(2):307–13.

Treatment of status migrainosus

Colman I, Friedman BW, Brown MD, *et al*. Parenteral dexamethasone for acute severe migraine headache: meta-analysis of randomised controlled trials for preventing recurrence. *BMJ*. 2008;336(7657):1359–61.

Fisseler FW, Shih R, Szucs P, *et al*. Steroids for migraine headaches: a randomized double-blind two-armed, placebo-controlled trial. *J Emerg Med*. 2011;40(4):463–8.

Kelly AM, Kerr D, Clooney M. Impact of oral dexamethasone versus placebo after ED treatment of migraine with phenothiazines on the rate of recurrent headache: a randomised controlled trial. *Emerg Med J*. 2008;25(1):26–9.

Singh A, Alter HJ, Zaia B. Does the addition of dexamethasone to standard therapy for acute migraine headache decrease the incidence of recurrent headache

for patients treated in the emergency department? A meta-analysis and systematic review of the literature. *Acad Emerg Med*. 2008;15(12):1223–33.

Wang SJ, Silberstein SD, Young WB. Droperidol treatment of status migrainosus and refractory migraine. *Headache*. 1997;37(6):377–82.

Oxygen treatment for cluster headache

Haane DYP, Dirkx THT, Koehler PJ. The history of oxygen inhalation as a treatment for cluster headache. *Cephalalgia*. 2012;32(12):932–9.

Acute treatment of headache during pregnancy and lactation

American Academy of Pediatrics Committee on Drugs. Transfer of drugs and other chemicals into human milk. *Pediatrics*. 2001;108(3):776–89.

Cunnington M, Ephross S, Churchill P. The safety of sumatriptan and naratriptan in pregnancy: what have we learned? *Headache*. 2009;49(10):1414–22.

Loder E. Migraine in pregnancy. *Semin Neurol*. 2007; 27(5):425–33.

Lucas S. Medication use in the treatment of migraine during pregnancy and lactation. *Curr Pain Headache Rep*. 2009;13(5):392–8.

Nezvalová-Henriksen K, Spigset O, Nordeng H. Triptan exposure during pregnancy and the risk of major congenital malformations and adverse pregnancy outcomes: results from the Norwegian Mother and Child Cohort Study. *Headache*. 2010;50(4):563–75. Erratum in: *Headache*. 2012;52(8):1319–20.

Pitfalls in drug therapy to prevent headaches

Decisions about preventive treatment for chronic headache problems are focused on answering the questions of *when, which, how,* and *for how long.* That is, when should preventive treatment be considered, which drug should be used, how should it be given, and for how long should therapy be continued? There is no single best answer to each of these questions, but there are some principles that can help guide decisions. These are listed in Table 8.1. Cases in this chapter illustrate the pitfalls that can be encountered in trying to optimize preventive drug therapy in some commonly encountered and challenging situations.

The major primary headache disorders of migraine, tension-type headache, and cluster headache occur in both episodic and chronic varieties. At either end of the frequency spectrum decisions about whether to use preventive treatment are relatively simple, but when headache frequency is variable or intermediate it can be difficult to know whether to recommend preventive therapy.

Decisions about which drug to use are also complicated. As several cases in this chapter illustrate, the choice of a particular preventive treatment depends heavily upon individual patient circumstances and concomitant illnesses. A particularly thorny problem in clinical practice is how to approach patients who have "tried everything." Is it ever appropriate to conclude that preventive treatment is ineffective? Treatment guidelines issued by authoritative groups such as

the American Headache Society (AHS) and American Academy of Neurology (ANN) categorize preventive medications according to the quantity and strength of scientific evidence supporting their use, but applying this in an individual patient's case may not be simple.

A man with frequent headaches who does not want daily medicine

Case

A 36-year-old man had a long history of episodic migraine without aura. He had a good response to sumatriptan but his physician was worried that he was using it too frequently. Two months after a follow-up visit at which he had received a prescription for 18 100 mg sumatriptan tablets with five refills, the patient called to request more sumatriptan. He said he was about to go on vacation, had used all of his recent prescription plus refills, and did not want to be without it and risk a headache while abroad. The physician approved a one-time refill of nine tablets, but asked the patient to come in for an appointment when he returned from vacation.

At that visit the physician told the patient that sumatriptan had not been studied for long-term daily use and that frequent use could paradoxically make headaches worse and lead to medication overuse headache. He recommended that the patient consider taking a daily medication to cut down on the frequency of his headaches. The patient admitted that he was taking sumatriptan "at least" three or four days a week, but said that it was working well and he had no side effects from it. Furthermore, he often had three or four days each week without headache. He did not like the idea of taking medication every day to treat a problem that was not daily.

Table 8.1. When to consider migraine prevention

- Three or more headache episodes per week
- Significant interference of headache with daily activity
- Acute medications ineffective, contraindicated, or overused
- Adverse effects from acute medications
- Patient preference for prevention
- Associated comorbidities: e.g. depression, anxiety, hypertension, insomnia
- Special circumstances: elderly, pregnant, pediatric populations

Was the physician right to urge the use of preventive medication for migraine?

There are several reasons to believe that the physician in this case was right in urging this patient to consider preventive therapy. This patient's pattern of frequent headache and excessive use of symptomatic medication for headache was not a recent development. The physician had long been worried about how much medication the patient was taking. If anything, the patient was probably underestimating his headache frequency, since he used 90 tablets of sumatriptan over a 60-day period. In these circumstances most doctors would have suspected medication overuse and probably would have discussed preventive treatment with the patient earlier. In hindsight, this case also highlights the importance of keeping track of headache frequency and medication use through headache diaries, more frequent office visits, or even pill counts.

It seems safe to assume that the patient's true headache frequency corresponded to at least 6–14 headache days per month. Patients in this intermediate frequency category are at high risk of developing even more frequent headaches over time. In the Frequent Headache Epidemiology Study, such patients were followed for a year. The risk of developing chronic headaches over that period was strongly related to baseline headache frequency. The risk of chronic headache increased exponentially at around one headache per week.

Based on this evidence, we discuss the use of prophylactic treatment for headaches once a patient with migraine or tension-type headache begins regularly having one or more headaches a week. This does not mean that everyone who has one headache a week must be on preventive treatment. Rather, it means that the use of preventive treatment should be considered. If a patient's headache frequency or medication use seems to be inexorably trending upwards, this is a natural point at which to consider the institution of preventive therapy.

Is daily medication the only thing that might reduce the risk of chronic migraine for this patient?

The Frequent Headache Epidemiology Study identified a number of other risk factors for the development of chronic headache in addition to baseline

Table 8.2. Risk factors for the development of chronic headache

Risk factor	Comments
Female sex	Not modifiable
Baseline headache frequency	Potentially modifiable with preventive medication that reduces headache frequency. Evidence is lacking to show that this has a long-term favorable impact on the natural history of headache
Overuse of medications to treat acute headache	Modifiable
Obesity	Modifiable; preliminary observational evidence suggests possible benefit of weight loss on headache frequency in migraine
Stressful life events	Modifiable through changes in environment and training in stress reduction and coping techniques
Depression	Modifiable through drug or other treatments
Snoring	Modifiable if snoring is related to upper airway problems or produces sleep apnea
Excessive caffeine consumption	Modifiable

Based on information from Scher AI, Stewart WF, Ricci JA, Lipton RB. Factors associated with the onset and remission of chronic daily headache in a population-based study. *Pain.* 2003;106:81–9.

headache frequency. These are listed in Table 8.2. Although headache sufferers with these characteristics were more likely to develop chronic headache, it remains unclear whether the relationship is causal. In other words, it is not clear whether being obese or experiencing stressful life events caused headaches to become chronic or whether some underlying factor was associated with both events. Because of this it is uncertain whether addressing the factors that can be modified will alter the natural history of headache.

There are, however, other important medical reasons to address many of these risk factors, and emerging evidence indicates that at least some of them may be causally related to the development of chronic headache. For example, several small studies have shown improvement in headache frequency in patients with chronic migraine who have lost weight following bariatric surgery.

As outlined in Table 8.2, risk factor modification can include recommendations to lose weight, perform regular physical exercise, learn relaxation techniques, maintain normal body weight, use treatments to reduce headache frequency, and treat snoring or sleep apnea if present.

Discussion

Patients at the low end of the headache frequency spectrum have occasional headaches that are widely dispersed in time. They usually prefer and benefit from treatment directed to individual attacks of headache. Most are reluctant to consider taking medication every day to cope with a problem that is intermittent. This is understandable, since even the best preventive drugs for migraine do not prevent all attacks, and most are associated with unintended adverse events. These range from minor nuisances to potentially serious or permanent problems. The trade-offs – slightly fewer headache days a month in exchange for a daily side effect – may not seem worth it to patients.

In contrast, patients with high frequency headaches have daily or near-daily headache. In most cases, they should strongly consider the use of preventive headache treatment. Even if an analgesic or triptan treatment for individual attacks works well, those drugs are not intended to be used on a daily basis. Too-frequent use of medications intended to treat individual episodes of headache can produce serious side effects such as gastric ulceration with nonsteroidal anti-inflammatory drugs, or tolerance or addiction in the case of barbiturate- or opioid-containing medications. Additionally, most drugs used to treat individual attacks of headache are also suspected of producing medication overuse headache when used too often. Decisions about whether preventive treatment is warranted can be difficult to make when patients report an intermediate headache frequency. In such situations it is useful for patients to keep an objective record of headache frequency in the form of a headache diary. That helps both patients and doctors identify the point at which headache frequency is so consistently high that it no longer makes sense to treat headaches individually.

Diagnosis

High frequency episodic migraine.

Tip

Patients with an intermediate frequency of headache should be closely monitored for excessive medication use and an increase in the number of headaches. The option of preventive therapy should be discussed once headache frequency is approximately once a week.

Selecting preventive treatment for a patient who has never used it

Case

A 27-year-old woman had been followed for several years with a diagnosis of migraine with typical visual aura. She was otherwise healthy and on no medications. Although triptans were effective for her headaches, she did not tolerate them because of unpleasant "triptan sensations" and fatigue. Fortunately, her individual headache attacks usually responded well to a combination of 10 mg of metoclopramide and 1000 mg of aspirin.

At a recent visit, however, her diaries showed that her headache frequency had gradually increased over the last year from an average of three headaches a month to six or seven attacks. Some attacks lasted several days and she was missing work because of them. She had recently gone to the emergency department for a headache that lasted three days.

Her neurologic and physical examination was normal. She had tried to reduce headache triggers such as erratic sleep patterns, caffeine use, and stress but had not been able to decrease her headache frequency. Because her doctor warned her about medication overuse headache, she had been careful not to use her abortive migraine treatment more often than two days a week. Instead, she had "toughed things out" but noted that "maybe that's how I ended up in the ED."

What does this patient's clinical course suggest and what treatment would you recommend?

This patient had experienced a steady, gradual increase in headache frequency, severity, and duration. She was experiencing disability as a result of headaches and is worried about losing her job. She had six or seven attacks of migraine a month, some lasting several days at a time. Her headache frequency was thus close to the cutoff of 15 days a month used to

Table 8.3. Summary of the 2012 American Headache Society and American Academy of Neurology treatment guidelines for the preventive treatment of episodic migraine

Level A: Established as effective
Should be offered to patients requiring migraine prophylaxis

Drug	Dose examples	Common side effects or problems
Divalproex/sodium valproate*	500–1000 mg/day	Known cause of birth defects; weight gain, fatigue
Metoprolol	47.5–200 mg/day	Fatigue, hypotension
Petasites (Butterbur)	50–75 mg bid	Classified as a nutritional supplement and not subject to the same level of FDA oversight or scrutiny
Propranolol*	120–240 mg/day	Fatigue, hypotension
Timolol*	10–15 mg bid	Fatigue, hypotension
Topiramate*	25–200 mg/day	Paresthesias, cognitive impairment, acute angle-closure glaucoma, renal stones

Level B: Probably effective
Should be considered for patients requiring migraine prophylaxis

Drug	Dose examples	Common side effects or problems
Amitriptyline	25–150 mg/day	Fatigue, dry mouth, weight gain
Fenoprofen	200–600 mg tid	Gastrointestinal side effects, platelet inhibition
Feverfew	50–300 mg bid; 2.08–18.75 mg tid for MIG-99 preparation	Classified as a nutritional supplement and not subject to the same level of FDA oversight or scrutiny
Histamine	1–10 ng subcutaneously twice a week	
Ibuprofen	200 mg bid	Gastrointestinal side effects, platelet inhibition
Ketoprofen	50 mg tid	Gastrointestinal side effects, platelet inhibition
Magnesium	600 mg trimagnesium dicitrate qd	Diarrhea
Naproxen/naproxen sodium	500–1100 mg/day for naproxen; 550 mg bid for naproxen sodium	Gastrointestinal side effects
Riboflavin	400 mg/day	Classified as a nutritional supplement (vitamin) and not subject to the same level of FDA oversight or scrutiny
Venlafaxine	150 mg extended release/day	Agitation

Level C: Possibly effective
May be considered for patients requiring migraine prophylaxis

Drug	Dose examples	Common side effects or problems
Candesartan	16 mg/day	Hypotension
Carbamazepine	600 mg/day	Fatigue, cognitive impairment, allergic reaction
Clonidine	0.75–0.15 mg/day; patch formulations also studied	Hypotension
Lisinopril	10–20 mg/day	Nonproductive cough, hypotension
Nebivolol	5 mg/day	Fatigue, hypotension
Pindolol	10 mg/day	Fatigue, hypotension
Flurbiprofen	200 mg/day	Gastrointestinal side effects, platelet inhibition
Mefanamic acid	500 mg tid	Gastrointestinal side effects, platelet inhibition
Coenzyme Q10	100 mg tid	Classified as a nutritional supplement and not subject to the same level of FDA oversight or scrutiny
Cyproheptadine	4 mg/day	Fatigue, dry mouth, weight gain

* FDA approved for migraine prevention.

distinguish episodic from chronic migraine. This pattern of gradually increasing headaches over time was consistent with the development of chronic migraine and is sometimes called "chronification." Furthermore, this patient had attempted to address lifestyle and other trigger factors that might have been contributing to her headache. She also had none of the potentially modifiable risk factors listed in Table 8.2. This is a situation in which the use of preventive treatment for migraine should be strongly considered. Her physician suggested that she consider the use of preventive treatment for migraine and prescribed divalproex sodium 250 mg twice daily, stating that this drug was US Food and Drug Administration (FDA) approved for migraine prevention and therefore a good treatment choice.

What are the choices for preventive treatment of migraine, and how do you choose among them?

Table 8.3 summarizes medications that have shown evidence of benefit in preventing migraine attacks. The evidence is best for Level A drugs, less strong for Level B drugs, and suggestive but least compelling for Level C drugs. Not all drugs with a high level of evidence are FDA approved for migraine prevention, which might be a factor in choosing a drug. Nondrug preventive treatments for migraine and other headache disorders are covered in Chapter 9, but several (such as biofeedback-assisted relaxation) have good evidence of benefit and could also be considered for this patient.

The choice of preventive treatment is often based on a patient's comorbid conditions or other medications. For example, in a patient with concomitant hypertension, a beta-blocker such as propranolol would be a good choice for migraine prevention. The patient described in this case had no other medical problems that might benefit from a particular drug, but she is already using aspirin for treatment of individual headaches. Thus, a nonsteroidal anti-inflammatory drug such as ibuprofen, ketoprofen, fenoprofen, or naproxen would not have been a desirable choice for preventive treatment.

The patient in this case returned three months later for a follow-up visit. Her headache diary showed a clear improvement in headache frequency, but she had gained 8 pounds and was concerned about weight gain: "I'm hungry all the time." She asked whether there

Table 8.4. Weight gain as a side effect of migraine preventive drugs

Associated with weight increase	Weight neutral	Associated with weight loss
Beta-blockers	Lisinopril, candesartan	Protriptyline
Divalproex sodium	Riboflavin (vitamin B2)	Topiramate
Most tricyclic antidepressants	Venlafaxine	

were other treatments that would help her headaches without producing weight gain.

Which preventive medications are less likely to produce weight gain or other undesirable side effects?

Patient preference for specific migraine drugs and adherence to treatment regimens is strongly influenced by drug side effect profiles. Certain adverse events, such as weight gain or reproductive toxicity, are particularly undesirable for young women, the group of migraine patients most likely to need preventive treatment for migraine. Unfortunately, weight gain is a common side effect of many migraine preventive treatments.

The association between migraine and weight is complex. There is no evidence that overweight or obesity increases the risk of developing migraine in the first place. In people who already have migraine, however, overweight and obesity are associated with an increased risk of migraine progression. Migraine is not, however, clearly associated with an elevated risk for becoming overweight or obese, at least in women.

Divalproex sodium is not only associated with weight gain, but is also a known cause of birth defects. It should be used with caution in women of reproductive potential, especially when there are other alternatives. It was probably not the optimal choice of preventive treatment for this patient.

Are there treatment choices that would reconcile the patient's desire to avoid weight gain with the physician's desire to use a Level A drug that is FDA approved for migraine prevention? Table 8.4 lists migraine drugs that are associated with weight gain, weight loss, or are "weight neutral." Only topiramate has Level A evidence supporting its use, is not associated with weight gain, and is FDA approved for migraine treatment. It may increase the risk of facial clefts in infants exposed during pregnancy, so this patient should be cautioned to use effective birth control measures.

Discussion

Specific patient factors should be taken into account in choosing preventive medication. Although it is generally preferable to start with drugs that have a high level of scientific evidence for their use, the side effect profiles of the drugs and patient preference should be considered.

Diagnosis

High frequency episodic migraine with typical visual aura.

Tip

Even drugs that are FDA approved for migraine prevention and rated Level A in treatment guidelines may be the wrong treatment choice for an individual patient. The optimal choice of preventive treatment for migraine requires a comprehensive assessment of comorbid medical conditions, patient side effect preferences, and the strength of evidence for each drug.

Preventive treatment for a patient who has "tried everything"

Case

A 38-year-old woman sought treatment for headaches she had experienced for years. She had received a diagnosis of chronic migraine. Following a careful history, review of her previous testing results, and physical examination her new physician concurred with that diagnosis. The patient had completed a written headache history form required by the practice. This showed that she has tried most typically used preventive and abortive treatments for migraine. When asked whether any had been helpful, she said she couldn't recall exactly, but then remarked that some of them "helped a little bit but obviously they weren't that good or I would still be on them." She was interested in pursuing nondrug approaches to headache, and asked if she was a candidate for the new "migraine surgery" she had read about in the newspaper.

Do you agree that this patient is refractory to commonly used migraine preventive medications?

While it is certainly possible that this patient is refractory to pharmacologic preventive treatment for migraine, the information she has provided is not sufficient to be certain. It is clear what drugs have been tried, but there is no information about the doses that were used or the duration of the treatment trials. It is also not clear what the patient means by "helped a little bit." For all of these reasons, it is not obvious that this patient with chronic migraine is truly treatment-refractory or that previous treatment trials have been inadequate.

Her new physician requested her previous treatment records and reconstructed her treatment history. This showed that while she had tried many of the typically used treatments for migraine, the doses used were uniformly subtherapeutic and the treatments were continued for only a few weeks before being discontinued. For example, the patient was treated for just three weeks with a dose of 20 mg of propranolol twice a day before it was discontinued and another medication begun. The physician suggested to the patient that the next step in her treatment was to retry some typical migraine preventive drugs, this time making sure to aim for the target dose of medication and continue each drug for two to three months. She also asked the patient to keep a careful record of her daily pain level in order to quantify any response to treatment.

How could the need for retrials of medication have been prevented?

There are only a limited number of therapies with good evidence of benefit for migraine prevention. It is important to make sure each drug selected is given a careful therapeutic trial. Meticulous, systematic regimens of treatment ensure that drugs are used appropriately and given every chance to work. This is important before concluding that one or all of them are ineffective.

It is very discouraging for patients to be told that they need to go back and retry medications that previously seemed ineffective, yet this is necessary when those drugs have not been used correctly. Adequate patient preparation for such trials is important. Before embarking on preventive treatment, we explore patient

Table 8.5. Principles of migraine prevention

- Choose preventive medications with comorbid conditions in mind
- Start with a low dose and increase slowly to target dose
- Continue target dose for at least 2 to 3 months
- Monitor with calendar or diary: goal is a 30–50% reduction in frequency or reduced intensity/use of abortive medication
- Consider combinations of preventive treatments in refractory patients
- Consider tapering or discontinuing medication after 4 to 6 months of good headache control

expectations about the benefits of preventive treatment. Many have unrealistic ideas about how effective these treatments are, and expect that they will quickly eliminate all headaches. We educate patients that the goal for preventive therapy is to reduce, not eliminate, headaches. We also stress that the treatment may take several months to become effective, and that the dose of medication may need adjustment. We emphasize the need to keep a headache calendar in order to identify the effects of treatment, since patient global recall of drug effectiveness is unreliable. The success of preventive therapy can be enhanced by adherence to several principles of treatment (Table 8.5).

Discussion

Treatment guidelines can aid in the choice of which preventive medication to use. Even in the best of circumstances most pharmacologic treatments to prevent migraine reduce the frequency of migraine attacks by about half. In some cases preventive therapy does not necessarily reduce headache frequency but instead makes individual headaches milder or improves the patient's response to abortive treatment. These modest benefits can be difficult to identify in a disorder like migraine which naturally waxes and wanes.

Then, too, most preventive drugs do not take effect immediately. It can be a month or two before treatment response is apparent. The dose of medication required to suppress headaches also varies from patient to patient; many of the drugs are commonly started at low doses in order to improve tolerability. If patients discontinue use before the target dose is achieved, the drug may appear to be ineffective. Thus, two or three months of treatment at a drug's target dose (or the highest tolerated dose) should be required before drawing conclusions about treatment benefits.

Diagnosis

Chronic migraine.

Tip

In a patient with apparent treatment-refractory headaches, it is important to verify that previous treatment trials have been of adequate dose and duration.

Another patient who has tried everything

Case

A 30-year-old female with a family history of migraine and a past history of menstrual-related migraine sought treatment for a two- to three-year history of disabling chronic migraine. Multiple treatments throughout her 20s had failed to produce improvement in her headaches, but she had found that with exercise and maintenance of a low stress level she could control her symptoms.

In her late 20s she began a stress-filled job in her family's large antiques business and experienced an increase in migraine frequency to 20 days per month. She was treated sequentially with amitriptyline, divalproex sodium, topiramate, verapamil, propranolol, venlafaxine, sertraline, and indomethacin. These drugs failed to provide meaningful improvement in headache frequency or severity. OnabotulinumtoxinA injections initially appeared to reduce the number of headache days per month to 15, but that improvement was not sustained.

The patient treated individual headaches with sumatriptan, which was partially effective, but her use of that drug was limited by insurance restrictions on the number of tablets she could get each month. The patient continued aerobic exercise but her headaches remained poorly controlled and her previous physician had told her that there was nothing more that could be done. He suggested that the patient reduce her work hours or quit her job.

Has this patient tried everything, and should she quit her job?

The patient's income was important to her family, so she hoped to avoid limiting or stopping work. Her disappointing response to previous prophylactic therapy is not unusual. Most preventive medications for migraine have modest benefits at best, and the benchmark for considering a drug trial a success is a 50%

reduction in headache frequency in 50% of subjects. Some patients do not achieve even this level of success, however. Thus, many patients in primary and specialty care report that they have "tried everything" to prevent headaches and have failed to benefit from treatment. In some cases previous treatment trials were of inadequate duration or a subtherapeutic dose of medication was used, and retrials of monotherapy must be pursued. Once the physician is satisfied that previous attempts at prophylaxis have been adequate, however, it is reasonable to consider using combinations of preventive medications.

Combination treatment or "rational polypharmacy" is the standard of care for other intractable illnesses such as treatment-resistant depression or hypertension, so it makes sense that it should also be used in refractory headache problems. When chosen carefully, combination treatment strategies may target different, complementary underlying causes of headache. As a general rule, drugs from the same therapeutic class should generally not be combined because of the risk of synergistic side effects. Rarely, some combinations can have serious side effects. The combination of divalproex sodium and topiramate, for example, has been reported to cause encephalopathy.

Combination therapy may also be wise in patients with multiple medical conditions such as depression and headache. Finally, combination therapy may allow the use of lower drug doses and reduce the chance of troublesome side effects. For example, a patient whose headaches are only controlled on a high dose of beta-blockers that produces fatigue might benefit from a lower dose of the drug in combination with a small dose of a tricyclic antidepressant.

How firm is the evidence supporting the use of combinations of preventive treatments for headache?

One disadvantage of combination therapy is the lack of evidence from clinical trials to inform treatment choices. Table 8.6 summarizes some commonly used combination treatments and the rationale for their use. Given the wide possible variety of different drug combinations and the small number of studies, there is insufficient evidence to evaluate the benefit of many treatment combinations. However, there is evidence of added benefit from the combination of nonpharmacologic therapies with some pharmacologic treatments.

Table 8.6. Some commonly used combinations of preventive treatments for migraine

Combination	Comments
Tricyclic antidepressant plus a beta-blocker	Patients who do not tolerate a full dose of either drug alone may do well on a combination of these two drugs in low or moderate doses
Topiramate plus beta-blocker	Topiramate may counteract mild weight gain that can be seen with beta-blockers
Topiramate plus antidepressant	Topiramate may counteract the sometimes substantial weight gain that can be seen with tricyclic antidepressants
Beta-blocker plus divalproex sodium	Different side effect profiles may improve tolerability
Beta-blocker plus other antidepressants, e.g. venlafaxine	This combination of medications generally does not produce synergistic side effects
Drug therapy plus nondrug therapy	There is substantial evidence that the combination of drug therapy (e.g. amitriptyline) and relaxation training is superior to either treatment alone
OnabotulinumtoxinA injections with any drug or nondrug therapy	OnabotulinumtoxinA generally does not produce systemic side effects so it is a good choice for combination therapy in patients with chronic migraine who have failed monotherapy. Note: it is only approved for prevention of chronic, not episodic, migraine

There is also evidence about at least one combination of treatments that does *not* work. A recent trial examined the benefits of adding long-acting propranolol 240 mg/day to topiramate 50–100 mg/day in patients with chronic migraine (average of 15 or more days of headache a month). There was no statistically significant difference between the two groups in treatment response: those in the combination group experienced an average drop of 4 headache days per month compared with 4.5 days per month in the group that received topiramate alone.

Since the superiority of some treatment combinations has been demonstrated in clinical trials, and since such treatments are commonly used in clinical practice, it is clearly important to conduct additional studies to examine this treatment strategy.

The successful therapeutic strategy for the patient in this case ultimately turned out to be a combination of four preventive drugs: amitriptyline, topiramate, venlafaxine, and onabotulinumtoxinA injections. Although the use of this many drugs in combination is unusual, it is sometimes necessary in patients with particularly refractory headaches. After six months on this therapy the patient was able to work full time without missing multiple days and was no longer overusing medication to treat individual headache attacks.

Discussion

The goal of combination therapy for prevention of headaches is better pain relief or fewer side effects or both. Ideally, the pain-reducing effects of the combination will be additive or even synergistic while side effects will not be. Combining treatments can increase the risk of adverse events, but this problem can be minimized by choosing the drugs carefully and by careful monitoring and adjustment of doses.

Diagnosis

Chronic migraine refractory to monotherapeutic preventive medications.

Tip

Before concluding that a patient has failed preventive treatment for migraine, combinations of preventive agents should be tried.

Preventive treatment in a patient with multiple medical conditions

Case

A 58-year-old woman sought treatment for headaches that started when she was a teenager. Until her late 20s, headaches occurred once a month, usually a few days before the onset of menstrual bleeding. They met diagnostic criteria for migraine. In her 30s the headaches increased in frequency. She was started on propranolol and headaches decreased to once a month. The drug was stopped a year later. In her early 40s the patient had developed rheumatoid arthritis. Despite treatment with nonsteroidal anti-inflammatory drugs, the condition progressed and she was treated with hydroxychloroquine and methotrexate. The patient also developed Raynaud's phenomenon, insomnia, and hypertension. Her blood pressure was well controlled on a thiazide diuretic but she had recently been switched to prazosin and given trazadone to help with sleep.

She reported that her headaches had again increased in frequency and were occurring twice a week. They still met criteria for migraine and her neurologic examination was normal. Her blood pressure was 142/92 mm Hg and she had changes consistent with rheumatoid arthritis on examination.

Are the patient's new medications or her elevated blood pressure producing headache?

The relationship of mild, chronic hypertension to headache is still debated, but most experts believe that modest elevations in blood pressure are unlikely to produce headache. Sudden, abrupt elevations in blood pressure, however, can certainly provoke headache. Such "malignant hypertension" is caused by severely elevated blood pressure and is associated with signs of end-organ damage. Malignant hypertension can occur with preeclampsia, cocaine intoxication, pheochromocytoma, following severe head injury, or a number of other conditions. Papilledema usually should be present to make a diagnosis of malignant hypertension, and the blood pressure is usually above 220/120 mm Hg.

In this case the patient's blood pressure is well below that associated with urgent or emergent levels of hypertension. She has a long-standing history of headaches that occurred even when her blood pressure was well controlled. It is not very likely that her blood pressure is contributing to her current headache problem, but her blood pressure *treatment* might be contributing to her headache problem. She was recently switched from a thiazide diuretic to prazosin. Prazosin is a postsynaptic alpha-adrenergic blocker that can cause substantial vasodilation, especially when it is first begun. Medications with strong vasodilatory effects commonly appear on lists of medications thought to aggravate or precipitate migraine. The patient has also recently been started on trazodone, another drug often identified as possibly aggravating pre-existing headache problems.

How do the patient's comorbid conditions affect the choice of treatment for her migraines?

Most drugs used for headache prevention were initially developed to treat other conditions, and their beneficial effects on headache were discovered serendipitously. In some cases the multiple effects of these treatments can be exploited to treat more than one condition with a single drug. For this patient, a calcium channel blocker such as verapamil could be considered as a way to treat three of the patient's medical problems: hypertension, migraine, and Raynaud's phenomenon. Updated treatment guidelines from the AAN and the AHS reviewed clinical trial evidence for the use of verapamil in the prevention of migraine, and concluded it was insufficient to make a recommendation for or against the use of the drug. Clinical experience, however, suggests there is a place for this drug in selected patients such as the one in this vignette, who stands to benefit on several fronts if treatment is successful.

On the other hand, vasoconstrictive medications such as triptans, ergotamine, dihydroergotamine, or isometheptene-containing compounds should probably be avoided in this patient, because they can elevate blood pressure. Hypertension should be well controlled before the use of these drugs is considered. Although the beta-blocker propranolol was previously effective for this patient's migraine, it is not a good treatment choice now that she has developed Raynaud's phenomenon.

Discussion

Headache that coexists with other medical complaints can be challenging to manage. Headache can be aggravated or caused by a wide variety of conditions that include rheumatologic conditions such as systemic lupus erythematosus or giant cell arteritis. In this patient, however, the headaches preceded the onset of rheumatoid arthritis by many years, suggesting no link between the two conditions. Similarly, her hypertension was not severe and was a long-standing condition. Her headaches had fluctuated in severity independently of her blood pressure control, suggesting that her mild hypertension was an unlikely explanation for her current headache exacerbation.

Many medications are suspected of causing or aggravating headaches. Patients with pre-existing headache disorders, such as the patient in this case, are probably most susceptible to this side effect. Vasodilators such as nifedipine, prazosin, and nitrates are probably the most common offenders. A careful review of this patient's medications suggested that the recent switch to prazosin might be responsible for both an increase in her headaches, perhaps related to its

vasodilating properties, and also for a decline in the control of her hypertension. The medication was discontinued and she was switched to verapamil, ultimately reaching a dose of 120 mg/day. Trazodone was replaced with melatonin. Her headaches decreased to her usual frequency of once a month, and her blood pressure and Raynaud's phenomenon were under good control.

Diagnosis

Migraine with superimposed headache attributed to medication.

Tip

In patients with headache and other medical conditions, it is important to determine whether the medical complaints are independent of the headache or related in some way, since headache can be an early manifestation of many diseases.

A woman on migraine prophylaxis who wants to become pregnant

Case

A 24-year-old woman with a history of frequent disabling migraines presented to a headache clinic to discuss the management of migraines during pregnancy. Her headaches had previously been under good control on a combination of propranolol and riboflavin for preventive therapy and she used sumatriptan to treat individual headache attacks. Her doctor had told her that she should be off all medications for several months before she tried to become pregnant. He also suggested that her migraines might be a contraindication to pregnancy. The patient wanted to have a child but was afraid that if she stopped her medications as recommended her headaches would be much worse and that she would be without treatment.

What is known about the effect of pregnancy on migraine, and does migraine increase the risk of poor pregnancy outcomes?

For most women with migraine, the news about pregnancy is good. Studies consistently show that about 70% of women with migraine experience some degree of improvement during pregnancy. This is most noticeable during the second and third trimesters and is most likely in women who do not have aura. Not all women improve, however: some experience no change in their headaches and a minority find that their headaches are worse. Some women with aura find that aura frequency and complexity may increase.

Migraine without aura does not appear to increase the risk of pregnancy complications or poor outcomes. Migraine with aura, however, is associated with an elevated risk of a number of pregnancy complications, including preeclampsia and peripartum stroke. Thus, women who have migraine with aura should be monitored carefully for the development of these problems. A particular clinical challenge is distinguishing worsening of migraine from an early case of preeclampsia, where headache can be an early and only symptom of the disorder.

What options are available for preventive treatment of migraine during pregnancy?

Most women with migraine are highly motivated to minimize the use of any medications during pregnancy, and they commonly try to limit medication use to individual attacks of headache. Appropriate abortive treatments for acute migraine are discussed in Chapter 7. If at all possible, it is desirable to avoid the use of preventive medication during the first trimester of pregnancy when most organogenesis is occurring. If headaches have not improved by the end of the first trimester this is a natural time at which to consider starting preventive treatment.

Table 8.7 lists commonly used migraine preventive medications and their FDA use-in-pregnancy ratings. For both topiramate and divalproex sodium there is good quality evidence of potential fetal risks. Topiramate is associated with orofacial clefts and divalproex with neural tube defects and cognitive deficits. Ergot derivatives such as methergine, angiotensin-converting enzyme inhibitors, and angiotensin receptor blockers should also be avoided in women who plan to become pregnant or who are not using effective birth control methods. The majority of commonly used migraine preventives are Category C drugs.

These ratings, however, do not always take clinical experience into account. For example, beta-blockers are in Category C (except atenolol, which is pregnancy Category D) yet have a long history of safe use during pregnancy. Because it has good evidence of efficacy,

Table 8.7. FDA use-in-pregnancy ratings for commonly used migraine preventive drugs[*]

Agent	FDA use-in-pregnancy rating
Amitriptyline	C
Botulinum toxin	C
Gabapentin	C
Nortriptyline	Not assessed
Propranolol	C
Topiramate	D
Valproate (divalproex sodium)	X for treatment of migraine
Verapamil	C
Steroids	C

[*] FDA use-in-pregnancy ratings: Category A: controlled human studies show no risk; Category B: no evidence of risk in humans but there are no controlled human studies; Category C: risk to humans has not been ruled out; Category D: positive evidence of risk in human or animal studies; Category X: contraindicated in pregnancy.

propranolol is therefore often considered the optimal choice when migraine preventive treatment is needed during pregnancy. In contrast, the clinical trial and other scientific evidence of efficacy is not as strong for many of the other "C" drugs, so it is more difficult to assess the balance of benefits and harms. We generally avoid the use of preventive medications that do not have substantial evidence of benefit for migraine. While it might be defensible to try such treatments in nonpregnant patients, the stakes are higher during pregnancy and we prefer to stick with Level A or Level B treatments (as rated in the 2012 AHS/AAN migraine prevention guidelines).

What about natural treatments such as herbs and vitamins or behavioral treatments? Are these safe to use in pregnancy?

Biofeedback-assisted relaxation therapy has good evidence of benefit for the prevention of migraine. Physical therapy is less well studied but likely to be safe. We generally encourage women with migraine who are planning pregnancy to consider learning biofeedback techniques prior to pregnancy so they are "on board" during the first trimester. In addition, the importance of staying well rested and well hydrated and minimizing daily stress should not be underestimated.

Worsening headaches can sometimes be effectively managed if patients cut back on home or work responsibilities.

Some preventive treatments for migraine are herbs or nutritional supplements. These are typically used in very large, supraphysiologic doses. These drugs are not subject to the same level of FDA scrutiny as prescription pharmaceuticals, and since they are purchased without a prescription patients do not interact with pharmacists. A worrying study done a number of years ago had researchers posing as pregnant women inquire at health food stores about "safe" treatments for headache and nausea. A surprisingly large proportion of women were advised by store workers to use products that are not recommended for use during pregnancy or that are known to be unsafe in pregnancy. Patients may assume that these "natural" treatments are likely to be safer than prescription pharmaceuticals, but in fact the safety of these substances in pregnancy is not known and we recommend they be avoided for this reason.

How long do patients need to be off of preventive medications before becoming pregnant?

Patients often ask how long before attempting pregnancy they need to discontinue their migraine medications, if medications are going to be discontinued. There is no evidence that a prolonged waiting period is required. The commonly used migraine preventive drugs do not accumulate in the body so once they have been stopped no meaningful fetal exposure will occur. Because the maternal–fetal blood supply is not connected until a week or so after fertilization, we sometimes suggest that patients who are tracking ovulation can take their medication until ovulation has occurred.

The patient in this case decided to start biofeedback-assisted relaxation training and gradually reduce the doses of her preventive medications before attempting pregnancy. If headaches were still troublesome at the end of her first trimester of pregnancy, she planned to restart propranolol and use acetaminophen to treat individual headaches.

Discussion

Migraine is highly prevalent during the reproductive years, so the management of headache in pregnancy is a common clinical challenge. Individually tailored management of migraine during pregnancy, emphasizing nonpharmacologic options, is safe and effective for many patients. Most patients with migraine cope well with pregnancy and are able to manage their headaches. Poor pregnancy outcomes are not common, so there is no good reason to discourage patients in good health from undertaking pregnancy. Given the epidemiology of migraine, the management of headache in the setting of pregnancy is a common occurrence.

Women with migraine should be encouraged to plan their pregnancies and to come for a preconception visit prior to attempting pregnancy. This is a useful opportunity to discuss a pregnancy treatment plan for headaches and to educate patients about the effects of pregnancy on migraine. It is also good practice to recommend that all women of childbearing potential take a multivitamin with folate, which has been shown to reduce the risk of neural tube defects.

In developing a migraine treatment plan for pregnancy, physicians and patients should weigh the potential benefits of treatment against known harms, taking an individual patient's situation into consideration. This is not always easy, since medications are not tested in pregnant women and data about pregnancy effects are thus sparse and imperfect, often based on post-marketing registry surveillance studies or other observational data. Certainly for women whose migraines are severe and lead to frequent protracted vomiting and dehydration, or cause significant emotional distress, the benefits of using pharmacologic therapy will usually be judged to outweigh the potential risks. Conversations about the harms and benefits of treatments during pregnancy should be documented in the patient's chart.

Diagnosis

Episodic migraine without aura; preconception planning.

Tip

Women with migraine should not be discouraged from attempting pregnancy and long medication-free intervals are not needed prior to pregnancy. Most women with migraine will be able to manage headaches during pregnancy and will have good pregnancy outcomes.

A middle-aged woman with chronic migraine and paresthesias

Case

A 39-year-old woman returned for a follow-up visit for migraine. She had a lengthy history of chronic migraine as well as asthma, Type II diabetes mellitus, hypothyroidism, Factor V Leiden deficiency, and a strong family history of venous thromboembolism. Her headaches had always been difficult to control. During her early 30s she had frequently missed work because of them. Eventually headaches improved on a combination of topiramate (50 mg twice daily) and propranolol (60 mg a day).

The patient did well for several years on this combination treatment. Two months before her current visit she underwent left shoulder manipulation and steroid injections in her elbow under anesthesia. She awoke from the surgery with shortness of breath and severe pain under her left breast. She was eventually diagnosed with an embolus in the left main pulmonary artery and was admitted to the hospital for anticoagulation and monitoring.

In the hospital, propranolol was discontinued because of low blood pressure. The patient's hospital stay was prolonged by the development of bilateral upper and lower extremity paresthesias. Topiramate was dismissed as a possible cause because the patient had been on the same dose of the drug for years without any problems. A neurology consultant identified no clear explanation for the paresthesias. Nerve conduction studies were performed and her doctors considered discontinuing her warfarin in order to perform electromyography (EMG) but ultimately decided against it. The patient asks you whether she should have an EMG.

What was the most likely cause of this patient's paresthesias?

This patient did have diabetes, a condition that can produce paresthesias and neuropathy, but it is unlikely that diabetic neuropathy and paresthesias would present so suddenly. Despite the fact that this patient had been on topiramate for years without troubling side effects, topiramate was the most likely cause for her bilateral paresthesias. When this was reviewed with the patient, she recalled that prior to her recent illness she had not always remembered to take her topiramate regularly and "might have missed some doses." In the hospital she received the medication as prescribed. After discharge, because she paid so much attention to taking her warfarin regularly, her adherence to the prescribed regimen of topiramate remained excellent. This effectively increased the amount of topiramate the patient was getting and resulted in a side effect that had not occurred at lower doses.

Paresthesias are the most common adverse event with topiramate treatment. In clinical trials for migraine, 47% of subjects randomized to the 100 mg/day dose of topiramate developed paresthesias compared with just 5% of those receiving placebo, and the risk of paresthesias was dose-related. In contrast, concentration difficulties and memory impairment, which are more widely recognized as topiramate side effects, occurred in just 5% and 6% of topiramate subjects, respectively, compared with 1% and 2% of subjects who received placebo.

Most side effects of topiramate occur during titration. One study concluded that if adverse events have not appeared after six weeks of treatment at a stable dose of the drug, they are unlikely to occur. In this case, however, the patient's dose of medication was not stable when she developed paresthesias. It had effectively been increased because of improved adherence to the prescribed dosing regimen. Because this explanation for her problem was so quickly discounted, the patient almost underwent risky discontinuation of anticoagulation in order to have an invasive procedure.

Can topiramate-associated paresthesias be prevented or treated?

Starting with a low dose of topiramate, such as 25 mg once daily, and working up slowly to the target dose (usually 100 mg/day) may help minimize adverse events and allow patients time to develop tolerance to them. Paresthesias often improve over time. If they do not, we find that many patients are willing to tolerate them in exchange for improved control of migraines, as long as they understand they are not dangerous and will remit when the drug is stopped.

Anecdotal evidence suggests that potassium supplementation may help reduce paresthesias. One expert suggests the use of 20–40 mEq of potassium chloride per day. Reducing the dose of the drug can also be helpful, and patients sometimes find that although a higher dose was needed to gain control of headaches, a lower dose works well once control is established. In some cases, however, a tolerable balance between benefits and side effects cannot be found and patients discontinue it.

A meta-analysis compared adverse drug events in trials of topiramate for migraine with adverse events in trials using the drug for epilepsy. The researchers found that the adverse event profile of topiramate differed in the two conditions. Migraineurs were more likely than subjects with epilepsy to experience a wide range of side effects and more likely to drop out of trials because of adverse events. For the 100 mg/day dose of topiramate, the risk ratio for paresthesias in migraineurs compared to epilepsy subjects was 2.7 (99% confidence interval: 1.80–3.97).

Discussion

This case reminds us that adherence to medications can never be assumed. The patient in this case was a nurse-practitioner and was certainly aware of the need to take medications as prescribed. Even motivated patients, however, find it difficult to take prescribed medications regularly, and adherence decreases as the number of daily doses increases.

Topiramate affects the activity of some types of glutamate receptors, gamma-aminobutyric acid (GABA) receptors, and voltage-gated sodium and calcium channels. It is also a carbonic anhydrase inhibitor and it is this pharmacologic effect that produces the reversible paresthesias seen with topiramate and other carbonic anhydrase inhibitors such as acetazolamide and zonisamide. Some researchers have suggested that the development of paresthesias is a favorable sign and indicates an enhanced likelihood that migraine prophylaxis will be successful.

Diagnosis

Chronic migraine; paresthesias due to topiramate.

Tip

When patients develop apparently new side effects while on a previously tolerated medication, it is worth exploring whether their compliance with recommended dosing has changed, or whether other medications have been added or discontinued that might affect the side effect profile.

Will preventive treatment work in a patient who is overusing abortive treatments?

Case

A 32-year-old man with chronic migraine was using over-the-counter analgesics on a daily basis. He reported that his headaches had gradually increased over the years, and that he had responded by using his prescribed and over-the-counter medications more frequently. He was taking as many ibuprofen tablets each day as allowed by the package instructions, along with several tablets a day of a combination analgesic containing acetaminophen, caffeine, and aspirin. He obtained temporary relief with these treatments but after an hour or so experienced the gradual return of a dull headache. He also typically awoke in the morning with a dull generalized headache.

The patient's neurologist advised him that he should be on preventive treatment for his headaches but that preventive therapy for migraine would not work while he was overusing short-acting medicines. He suggested abrupt discontinuation of these medications, followed by a medication-free period of a month. The doctor told the patient he probably had medication overuse headache and that it was important to see if headaches improved when the overused medications had been removed. The doctor told the patient that he had done everything he could and that "the ball is in your court." The patient was afraid that he would be unable to work if he discontinued his headache medications. His doctor then said that he could offer no further advice and the patient left care.

Does this patient have medication overuse headache?

It can be difficult to distinguish chronic migraine from medication overuse headache, but it seems likely that medication overuse is contributing to this patient's pattern of chronic headaches. Medication overuse occurs when a susceptible person uses excessive amounts of symptomatic medication. Susceptibility to medication overuse headache probably varies, and there are many patients in whom the development of daily headache clearly precedes the medication use. With medication overuse headache, headache severity and frequency and medication use increase in lock-step, so that patients may feel they are trapped in a never-ending cycle of more medication and more headaches. This patient's headaches have worsened in close proximity to his increased use of medication.

The concept of medication overuse headache is controversial, and diagnostic criteria change frequently. Several clinical features, however, are useful clues to the possibility that medication is making a headache worse. First, the headache has either begun or worsened substantially in the setting of daily or near-daily use of analgesic medications such as triptans, ergot derivatives, opioids, or combination analgesics. (Nonsteroidal anti-inflammatory drugs are not universally believed to produce medication overuse headache.) Second, the headache usually improves and sometimes even resolves when the offending medication is stopped. This latter criterion is particularly controversial, however, since some experts suspect that medication overuse can occasionally trigger an irreversible headache increase. We also find it useful to inquire about whether headaches are present upon awakening or waken a patient from sleep, which was the case with this patient. Overnight is the longest period of time many patients are without their medication, and their rest is often disturbed by withdrawal headache.

Is it always necessary to remove a medication that is suspected of producing medication overuse headache before instituting preventive treatment of migraine?

Clinical experience suggests that many patients who are overusing symptomatic medication do obtain benefit from migraine preventive medications. Once headache frequency decreases, those patients may be able to decrease their use of symptomatic medication and experience substantial additional improvement in headaches. This clinical impression has been bolstered by several recent clinical trials in which even patients who were overusing analgesic medications responded to onabotulinumtoxinA or topiramate treatment for chronic migraine.

While it is often desirable for a patient with refractory migraine to decrease the use of symptomatic medication, the specifics of the clinical situation, as with this patient, may make abrupt discontinuation imprac-

tical. Additionally, abrupt discontinuation of certain medications can produce a discontinuation syndrome that is unpleasant or even dangerous: for example, too-rapid elimination of barbiturate medications can provoke seizures while abrupt opioid withdrawal may produce a flu-like syndrome. Before insisting upon "cold turkey" and rapid withdrawal of symptomatic medications, we prefer to "meet patients half-way" by instituting preventive therapy first followed by slow reduction in the overused medication.

Discussion

Despite the fact that preventive medication may be helpful even in patients who are overusing symptomatic medications, it is still important to address the problem of medication overuse. For some patients preventive treatment will not be fully effective until the problem of overuse has been addressed. The process of medication reduction can sometimes be expedited with the use of a burst and taper of steroids (e.g. methylprednisolone) or (if an infusion center is available) with repetitive intravenous dihydroergotamine given for several days during medication withdrawal.

Diagnosis

Medication overuse headache in the setting of chronic migraine.

Tip

Abrupt discontinuation of overused symptomatic medication is not always necessary to ensure response to preventive treatment.

A woman on migraine treatment who has a fall

Case

A 56-year-old woman was seen for evaluation of headaches that had started in her early teens. The headaches were unilateral, throbbing, and of severe intensity, with associated nausea but no photo or phonophobia. She did not experience aura. Headaches typically lasted six to eight hours. They had occurred roughly twice a month until about a year ago, when headache frequency increased in the setting of a new, more demanding job. She was experiencing two to three headaches a week. Investigation, including an

MRI scan of the head, had been normal. A variety of migraine preventive treatments had been tried, including propranolol, divalproex sodium, and topiramate, but the patient had not tolerated them.

She reported that she was very sensitive to drug side effects. On propranolol she was fatigued, on topiramate and divalproex she had memory problems, and on amitriptyline she gained weight. Because the patient was very worried about sedation, cognitive impairment, and fatigue, she was given a prescription for lisinopril, a drug that is typically not associated with those adverse events.

Three weeks after beginning treatment with 10 mg of lisinopril, the patient awoke in the middle of the night and got out of bed to use the bathroom. She stumbled and fell, sustaining a mild head trauma. In the emergency department her blood pressure was 104/68 mm Hg. She was told that orthostatic hypotension from the lisinopril might have caused her fall and was advised to stop the drug.

Was this patient's fall caused by her migraine treatment?

Many things, including tripping over furniture or a rug, missing her footing in the dark, or even an acute neurologic event, could have caused this patient's fall. Still, it is hard to ignore the temporal association between the fall and the initiation of an antihypertensive medication for migraine. The patient took her once-daily dose of lisinopril at bedtime, so its maximal effect on blood pressure probably occurred during the night. A syncopal or presyncopal event related to orthostatic hypotension is therefore high on the list of possible explanations for her fall. The patient in this case did not recall any presyncopal symptoms because she was groggy and sleepy.

Could this have been prevented?

Although the patient was started on a relatively low dose of lisinopril, starting at even smaller doses might be reasonable when there is a possibility of side effects. Some patients, however, will forget to increase the dose as instructed or will become impatient with a perceived lack of effect at lower doses. They may prematurely discontinue therapy.

In our experience, though, most patients are able to follow a simple titration schedule starting at a low dose and increasing each week until the target dose is reached. When the reasons for this "start low, go slow" approach are explained, many patients are grateful that the physician is attempting to prevent the development of side effects (which are a significant concern to patients who may be otherwise healthy). We have learned the hard way, however, that any patient being started on antihypertensive treatment for migraine should be cautioned about the possibility of orthostasis and presyncopal symptoms.

Rapid movement from lying to sitting or standing is a common activity, but also a considerable physiologic stress. Syncope can occur with immediate, transient drops in blood pressure or from delayed orthostatic hypotension, which can occur as late as 15 minutes after a change in posture.

The risk of orthostatic drops in blood pressure appears to increase with age, so older patients should be particularly cautioned to take care when getting out of bed or rising quickly from a sitting position.

Discussion

Although antihypertensives are among the best tolerated migraine preventative medications, there are several side effects that can limit use. As may have occurred in this case, medication-related hypotension and bradycardia may contribute to symptomatic orthostasis. Syncope or near syncope due to orthostatic hypotension can affect patients of any age. The side effects of orthostasis and bradycardia should be of particular concern in older patients, who are at greater risk for falls and for negative sequelae of falls.

Although syncope or presyncope is a side effect with great potential for harm, antihypertensives can also produce other adverse events. Exercise intolerance may be seen with both beta-blockers and calcium channel antagonists, although more commonly with the former. Beta-blockers have been suspected of aggravating depression, although this is controversial. In any case, patients are likely to recognize this if cautioned about the possibility ahead of time. Beta-blockers also may worsen active asthma or Raynaud's disease. Calcium channel antagonists, on the other hand, may produce constipation or pedal edema, as well as generalized fatigue.

Although the phenomenon has not been systematically studied, we have found that many patients with migraine are unusually susceptible to medication side effects. In most patients, it is prudent to start preventive medications at quite low doses and increase slowly as tolerated. For example, lisinopril could be started at 5 mg nightly and increased to 10 mg after a week. Propranolol could be started at 20 mg nightly, and the dose then increased by 20 mg every week or two if no side effects develop. This strategy of slow up-titration is also recommended for patients with a history of childhood asthma. Verapamil can be started at 40 mg nightly. Patients can also be asked to monitor their blood pressure and heart rate between visits, although they should be cautioned that this is to assess for side effects and not for drug benefit. There is no clear correlation between heart rate or blood pressure and headache benefits.

Although some patients are unusually sensitive to the side effects of antihypertensives, this reaction is somewhat idiosyncratic. In fact, most patients with low baseline blood pressure do very well when placed on blood pressure medicines for the treatment of migraine. Antihypertensives are frequently well tolerated by patients concerned about possible sedation or cognitive side effects with other migraine preventives, and are an important tool in the migraine armamentarium. The key is to start low and go slow, advice commonly given when starting any medication for older patients, but worth remembering for younger patients as well.

Diagnosis

Migraine; orthostatic syncope possibly due to lisinopril.

Tip

Orthostatic hypotension is a possible complication of migraine prophylaxis with antihypertensive drugs. Susceptibility to this side effect may increase with age, so starting with low doses and warning patients about falls are important.

An older woman with blurry vision on amitriptyline

Case

A 66-year-old woman with a long-standing history of migraine without aura reported an increase in headache frequency which she attributed to family stress from her daughter's divorce. She had begun to care for her young grandchild, and described this as "simultaneously delightful and stressful." She asked about starting a preventive medication "to get me over the hump" until she could adjust to the demands of her new routine. She was healthy except for borderline increased intraocular pressures, and her blood pressure was 108/74 mm Hg. Her physician considered prescribing topiramate but knew that it might raise intraocular pressures and precipitate glaucoma, so instead he prescribed amitriptyline. The patient's headache decreased in frequency, but two months later the physician received a call from the emergency department. The patient had presented several hours ago with acute bilateral loss of vision and eye erythema. Ophthalmologic evaluation showed acute angle-closure glaucoma.

What happened?

Topiramate is the migraine preventive most commonly associated with increased intraocular pressure. Topiramate may precipitate secondary acute angle-closure glaucoma due to cilio-choroidal effusion, which displaces the lens and ciliary body. This can sometimes be bilateral. It is less commonly realized that tricyclic antidepressants or antipsychotic medications (such as promethazine, which is sometimes used for headache-associated vomiting) can also produce angle-closure glaucoma.

The anticholinergic actions of tricyclic antidepressants and some antipsychotic medications produce mydriasis, which can precipitate angle closure in susceptible patients. Thus, all of these drugs should be avoided in patients known to have narrow angles. In contrast, patients with open-angle glaucoma are usually able to take these medications without adverse events. Many patients are not aware of the difference between the two types of glaucoma, so consultation with the patient's optometrist or ophthalmologist is useful if either drug is considered for patients who report a history of intraocular pressure abnormalities.

Discussion

Many medications used to prevent headaches can occasionally be associated with ocular adverse events. Lithium can produce eye irritation and keratoconjunctivitis, probably because of effects on sodium transport. In addition to producing angle-closure glaucoma in predisposed patients, tricyclic antidepressants (and even selective serotonin reuptake inhibitors [SSRIs]) cause mydriasis and accommodation problems that may result in blurred vision. This is often transient.

Ocular dystonias, eye movement disturbances and changes in color or contrast discrimination have rarely been associated with the use of topiramate or SSRIs.

Diagnosis

Acute angle-closure glaucoma from amitritpyline.

Tip

Potentially serious ocular complications are well recognized with topiramate therapy but can also occur with other commonly used migraine preventive drugs, particularly tricyclic antidepressants.

A woman with migraine worried about the long-term safety of topiramate

Case

A 33-year-old woman presented to establish care with a local neurologist after recently moving to the area. She had a long-standing history of migraine without aura and had been started on topiramate five years ago by her previous headache specialist. Trials of several other preventive treatments had not been successful, but with topiramate her headaches decreased from a frequency of three times a week to three times a month. Her breakthrough headaches were effectively treated with a triptan. She did not want to change her treatment regimen, but she wanted to know if it was safe to take topiramate long term.

What is known about the long-term risks of chronic topiramate treatment?

Both cognitive side effects and paresthesias are common side effects of topiramate. They often lead to treatment discontinuation, but they are entirely reversible. Even the rare but feared complication of acute angle-closure glaucoma usually resolves if the drug is discontinued promptly. The incidence of nephrolithiasis in patients taking topiramate was approximately 1% per year in clinical trials; thus, the cumulative risk increases with duration of therapy but there is no evidence that the risk of kidney stones persists after the drug is stopped. In contrast, bone loss is painless and insidious, and the pharmacologic profile of topiramate does suggest that this may be an irreversible complication of long-term topiramate treatment.

Several lines of evidence suggest topiramate may produce bone loss. Bone loss is a known complication of many antiepileptic drugs. The risk has been best studied with older antiepileptic drugs such as divalproex sodium. Less evidence has accumulated about the risk of bone loss with newer antiepileptic agents such as topiramate. However, a recent pilot study evaluated biochemical and radiologic tests of bone metabolism in women with migraine taking topiramate, and found osteopenia in 53% of them. The risk seemed to be associated with duration of use but not dose.

A risk of bone loss with long-term topiramate treatment is plausible because it is a carbonic anhydrase inhibitor. The mild metabolic acidosis it produces may have an effect on bone metabolism and turnover. This is concerning because migraine is a condition of long duration and most patients requiring long-term prophylaxis for it are women.

Discussion

The package insert for topiramate recommends obtaining baseline and periodic serum bicarbonate levels in patients using topiramate, based on a correlation between chronic metabolic acidosis and fatigue. It is unclear, however, whether serum bicarbonate levels can be used to indicate a risk for bone loss. A number of strategies have been proposed to minimize or prevent bone loss in patients treated with antiepileptic drugs. At present, however, evidence is insufficient to make strong recommendations for these proposals, which include:

- Measurement of bone mineral density at the start of treatment and periodically on an individualized basis.
- Monitoring of vitamin D (25-OHD) levels so that vitamin D supplementation can be adjusted on an individualized basis.
- Recommendations for adequate calcium intake and vitamin D supplementation with 400–2000 IU/day as prophylaxis.

Many patients have questions about the long-term safety of migraine preventive treatment. This is understandable because most people with migraine are otherwise healthy. Migraine itself confers little long-term health risk, unlike other conditions such as epilepsy for which long-term preventive treatments might be used. Thus the balance of benefits and harms of long-term treatment with drugs such as topiramate will be weighed differently depending upon whether they are used for migraine or epilepsy.

Diagnosis

Chronic migraine.

Tip

Most of the troublesome side effects of topiramate are reversible when treatment is stopped, but patients should be cautioned about the possibility of long-term treatment-related bone loss.

A woman worried about whether her contraceptive will work when she is on topiramate

Case

A 21-year-old woman with chronic migraine called her physician to report that she had missed her last menstrual period. She was taking an oral combination hormonal contraceptive for contraception and menorrhagia. Six months ago she had started topiramate. When she went to the pharmacy to fill the prescription, the pharmacist told her there was an interaction between topiramate and oral contraceptives that might increase her risk of becoming pregnant. At the time, her physician had reassured both her and the pharmacist that this interaction was not clinically important with typical anti-migraine doses of topiramate. However, in view of her missed period the patient was concerned that perhaps the pharmacist had been right, and that she might now be pregnant. Although the physician had used these two medications in many patients over the years, she was also worried.

What is the interaction between topiramate and combination hormonal contraceptives?

Topiramate decreases serum concentrations of ethinyl estradiol, the active estrogen component in many combined hormonal contraceptives. Studies show that the blood concentration of ethinyl estradiol is reduced by an average of 18% in women who are also taking topiramate 200 mg daily. The decline in estrogen levels depends upon the dose of topiramate: estrogen levels decreased by an average of 21% when used with a daily dose of 400 mg of topiramate, and 30% with a dose of 800 mg/day. This interaction is substantial enough to interfere with the contraceptive efficacy of the newer low estrogen dose combination contraceptives that are now in common use.

When used for migraine prophylaxis, however, topiramate is rarely given in doses above 150 mg/day; a more typical dose is 100 mg/day. One study showed that healthy volunteers taking topiramate at doses of 50–200 mg/day did not experience statistically significant decreases in ethinyl estradiol concentrations. On the basis of these data, which are described in the package insert, it is very unlikely that topiramate prescribed at doses less than 200 mg/day will decrease the efficacy of combination estrogen–progestin contraceptives. For patients who might be imperfectly compliant with oral contraceptive regimens, however, one might consider the use of a combination hormonal contraceptive with a slightly higher dose of ethinyl estradiol. In this case, the patient had a negative pregnancy test and a normal menstrual period two weeks later. The patient decided to continue topiramate, but changed to a combination hormonal contraceptive with 30 μg of ethinyl estradiol "for peace of mind."

Diagnosis

Chronic migraine.

Tip

At doses less than 200 mg/day, topiramate does not interfere with contraceptive efficacy.

An older man treated for tension-type headache who has a seizure

Case

A 66-year-old man with history of hypertension, hyperlipidemia, and peptic ulcer disease was referred to the headache clinic to discuss treatment for his migraines. Headaches had become more frequent over the last year, and he attributed this worsening to emotional stress and worry about his other health problems. His doctor had started him on amitriptyline 25 mg at bedtime, and his headache frequency had decreased from three times a week to once a week. He

Table 8.8. Some headache treatments that may lower the seizure threshold

Category	Drug Example
Antidepressants	Tricyclic antidepressants SSRIs and selective serotonin–norepinephrine reuptake inhibitors (SNRIs)
Local anesthetics (if systemic absorption occurs)	Lidocaine Bupivacaine Procaine
Analgesics	Fentanyl Meperidine Pentazocine Propoxyphene Tramadol
Neuroleptics	Clozapine Phenothiazines Butyrophenones
Other	Anticholinergics Anticholinesterases Antihistamines Baclofen Hyperbaric oxygen Lithium

also reported improved sleep. At this visit he reported continued worry about the migraines he still had, however, because he had not found any effective treatment for the infrequent but very severe events. Triptans were contraindicated because he had coronary atherosclerosis, and he could not take anti-inflammatory drugs such as aspirin because of a previous problem with gastric ulcers. His physician thus prescribed tramadol. Three weeks later the patient was admitted to the hospital for evaluation after suffering a witnessed, generalized tonic–clonic seizure.

What happened?

Medications that lower the seizure threshold are thought to cause about 6% of new-onset seizures. Many medications associated with an increased risk of seizures are used to treat migraine and some are listed in Table 8.8. The epileptogenic effects of medication are not often taken into consideration when prescribing treatment for patients with no prior history of or risk factors for seizure. In clinical practice, drug-induced seizures are rare in patients who are using a single medication that lowers seizure threshold. In contrast, the risk of inadvertent seizures is higher in patients who are prescribed a combination of such medications. Older patients may be particularly vulnerable.

Discussion

Certain medications are more frequently associated with drug-induced seizures than others. In a recent retrospective analysis, the drugs most frequently associated with seizure induction were bupropion (23%), diphenhydramine (8.3%), tricyclic antidepressants (7.7%), tramadol (7.5%), amphetamines (6.9%), isoniazid (5.9%), and venlafaxine (5.9%). Since a large number of the events analyzed in this study were described as suicide attempts, it is probably that the risk is dose related as well as drug related. Overall, about 18% of seizure cases involved the use of more than one medication known to lower the seizure threshold.

Diagnosis

Probable medication-induced seizure in a patient taking multiple medications with epileptogenic side effects.

Tip

The use of multiple epileptogenic medications should be avoided when possible, especially in older patients.

A fatigued patient on two blood pressure medicines

Case

A 47-year-old woman was being treated for intractable chronic migraine. She had previously experienced a small reduction in headache frequency with propranolol and had remained on a dose of 120 mg a day. Multiple other trials of preventive medications had failed to produce improvement, so verapamil was added at a dose of 40 mg orally three times a day. At her follow-up visit she reported profound fatigue, which she attributed to her medications. She was having trouble getting out of bed and getting to work. On examination, her blood pressure was 95/62 mm Hg and her pulse was 48 beats per minute.

What was the likely cause of her fatigue?

Nonselective beta-adrenergic blockers, including propranolol, inhibit sympathetically mediated increases in heart rate and cardiac contractility. Calcium channel antagonists such as verapamil reduce atrioventricular nodal conduction and cause peripheral vasodilation.

Used together, these medications may produce a synergistic decrease in cardiac conduction, heart rate, and contractility. This can lead to symptoms such as fatigue that are caused by bradycardia and reduced cardiac output. Peripheral edema also may develop as a result of vasodilation.

Caution should be exercised when prescribing two migraine preventive medications with overlapping mechanisms of action. Another example of migraine preventive medications where a deleterious overlap in effect might be expected in combination would be the use of beta adrenergic blockers with angiotensin-converting enzyme inhibitors or angiotensin receptor blockers (such as lisinopril or candesartan, respectively). This combination would also be likely to lower blood pressure significantly and perhaps produce fatigue or syncope.

Combinations of antiepileptics used for migraine prevention may also produce synergistic adverse events. Concurrent use of sodium valproate and topiramate, for example, may increase the risk of hyperammonemia. The concurrent use of valproate and lamotrigine may increase the risk of development of Stevens–Johnson syndrome. In contrast, gabapentin can often be combined with other antiepileptic drugs without causing intolerable side effects. Its usefulness for migraine prevention, however, is not settled. Recent guidelines for preventive migraine therapy issued by the AAN and the AHS concluded that current evidence is insufficient to recommend for or against use of gabapentin for migraine prophylaxis. Nonetheless, as with other drugs in that category, the drug is still in widespread use for migraine prophylaxis based on clinical impressions of benefit.

Discussion

The use of medications in combination has been suggested in the management of refractory migraine and in most instances is considered safe and well tolerated. The potential complications of such combinations, though, should be borne in mind. Anticipating drug side effects is important. Many potential synergies can be suspected based on what is known about a drug's mechanisms of action. Since most drugs have multiple actions, however, this is not always the case. Table 8.9 lists combinations of preventive medications that should be used with caution due to the potential for overlapping side effects.

Table 8.9. Combinations of preventive headache medications that should be avoided

Combination	Comment
Any combination of antihypertensives	An exception could be made for patients with treatment-resistant hypertension
Two or more antiepileptic drugs	Gabapentin might be an exception to this rule because it is generally well tolerated both alone and when used with other drugs
Topiramate and propranolol	A recent randomized trial demonstrated no benefit for the combination compared with topiramate treatment alone
Two or more antidepressants	In addition to synergistic side effects of agitation or somnolence, there is a risk of serotonin syndrome with this combination. Psychiatrists occasionally use a full dose of an SSRI or SNRI with a small dose of a tricyclic antidepressant at night to help with sleep

Diagnosis

Profound fatigue related to drug-induced hypotension and bradycardia.

Tip

Avoid prescribing drugs with overlapping side effect profiles.

How about Botox for episodic migraine?

Case

A 42-year-old woman had a 20-year history of migraine without aura, with headaches consistent with migraine occurring about eight days a month for the last three years. On the advice of a friend she began treatment for her headaches with intramuscular injections of 155 units of onobotulinumtoxinA every three months. After one year of therapy she had not noted significant improvement. She presented for a second opinion at a headache center; she suspected that the lack of improvement was due to an inadequate dose of botulinum toxin. She requested that the headache center take over the treatment and requested a letter to her health insurance company in support of continued therapy using 300 units of the drug every three months. She was not overusing analgesic medications and her past medical history was otherwise notable only for a mild anxiety disorder. Her neurologic examination was normal and her body mass index (BMI) was 33.

Is onabotulinumtoxinA the best therapeutic recommendation for this patient's pattern of headache?

Although the use of onabotulinumtoxinA is supportd by an FDA indication for chronic migraine, it is not approved for treatment of episodic migraine. A large number of randomized clinical trials have failed to show benefit in episodic migraine and AAN treatment guidelines currently label onabotulinumtoxinA therapy as "probably ineffective" for treatment of episodic migraine. The likely explanation for the lack of benefit of this therapy in the patient described in this case is that this is simply the wrong choice of treatment for her condition.

It may have seemed logical to use onabotulinumtoxinA therapy; one argument might have been that this was a safe therapy for use in a motivated patient with high frequency migraine who might have been in the process of transformation to a chronic pattern. Why not, it could be asked, just skip all the systemically active preventive medication trials with their possible associated side effects and jump all the way to onabotulinumtoxinA treatment? There are several problems with this approach. The first, as noted, is that there is high quality evidence that the drug is not effective for episodic migraine. Why this is so is not entirely clear, but may be tied to its mechanism of action and the processes that come into play when migraine transforms from an episodic to a chronic form. In part, the mechanism of action of onbotulinumtoxinA in chronic migraine may relate to peripheral inhibition of neurotransmitter and neuropeptide (e.g. substance P, calcitonin gene-related peptide [CGRP], glutamate) release which is related to inhibition of central sensitization. In episodic migraine patients, whose disorder is unlikely to involve sustained central sensitization, onabotulinumtoxinA may not work.

What therapy should be offered to the patient?

This patient should be advised that onabotulinumtoxinA therapy has been shown to be ineffective for her condition. Instead, a combination of abortive and preventive medications should be considered, perhaps combined with lifestyle management including exercise and weight control, along with attention to any comorbid conditions such as anxiety that may be aggravating her headaches.

Discussion

The FDA approved onabotulinumtoxinA for treatment of chronic migraine in 2010. International Classification of Headache Disorders (ICHD)-3 beta criteria for chronic migraine require the presence of more than 15 headache days a month, with a headache day defined as one with headache for more than four hours. Headaches must have features of migraine, or be relieved by the use of a migraine-specific drug (triptans or ergots) on at least eight days a month.

The approved treatment protocol for onabotulinumtoxinA for chronic migraine is the administration of 155 units intramuscularly in 31 fixed sites. The drug is diluted with saline, and individual injections of 5 units are made in the muscles depicted in Figure 8.1.

Subsequent analysis further suggests that patients with concomitant medication overuse derive a similar benefit from onabotulinumtoxinA therapy to those without, and that in many patients the clinical effect increased over subsequent injection cycles. Reported adverse events overall leading to study discontinuance were low (3.8%) in the clinical trial treatment groups.

Neurotoxins appear to be taken up in peripheral motor neurons, where they disrupt the protein complex that facilitates vesicle fusion and release from the axonal endplates. Neurotoxins also may affect sensory neurons by inhibiting release of proinflammatory mediators at several sites within the neuron. More specifically, onabotulinumtoxinA could suppress neurogenic inflammation near the scalp or facial injection site by preventing the release of the neuropeptides CGRP and substance P from free nerve endings that provide sensory innervation to the skin and muscles. In addition, neurotoxins may exert central effects by blocking the release of CGRP and glutamate from nociceptive nerve fibers in the spinal cord, leading to a suppression of stimulation of second-order neurons that are theoretically associated with the maintenance of central sensitization and pain.

The exact mechanism of onabotulinumtoxinA in chronic migraine is unknown, and perhaps multiple mechanisms are involved, as above, including: inhibition of neurotransmitter release from both motor neurons and sensory nociceptive neurons, leading to

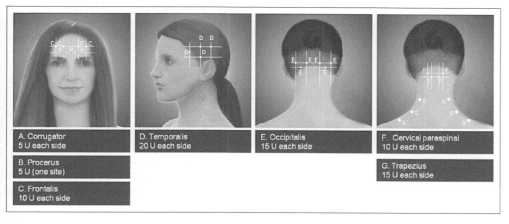

| A. Corrugator 5 U each side | D. Temporalis 20 U each side | E. Occipitalis 15 U each side | F. Cervical paraspinal 10 U each side |

B. Procerus 5 U (one site) | | | G. Trapezius 15 U each side |

C. Frontalis 10 U each side |

Figure 8.1 Paradigm for injection of onabotulinumtoxinA for chronic migraine.

a reduction in both peripheral and central sensitization; direct antinociceptive effects through blockage of CGRP and glutamate release; and lastly possibly a direct muscle relaxant effect that may also play a role in headache management in some patients. The most likely mechanism of action is that the preventive effect of onabotulinumtoxinA in chronic migraine is due to its ability to inhibit motor neuron overactivity and sensory neuron hyperexcitability, leading to suppression of peripheral and central sensitization.

One barrier to use of onabotulinumtoxinA is cost, although this may be partially offset by savings through reduced usage of expensive abortive agents such as triptans and by fewer emergency department visits by those who respond to the treatment. Preapproval from the patient's health insurer is often required, a process that adds work and can significantly delay the initiation of therapy. OnabotulinumtoxinA is not interchangeable with other botulinum neurotoxins and at the time of this writing is the only FDA-approved neurotoxin for chronic migraine.

Diagnosis

Episodic migraine without aura.

Tip

Though useful in chronic migraine, onabotulinumtoxinA (Botox) is not indicated for and is not useful in the treatment of episodic migraine headache. Its use should be restricted to patients with well-documented chronic migraine.

A young woman with headache after head trauma

Case

A 19-year-old woman presented to the headache clinic with her mother to discuss persistent headaches after head trauma. The initial head injury had occurred one year ago while she was playing soccer and hit the shoulder of another player with her head. There was no loss of consciousness but she immediately developed dizziness, nausea, holocephalic headache, and balance difficulties. She was taken off the field and evaluated by her team trainer, who diagnosed her with a concussion. The concussive symptoms improved over the next three months without medication and she was able to return to play.

Several months later, during a spring-break trip, she sustained a second head trauma while off-roading on an all-terrain vehicle (ATV). She was not wearing a helmet and her ATV overturned, resulting in head trauma with loss of consciousness for around a minute. Her symptoms, including headache, immediately returned and have been persistent since. The headaches are present daily, usually better in the morning and worse in the evening. Activity, concentration, trying to read, sustained visual focus, loud noise, and bright lights all worsen the headache. The pain may reach 8/10 and can be pulsing or throbbing, though still holocephalic. She denies any aura. She has been tried on amitriptyline without any benefit.

What factors predisposed this patient to the development of post-traumatic headache?

In a recent multicenter study done to determine factors associated with headache after traumatic brain injury (TBI), the most significant risk factor for post-traumatic headache (PTH) was a pre-injury diagnosis of migraine or other headaches. Penetrating-type TBI and female sex were also associated. In a pediatric study, adolescents were more likely to develop post-concussive headache than younger children. Other factors associated with development of chronic PTH include mild (rather than moderate or severe) head trauma and low educational and socioeconomic status. While not formally studied as a risk factor for headache, repeat head trauma often causes more severe post-concussive symptoms.

Upon further questioning, the patient denied a history of headache prior to the injury. She was very prone to motion sickness both as a child and through her adolescent years, however, and she had a strong family history of migraine. Both of these factors suggest an underlying predisposition to headache. This, in combination with her age, sex, and multiple head traumas, may have contributed to the risk of developing PTH.

What treatment options are available for this patient?

There is very little high quality evidence on which to base treatment of PTH. Prophylactic therapies for PTH have not been compared in randomized controlled trials, but open-label studies suggest benefit from amitriptyline, topiramate, valproate, and propranolol. Case reports have also described improvement after botulinum toxin treatments. We approach PTH as though it were the underlying headache disorder it most resembles, treating migrainous headaches with migraine preventatives, cluster-like headaches with verapamil, etc. This approach extends to symptomatic treatment, and in our experience patients who have migrainous PTH exacerbations may respond well to triptan therapy.

In this case, the patient had headaches with migrainous features and the care plan was modeled after treatment of migraine. She was started on topiramate with partial improvement, and had nearly complete resolution after the addition of low-dose propranolol. A trial of sumatriptan was also successful for management of individual severe headaches.

Discussion

The incidence of TBI is increasing in many populations, particularly among soldiers returning from combat and young athletes. Increased recognition of TBI in athletes may also be contributing to the rise in diagnosis. Headache is the most common symptom accompanying concussion, is often the first post-concussive symptom to develop, and is typically the last to resolve. PTH does not have any specific clinical criteria, and the diagnosis is made based on a temporal relationship to head trauma. Currently, the diagnosis is made if the headache develops within seven days of head or neck trauma, although many providers who work with TBI patients describe development of headache with a longer delay. This is a subject of some debate in the headache community.

A headache meeting the clinical criteria for migraine is the most commonly described phenotype, but headaches resembling tension-type headache, cluster headache, occipital neuralgia, and cervicogenic headache have also been described after head trauma. The headache may also be nonspecific, not fully resembling any primary headache disorder. Diagnosis can be complicated in younger patients as the first presentations of many primary headache disorders typically occur at this age. In our experience, mild head trauma may be a precipitating event for the emergence of an underlying primary headache disorder.

There are no data to suggest when to start prophylactic treatment for PTH. Some providers feel that starting treatment early, after a few weeks of headache, may return the patient to function more quickly. This approach may delay return to play/work, however, as the current guidelines for returning to full activity require that the patient is asymptomatic off medications. Other providers wait for several months of persistent headache prior to starting preventive treatment. If the patient is still having bothersome headache several months after the injury, preventive therapy is indicated.

As this case illustrates, patients with repeated head trauma may experience more severe post-concussive symptoms with each successive head trauma. Patients should be educated about the risks of successive head traumas and advised to wear helmets. After a second concussion, a discussion about whether to return to playing contact sports may be warranted.

Diagnosis

Chronic post-traumatic headache after mild head injury.

Tip

Post-traumatic headache is more likely to occur after mild head injuries and with repeat head injuries. Treatment is aimed at the headache type it most resembles.

Further reading

When to start prevention in patients with frequent headaches

Buchanan TM, Ramadan NM. Prophylactic pharmacotherapy for migraine headaches. *Semin Neurol.* 2006;26(2):188–98.

Weight gain and migraine

Blumenfeld AM, Bloudek LM, Becker WJ, *et al.* Patterns of use and reasons for discontinuation of prophylactic medications for episodic migraine and chronic migraine: results from the second international burden of migraine study (IBMS-II). *Headache.* 2013;53(4): 644–55.

Vo M, Ainalem A, Qiu C, *et al.* Body mass index and adult weight gain among reproductive age women with migraine. *Headache.* 2011;51(4):559–69.

Winter AC, Wang L, Buring JE, Sesso HD, Kurth T. Migraine, weight gain and the risk of becoming overweight and obese: a prospective cohort study. *Cephalalgia.* 2012;32(13):963–71.

Young WB, Rozen T. Preventive treatment of migraine: effect on weight. *Cephalalgia.* 2005;25(1):1–11.

Principles and guidelines for migraine prevention

Loder E, Burch R, Rizzoli P. The 2012 AHS/AAN guidelines for prevention of episodic migraine: a summary and comparison with other recent clinical practice guidelines. *Headache.* 2012;52(6):930–45.

Rizzoli, P. Acute and preventive treatment of migraine. *Continuum (Minneap Minn).* 2012;18(4):764–82.

Silberstein SD, Holland S, Feitag F, *et al.* Evidence-based guideline update: pharmacologic treatment for episodic migraine prevention in adults: report of the Quality Standards Subcommittee of the American Academy of Neurology and the American Headache Society. *Neurology.* 2012;78:1337–45.

Refractory migraine

Peterlin BL, Calhoun AH, Siegel S, Mathew NT. Rational combination therapy in refractory migraine. *Headache.* 2008;48(6):805–19.

Silberstein SD, Dodick DW, Lindblad AS, *et al.* Randomized, placebo-controlled trial of propranolol added to topiramate in chronic migraine. *Neurology.* 2012;78:976–84.

Combination treatment of migraine

Domingues RB, Silva AL, Domingues SA, Aquino CC, Kuster GW. A double-blind randomized controlled trial of low doses of propranolol, nortriptyline, and the combination of propranolol and nortriptyline for the preventive treatment of migraine. *Arq Neuropsiquiatr.* 2009;67(4):973–7.

Holroyd KA, Cottrell CK, O'Donnell FJ, *et al.* Effect of preventive (beta blocker) treatment, behavioural migraine management, or their combination on outcomes of optimised acute treatment in frequent migraine: randomised controlled trial. *BMJ.* 2010;341: c4871.

Paresthesias on topiramate

Lee ST, Chu K, Park JE, *et al.* Paresthesia as a favorable predictor of migraine prophylaxis using topiramate. *Eur J Neurol.* 2007;14(6):654–8.

Luykx J, Mason M, Ferrari MD, Carpay J. Are migraineurs at increased risk of adverse drug responses? A meta-analytic comparison of adverse drug reactions in epilepsy and migraine. *Clin Pharmacol Ther.* 2009;85(3): 283–8.

Silberstein SD. Control of topiramate-induced paresthesias with supplemental potassium. *Headache.* 2002;42(1):85.

Medication overuse headache

Hagen K, Albretsen C, Vilming ST, *et al.* Management of medication overuse headache: 1-year randomized multicentre open-label trial. *Cephalalgia.* 2009;29(2): 221–32.

Tepper SJ. Medication-overuse headache. *Continuum (Minneap Minn).* 2012;18(4):807–22.

Orthostatic hypotension

Mussi C, Ungar A, Salvioli G, *et al.* Orthostatic hypotension as cause of syncope in patients older than 65 years admitted to emergency departments for transient loss of consciousness. *J Gerontol A Biol Sci Med Sci.* 2009;64(7):801–6.

O'Mahony D, Foote C. Prospective evaluation of unexplained syncope, dizziness, and falls among community-dwelling elderly adults. *J Gerontol A Biol Sci Med Sci.* 1998;53(6):M435–40.

Angle-closure glaucoma from amitriptyline

Boentert M, Aretz H, Ludemann P. Acute myopia and angle-closure glaucoma induced by topiramate. *Neurology.* 2003;61:1306.

Bouassida W. Drug-induced acute angle closure glaucoma. *Curr Opin Ophthalmol.* 2007;18:129–33

Long-term side effects of topiramate

Ali II, Herial NA, Orris M, Horrigan T, Tietjen GE. Migraine prophylaxis with topiramate and bone health in women. *Headache.* 2011;51:613–16.

Láinez MJ, Freitag FG, Pfeil J, *et al.* Time course of adverse events most commonly associated with topiramate for migraine prevention. *Eur J Neurol.* 2007;14(8):900–6.

Mikati MA, Ataya N, El-Hajj Fuleihan G. Re: Epilepsy-associated bone mineral density loss should be prevented. *Neurology.* 2009;72(10):943; author reply 943–4.

Pack AM, Morrell MJ. Adverse effects of antiepileptic drugs on bone structure: epidemiology, mechanisms and therapeutic implications. *CNS Drugs.* 2001;15(8):633–42.

Topiramate and oral contraceptive efficacy

Reddy DS. Clinical pharmacokinetic interactions between antiepileptic drugs and hormonal contraceptives. *Expert Rev Clin Pharmacol.* 2010;3(2):183–92.

Drug-induced seizures

Ruffmann C, Bogliun G, Beghi E. Epileptogenic drugs: a systematic review. *Expert Rev Neurother.* 2006;6(4):575–89.

Synergistic side effects and drug-induced headache

Brouwers L, Iskar M, Zeller G, van Noort V, Bork P. Network neighbors of drug targets contribute to drug side-effect similarity. *PLoS One.* 2011;6(7):e22187.

Chakor RT, Bharote HS. Topiramate-valproate-induced encephalopathy in migraine. *Headache.* 2012;52(8):1321–2.

Chen HC, Tsai SJ. Trazodone-induced severe headache. *Psychiatry Clin Neurosci.* 2011;65(7):681–2.

Garcia-Serna R, Mestres J. Anticipating drug side effects by comparative pharmacology. *J Expert Opin Drug Metab Toxicol.* 2010;6(10):1253–63.

OnabotulinumtoxinA for chronic migraine

Blumenfeld A, Evans RW. OnabotulinumtoxinA for chronic migraine. *Headache.* 2012;52:142–8.

Blumenfeld A, Silberstein SD, Dodick DW, *et al.* Method of injection of onabotulinumtoxinA for chronic migraine: a safe, well-tolerated, and effective treatment paradigm based on the PREEMPT clinical program. *Headache.* 2010;50:1406–18.

Durham PL, Cady R. Insights into the mechanism of onabotulinumtoxinA in chronic migraine. *Headache.* 2011;51:1573–7.

Evans RW. A rational approach to the management of chronic migraine. *Headache.* 2013;53:168–76.

Post-traumatic headaches

Erickson JC, Neely ET, Theeler BJ. Posttraumatic headache. *Continuum (Minneap Minn).* 2010;16(6 Traumatic Brain Injury):55–78.

Lucas S. Headache management in concussion and mild traumatic brain injury. *PM R.* 2011;3(10 Suppl 2):S406–12.

Walker WC, Marwitz JH, Wilk AR, *et al.* Prediction of headache severity (density and functional impact) after traumatic brain injury: a longitudinal multicenter study. *Cephalalgia.* 2013;33(12):998–1008.

Pitfalls in nonpharmacologic treatment of headache

Although medications are the mainstay of headache treatment, nonpharmacologic treatments are often pursued as alternatives by both patients and practitioners. "Nonpharmacologic treatment" is a term often used to refer to a heterogeneous group of therapies. These range from adjunctive integrative therapies such as vitamins, supplements, mind–body practices, and behavioral therapies to potentially invasive procedures including surgery or nerve blocks.

Interest in nonpharmacologic treatments of all kinds is increasing in both popular culture and among providers. As more evidence about these treatments emerges they are becoming more mainstream and patients feel more comfortable asking for or about them. Many of these treatments have useful roles in headache management. They can be helpful for patients who do not tolerate medications or are averse to the idea of taking medications, and can also be useful adjuncts for those already using pharmacologic therapy.

While these therapies may seem benign, they are not without risk. In fact, the risks of the non-medication treatments are often overlooked because these treatments are perceived as safer and less likely to cause adverse events than traditional medical therapy. In many cases, however, there is a lack of good data about safety, and nonpharmacologic medications that are classified as dietary supplements are exempted from strong regulatory oversight by the US Food and Drug Administration (FDA). These things should lead to considerable caution on the part of doctors in recommending some of these interventions to patients. Most of all, nonpharmacologic interventions should not be assumed to be risk free, but instead should be evaluated in a similar fashion to any other intervention. In general, however, these treatments are well tolerated.

In this chapter, we will discuss the indications and pitfalls of some commonly used nonpharmacologic treatments for headache. Surgical interventions sometimes considered for migraine treatment are also discussed here. We will start, however, by considering the role of trigger avoidance in headache management – perhaps the most basic nonpharmacologic intervention of all.

A young woman with dietary triggers for headache

Case

A 23-year-old woman presented for a second opinion regarding her headaches. She had had headaches that met criteria for migraine without aura about twice a week since she was a young teenager. Initially these were well managed with nonprescription analgesics such as acetaminophen or ibuprofen, but over the last several years these had stopped working. A previous physician had started her on a triptan but also told her that her headaches were likely due to environmental factors, specifically her diet. Since that visit about one year ago, she had eliminated multiple foods, including lactose, gluten, soy, tree nuts, alcohol, and chocolate. Although none of these changes had substantially reduced the frequency of her headaches, the patient was afraid to reintroduce any of these foods lest her headaches worsen. She was very distressed in the office and stated that she is losing weight because she did not know what she could eat, and that her dietary restrictions prevented her from going out with her friends. On exam she was very thin but the neurologic exam was normal.

What is the relationship between dietary factors and migraine?

The possible effect of specific foods or even entire diets on frequency of migraine is a topic of much interest to both headache practitioners and patients. Up to 46% of migraine patients identified dietary triggers in one study, and another found that 75% of patients with chronic headache reported they were aware of possible connections between food intake and headache.

There are several possible mechanisms by which a certain food could be associated with migraine: direct toxic or metabolic effect, vasodilation, and allergic response are all plausible biologic explanations, while conditioned taste aversion, expectation and self-fulfilling prophecy, or confounding factors (such as when stress triggers both consumption of a certain food and headache, thus causing the appearance of the food triggering the headache) are behavioral explanations. The role of anchoring cannot be overstated, as patients will almost always have eaten something in the 24 hours prior to having a migraine, thus making diet an easy target when searching for a cause.

Fasting is a well-established trigger for migraines. This is often seen in patients who fast for religious reasons, including the observance of Yom Kippur or Ramadan. Patients who habitually skip meals may find that eating more regular meals may help to reduce headache frequency.

In this case, it seems unlikely that any individual dietary trigger is responsible for her headaches. This case illustrates the potential harm in placing undue emphasis on dietary triggers in migraine.

What is the quality of evidence about dietary triggers for migraine and what is the best advice for this patient?

Given the subjective experience of patients and the emphasis given to dietary triggers in popular literature, controlled studies are surprisingly inconclusive and by and large do not support any universal statements about the relationship between diet and migraine. Alcohol, chocolate, and cheese are the dietary triggers most commonly reported by migraineurs. In one placebo-controlled dietary challenge study, subjects who identified chocolate as the dietary trigger were fed bars containing chocolate or a closely matched placebo, and headaches in fact were more likely to occur in the group fed chocolate. No study has found that cheese or its hypothesized triggering agent, tyramine, reliably causes migraine. Red wine, however, does have some evidence to support activity as a migraine trigger. In a study comparing red

wine with disguised vodka, 9 of 11 patients who drank red wine developed a headache while none of the 8 who drank vodka did. As limited as these studies may seem, there is even less evidence for any influence of gluten or lactose. No studies examining the effect of a gluten- or lactose-free diet on headache have been performed.

In this case, the patient could be counseled about the lack of clear evidence for a relationship between diet and migraine. It may be helpful, however, to provide anecdotal support for the idea that certain foods seem to reliably trigger headaches in some patients. She need not be hostage to her diet, however. She could try gradually reintroducing foods one at a time, keeping a headache diary to assess the effect on headaches.

Discussion

There is clearly tremendous interest in dietary precipitants of headache and migraine, both among patients and among physicians. A "migraine diet" of some kind is a common component of many popular lay programs for treatment of migraine. The rise of public awareness about food intolerance and allergies, along with widespread acceptance of elimination diets also contributes to interest in this approach to management of medical conditions. A possible dietary effect on migraine is biologically plausible, especially for substances that have direct or indirect effects on vascular tone or levels of biogenic amines that might be involved in migraine. The evidence, however, is scant, making an evidence-based recommendation about dietary triggers in migraine challenging.

It should also be noted that recommending the elimination of multiple food groups from the diet is not entirely benign. A lack of specific nutrients may result, or, as in this patient, an overall lack of adequate caloric intake. Because the list of potential dietary migraine triggers is vast, large food groups become suspect to the patient. Over time this can encourage secondary anxiety around dietary choices, which in and of itself may contribute to worsened headache. Placing undue emphasis on dietary triggers of migraine may also have the unintended effect of making patients feel that they are entirely responsible for the frequency of their headaches. The balance between supporting a healthy lifestyle by avoiding known triggers and placing too much emphasis on environmental factors is a fine one.

If a patient expresses interest in an elimination diet, it may be helpful to give a systematic framework within which to conduct such trials. They may be encouraged to keep a diary for a time, identify a list of possible triggering foods, and then track headache frequency with the diary while eliminating each food for several weeks at a time. If no improvement in headaches is seen, the food can be reintroduced. This approach may help to identify triggers while preventing cumulative loss of whole food groups from the diet.

Diagnosis

Episodic migraine without aura with possible dietary triggers.

Tip

Evidence is lacking to support a clear role for many foods commonly assumed to be triggers of migraine. Physicians should be cautious about recommending highly restrictive dietary regimens for migraine, and avoid placing undue emphasis on dietary triggers.

A young woman with frequent headaches attempting pregnancy

Case

A 29-year-old woman presented for evaluation of migraine headaches since age 19, which had occurred about once a month until six months ago when they increased in frequency. The migraines seemed to be provoked by stress, let down from stress, lack of sleep, skipping meals, and caffeine. She worked as a medical assistant and had started school to train as a physician assistant around the time that the headaches worsened. Her quality and duration of sleep had declined. At the time of evaluation the headaches were occurring about twice a week, and she had started to miss work occasionally because of them.

She had been treating her headaches only with acetaminophen because she was planning to attempt pregnancy in the next several months. Her exam was normal and she had a negative MRI and blood work ordered by her primary care physician.

Is this patient's description of headache triggers likely to be accurate?

Most patients with migraine (between 75% and 95%) report having headache triggers, or precipitants that bring on a headache. The research on triggers is, however, surprisingly thin. Researching triggers is difficult as it is very difficult to isolate single triggers in real life. Studies attempting to verify specific triggers such as changes in barometric pressure have been negative. Further complicating the question of triggers is the phenomenon of "anchoring," which occurs when patients (or doctors!) connect an outcome with a recent event. Those two conditions become connected in the patient's mind and evidence to support this connection is unconsciously sought. Therefore, someone may have a headache after eating tomatoes and from then on pay more attention to headaches that occur after eating tomatoes.

Despite the lack of evidence, however, some events are clearly linked to the development of headaches in some patients. In this case, the patient noted a clear correlation between drinking coffee and developing a headache within the next hour. When a trigger is reliably reproducible, as in this example, the trigger is likely to be accurate.

Is there a role for trigger avoidance in this case?

Just as there is poor evidence for individual triggers for headache, there are also very few data about the role of trigger avoidance in the management of headache. Despite this lack of evidence, however, we have seen repeatedly in our clinic that patients often improve when some effort at trigger management is undertaken. Some triggers can be addressed with behavioral changes, such as sleep hygiene (see Table 9.1), eating regular meals, and avoidance of situations likely to involve strong sensory input (the perfume counter at a department store, for example). Some triggers, however, cannot be avoided, particularly including hormonal variation. For some patients, avoidance of some life stress is simply not feasible. Trigger management alone is therefore unlikely to be an adequate preventative strategy in cases of severe or frequent headache, but in less frequent or milder headache disorders it may be sufficient. In a setting where preventive medication therapy is not desired, these and other behavioral interventions are at least a good place to start. In

Table 9.1. Sleep hygiene principles

Maintain a regular sleep schedule, including a regular bedtime and waking time

Do not sleep more than is necessary to feel rested. Do not stay in bed long after waking up

Do not "force" sleep. If unable to sleep after 20 minutes, get out of bed and do something calming

Avoid caffeine after 2 p.m. and alcohol in the evenings

Avoid smoking, especially at night

Do not go to sleep on an empty stomach or just after eating

Keep a daily exercise schedule, but avoid exercise within 4 hours of bedtime

Let go of worries before bed. It may help to take a warm bath before bed

Avoid electronics including TV before bed or in the bedroom

this case, quality and duration of sleep was addressed with sleep hygiene and her headaches decreased in frequency to about once a week. These were relatively well managed with acetaminophen.

Discussion

We distinguish between migraine *triggers*, which increase the probability of a migraine attack in the short term (usually < 48 hours) and migraine *aggravating factors*, which are associated with a longer-term (usually weeks to months) increase in the severity or frequency of attacks. The most commonly reported triggers, in addition to stress/tension, are menstruation in women, sensory input (bright lights, loud sounds, strong odors), lack of sleep, and skipping meals. It also seems likely that triggers may be additive, in that one trigger alone may not be sufficient to cause headache but multiple simultaneous triggers (such as exposure to a strong odor while sleep deprived) may provoke a headache.

The idea that avoidance of triggers is an effective method of migraine prevention is an old one, and we see many patients who have been told that if they could only identify and eliminate their headache triggers, their headaches would resolve. This idea seems to follow good old-fashioned common sense: if something gives you a headache, do not do it. There are currently no data to suggest that this is an effective strategy for migraine prevention, however. Placing undue emphasis on trigger avoidance may even be detrimental to the patient's care. It has been suggested that trying to manage migraines through trigger avoidance can lead to a restriction of activities and increased

life stress. This increased stress could paradoxically increase headaches, as the most commonly reported headache trigger is typically "stress/tension."

Diagnosis

Episodic migraine.

Tip

Patient recall of triggers is not always reliable. Trigger management alone is often not sufficient treatment for frequent or severe headache disorders.

A woman with frequent headaches and multiple allergies

Case

A 39-year-old woman presented for evaluation of headaches occurring about three times a week. The headaches often met criteria for tension-type headache but several times a month she would have more severe migrainous headaches. The headaches had been increasing in frequency over the last year, which she associates with increased stress related to her mother-in-law becoming ill and moving into their home for an increased level of care. She also had two young children. She reported a large number of medication allergies and sensitivities including several previously tried headache preventatives. At the visit, she stated that she didn't want to pursue further preventive trials because "I do very badly with medications and they don't work for me anyway."

What nonpharmacologic options are available to this patient?

The term "nonpharmacologic" may refer to several types of therapeutic interventions, including behavioral strategies, complementary modalities, and herbs and supplements. These last are discussed later in this chapter. Of the treatments that do not involve ingesting a substance of some kind, behavioral treatments, which include biofeedback, cognitive behavioral therapy, and relaxation training have been the most studied. Complementary treatments (also called complementary and alternative, alternative, or integrative therapies) include acupuncture, chiropractic care, craniosacral therapy, and massage. Table 9.2 lists some nonpharmacologic interventions.

Table 9.2. Nonpharmacolgic therapies

Behavioral:
– Relaxation training
– Biofeedback
– Cognitive behavioral therapy

Complementary and alternative:
– Craniosacral therapy
– Acupuncture
– Chiropractic care
– Massage

The primary limitation for access for many patients is cost, as these therapies are rarely covered by insurance. Despite the greater volume of data for behavioral therapies, there are typically fewer practitioners trained in modalities such as biofeedback or relaxation training than there are practitioners of acupuncture, chiropractic care, or massage. Access to these behavioral treatments may also therefore be limited by access to providers. The effort required to learn a behavioral treatment may also be a barrier to use.

For this patient, who is motivated and willing to pay for treatments not covered by her insurance, nonpharmacologic therapies could be recommended on the basis of efficacy.

How successful are these interventions likely to be?

Behavioral treatments used for treatment of migraine are the most studied nonpharmacologic treatments. A comprehensive review of meta-analyses and evidence-based reviews included studies of all three types of behavioral treatments. This review found that all three forms of behavioral therapy are associated with a 30–60% reduction in headache activity. Likewise, the US Headache Consortium in 2000 gave a Grade A recommendation to relaxation training, thermal biofeedback combined with relaxation training, electromyography (EMG) biofeedback, and cognitive behavioral therapy, indicating that all of them "may be considered as treatment options for prevention of migraine."

Acupuncture has also been shown to be effective for prevention of migraine. A 2009 Cochrane review found that compared with no preventative treatment or routine care, acupuncture reduced headache frequency, overall headache days, and headache scores at three to four months. In the one trial with long-term follow-up, this effect seemed to dissipate by nine months after cessation of treatment. There was

no difference in improvement seen when comparing groups who received true vs. sham acupuncture. Compared with pharmacologic treatments, acupuncture had slightly better outcomes and fewer side effects. There are very little data available regarding the efficacy of craniosacral therapy.

Systematic reviews show spinal manipulation produces some improvement of migraine headache compared with drug treatment, but the level of evidence was rated as modest. There have been only a handful of very small studies of the efficacy of massage for headache, though these did show some benefit.

While it is difficult to say which treatment will be the most successful in a given individual, thermal biofeedback combined with relaxation training and/or cognitive behavioral therapy may be the most helpful interventions.

Discussion

Behavioral treatments for management of headache have been in use for at least 40 years. The three types most often used and studied are cognitive behavioral therapy, relaxation training, and biofeedback. Cognitive behavioral therapy is conducted by a licensed therapist and is short term, goal directed, and predicated on the idea that changing dysfunctional thoughts can change emotions and on reducing behaviors or environmental events that reinforce negative thoughts. As applied to headache, it is often used as a tool for identifying and managing sources of stress. Emphasis is placed on empowering an individual to choose their thoughts and behaviors (internal locus of control). A therapist with the goal of inducing global relaxation or the "relaxation response" does relaxation training. This may be done as a guided exercise or may be enhanced by biofeedback. Biofeedback allows the patient to control physiologic parameters through awareness of those parameters. Parameters used include muscle tone (measured by EMG), temperature, and heart rate. This may also help patients to learn how to relax certain muscles, lower their heart rate, or induce relaxation.

The rationale for various complementary and alternative therapies varies. It is sometimes difficult to generalize about them as there is a lot of heterogeneity within specific modalities. Acupuncture was developed in ancient China and involves placing needles into the skin at certain prespecified points. It is one of the most commonly used complementary and

Table 9.3. Who will benefit from behavioral treatments?

Patients who
- Have poor or inadequate response to treatment with medication
- Have contraindications to pharmacologic treatments for medical reasons
- Do not tolerate pharmacologic treatments well
- Express a preference for nonpharmacologic treatments
- Are prone to overusing acute medications or have medication overuse headache
- Have a high burden of stress or would benefit from improved stress coping strategies
- Are pregnant or planning to become pregnant

alternative treatments, and is frequently used for treatment of headache. Of the roughly 4% of the US population who reported ever being treated with acupuncture, 10% of them had been treated for headache. Craniosacral therapy is a gentle hands-on modality that purports to make changes to pulsations of the intracranial fluid by manipulation of the cranium and sacrum.

Chiropractic care and massage are usually focused on addressing musculoskeletal abnormalities which are hypothesized to cause headache. Although the literature has not formally addressed this issue, we have anecdotally seen many patients whose headaches worsen after these treatments. Massage or manipulation of the cervical area particularly may provoke headache. Other patients, particularly those whose headaches seem strongly related to cervical and shoulder tension, may derive some benefit from massage. Evidence about the relationship between vertebral artery dissection (VAD) and chiropractic cervical manipulation is contradictory, but at this time we advise our patients to avoid high velocity rotational manipulation of the neck.

Not all patients are equally likely to benefit from a nonpharmacologic intervention. A review of behavioral therapies found that between 40% and 70% of patients did not respond to these therapies, and that medication overuse headache, chronic daily or unremitting headache, and cluster or post-traumatic headaches are all more likely to be refractory to these treatments. The US Headache Consortium defined a group of patients who are likely to benefit from nonpharmacologic therapies, as shown in Table 9.3.

The patient in this case met several of the US Headache Consortium criteria for patients who would benefit from behavioral therapies. She was recommended to undergo training for biofeedback, which she was able to do. She was also referred for cognitive

behavioral therapy. With this, her headaches improved to about once a week. Although she would have preferred to have fewer headaches, she felt this headache frequency was manageable.

Diagnosis
Mixed tension-type and migraine headaches.

Tip
In patients who cannot or do not want to use pharmacologic treatment, nonpharmacologic treatments may be helpful preventive strategies.

A woman interested in natural treatments for migraine

Case
A 33-year-old woman presented to the office with a history of migraines with aura since age 16. They had occurred about twice a month until earlier in the year, when frequency gradually increased. She was not able to identify any precipitating factors. At the time of the visit she was having headaches at least once and sometimes twice a week. The headaches were unchanged in character from her previous migraines. Her neurologic examination was normal and no further workup was felt necessary. Preventive medications were offered, but she said "I don't want to go on a medication every day. Isn't there something natural I can take?"

What vitamins or supplements might be recommended?
The three most commonly studied vitamins or supplements for the prevention of migraine are magnesium, vitamin B2 (riboflavin), and coenzyme Q10 (CoQ10). Several placebo-controlled trials have examined the efficacy of magnesium with conflicting but largely positive results. The doses tested were 360 to 600 mg/day. Magnesium is generally well tolerated, with gastrointestinal symptoms being the most common and diarrhea being the most frequently described limiting factor. This may depend to some extent on the magnesium salt used. Magnesium should not be used in patients with renal failure.

Riboflavin has also been tested in controlled trials and generally has very few side effects other than turning urine bright yellow. Riboflavin, like magnesium,

Table 9.4. Vitamins, supplements, and herbs used in the prevention of migraine

Vitamins and supplements	Doses	Side effects	Notes
Magnesium	400–600 mg/day	Gastrointestinal upset, diarrhea	Oxide and chelates may be better tolerated. May require several months for efficacy. Useful for migraine with aura and in pregnancy
Vitamin B2 (riboflavin)	400 mg/day	Turns urine fluorescent yellow	Not studied in pregnancy. May require up to 3 months for efficacy
Coenzyme Q10	150 mg/day	Insomnia if taken at night	Less evidence for efficacy; expensive
Herbs			
Feverfew	150 mg daily	Mouth ulcerations, gastrointestinal upset	Not safe in pregnancy
Butterbur (*Petasites*)	75 mg bid	Burping	Not safe in pregnancy. Quality control of preparation essential given toxicity of whole plant extracts

likely needs to be taken for several months for benefit to be seen. CoQ10 has little data to support its use in the adult population of migraineurs, although there is some evidence in the pediatric literature. It seems well tolerated aside from causing possible insomnia if taken at night.

Magnesium and riboflavin may be good options to recommend to the patient described in the vignette. Magnesium may be particularly effective in patients with aura, yet another reason to recommend it to this patient.

Would herbal treatments be helpful?

Feverfew and butterbur (genus *Petasites*) are two herbs that have been studied for migraine prevention. In the recent American Headache Society/American Academy of Neurology (AHS/AAN) guidelines, butterbur received a Category A rating, suggesting that it "should be offered" to patients. Feverfew received a Category B rating ("should be considered") in the AHS/AAN guidelines. The dose of butterbur is typically 75 mg given orally twice daily and feverfew is typically dosed at 150 mg orally daily. There are safety concerns about the possible presence of alkaloids in butterbur and neither of these herbs should be considered safe during pregnancy. This may limit recommendations for their use in this woman of childbearing age.

Both of these treatments are generally well tolerated. One sometimes bothersome effect of butterbur is eructation (burping). Feverfew can cause mouth soreness and ulcerations, stomach upset, and abdominal pain. Because of their benign tolerability profile, patients often seek these herbal treatments. Lastly, for treatment of nausea in this patient, ginger tea or ginger supplements might be recommended.

Discussion

Vitamins, supplements, and herbal treatments commonly used for migraine are summarized in Table 9.4. These treatments may be useful for patients who would like to avoid "medications" on a daily basis. Because the FDA has limited regulatory oversight of herbal treatments and supplements, there can be a great deal of variation in the strength of the active ingredients. The amount of active ingredient in feverfew preparations, for example, has been shown to vary by 400% among different formulations. Different magnesium salts may also have differing effects, as some are absorbed more completely than others. For this reason, it can be difficult to know exactly what substances a patient is taking when they purchase and use one of these treatments.

Many of the trials of magnesium for prevention of migraine have shown some benefit on migraine, with one negative trial and one equivocal trial. Certain magnesium salts are not well absorbed and may not be effective, though no study has compared efficacy between the different magnesium salts. In our practice, we typically recommend 400–500 mg daily and caution that it may take several months for effects to be seen. We find magnesium chelate and oxide to be generally well tolerated. The clearest indication for magnesium is probably in patients who have migraine with aura, or in patients in whom aura is the predominant symptom. Magnesium is also considered a good choice during pregnancy. Patients who have low serum or red blood cell magnesium may also be particularly responsive.

Riboflavin (vitamin B2) and CoQ10 are mitochondrial cofactors. CoQ10 has been somewhat better studied in the pediatric literature. One trial compared a combination of riboflavin, magnesium, and fever-few (marketed as Migralief) with riboflavin alone and with placebo. Both the riboflavin and the combination group saw improvement in migraine days and other endpoints. In our clinic, we often recommend magnesium and riboflavin 400 mg daily given together. Riboflavin has not been studied in pregnancy and we do not recommend its use in pregnancy. Because CoQ10 is a costly supplement with limited evidence of benefit, we do not recommend it to patients in our clinic. Adverse events are, however, low and there have been no reported safety concerns, so we do not discourage its use if patients are interested.

Although herbal treatments are available without a prescription, there are safety concerns. In addition to being associated with significant fetal risk, *Petasites* requires another safety caveat: the rhizomes and stalks of the plant contain hepatotoxic and carcinogenic pyrrolizidine alkaloids. Concentrations of these alkaloids are lowest in the leaves. Because of this, *Petasites* should be obtained from a reputable manufacturer who can guarantee lack of toxicity. Feverfew has not been studied in pregnancy and should be avoided given its herbal medicine use to induce labor and promote uterine contractions.

Diagnosis

Episodic migraine with aura.

Tip

Although available without a prescription, the long-term safety of herbal treatments and supraphysiologic doses of vitamins has not been well studied. They may be helpful for patients who are averse to taking prescription medications, however.

A middle-aged man with pain in the neck

Case

A 38-year-old data entry technician was seen with complaints of refractory neck and head pain. He reported that his pain began about three years ago when his work station was equipped with a new monitor and computer system. The placement of the monitor required him to turn his head to the left to see it, while the data he entered into the computer were on cards and pieces of paper that were placed to his right.

The patient noted that his pain was left-sided and radiated to the back and front of his head on the left. It was constant, not throbbing, and rated on average 4–5 on a 0–10 pain scale. He had no other associated symptoms such as nausea, photo or phonophobia. Initially the pain was intermittent and cleared after the patient left work and was able to change his posture and relax. For the last few months, however, it had increased in frequency and was often present after he left work. He was using over-the-counter ibuprofen with some relief.

The patient's physical and neurologic examinations were normal with the exception of decreased neck mobility, tenderness, and tightness and increased tone of the left neck and shoulder muscles. Neck X-rays showed minimal degenerative changes of the spine. He was diagnosed with migraine and given rizatriptan to use when the pain was severe. He returned several weeks later to say that the rizatriptan was not helpful and his pain was unchanged.

Was a diagnosis of migraine warranted?

This patient did have unilateral head pain of moderate intensity, but he had no other migrainous symptoms. Furthermore, his pain did not respond to a reasonable dose of a specific anti-migraine drug. Based on this patient's history, his pain was most likely originating in structures in the neck. His problem appeared shortly after the installation of a new computer system at work that required him to sustain a nonphysiologic head posture frequently and for long periods of time. A cervical origin for his pain was suggested by examination findings of reduced neck mobility and increased muscle tenderness and tone in the area of the affected muscles. His X-ray findings showed only minimal arthritic changes that were unlikely to be the cause of his pain.

The existence of "cervicogenic headache" is controversial, and there is disagreement about how a cervical cause of headache should be diagnosed, with several sets of diagnostic criteria in use. Most experts suggest that a diagnosis of cervicogenic headache can be made when pain is plausibly related to a neck source and experienced in the head or neck. This requires demonstration by imaging or other methods such as clinical examination of a disorder in the spine or adjacent soft tissues that is known to be a cause of head pain. The connection between this lesion and the pain should be demonstrated by pain relief with diagnostic blockade of the nerve supply of the suspected causative structure, as well as clinical signs that implicate the neck as a pain source.

There are plausible biologic explanations for the radiation of pain from neck structures into the head. The upper three cervical spinal nerves synapse with second-order neurons in the trigeminocervical nucleus of the upper spinal cord, which also receives input from first-order trigeminal neurons. "Crosstalk" between these converging neurons in the trigeminocervical complex may result in neck problems producing head pain, and vice versa.

What treatment should be suggested for this patient?

The authors of a recent systematic review of manual therapies for cervicogenic headache located only seven studies. These studies tested a variety of manual techniques for patients with head pain originating in the neck, including physical therapy, spinal manipulation, and jaw mobilization techniques. Unfortunately, the quality of included studies was low, with only one including a "no treatment" control group. The authors concluded that although there was a suggestion that physical therapy and manipulative therapy might be helpful for cervicogenic headache, further research was needed to substantiate any benefits. A recent randomized controlled trial of exercise and manipulative therapy for cervicogenic headache showed benefits for both of the individual treatments compared with a control group. The combination of the two treatments, however, was not clearly superior to either treatment alone.

In the absence of consensus about the best method of treatment, our practice is to begin with symptomatic treatment such as muscle relaxants and refer patients for physical therapy. We encourage the use of time-limited active physical therapy interventions such as postural training and exercises to improve cervical muscle mobility and strength. Passive techniques such as massage or ultrasound may offer temporary pain relief to some patients, but they can foster the development of dependence on continued physical therapy that is not in the patient's best long-term interests.

In this case, the occupational environment was likely contributing to the patient's problem. The physical therapist visited the patient's workplace and suggested rearrangement of his work station and alteration of the flow and processes of his work. At a follow-up visit the patient was no longer bothered by substantial neck pain. Some physicians would refer patients like this who do not respond to conservative measures for local anesthetic blocks of the C2 nerve root, but in our experience this invasive procedure is rarely necessary. We do, however, sometimes use greater occipital nerve blockade in these patients.

Discussion

Cervicogenic headache is a cause of unilateral head and neck pain, usually without any side shift. The pain is moderate to severe but otherwise lacks typical associated features of other unilateral headache disorders. Specifically, it is not associated with nausea, vomiting, or photo or phonophobia, which can help distinguish it from migraine. It is not associated with autonomic features, which can help distinguish it from cluster headache. It is usually provoked by neck movement or posture. A plausible cervical source of pain, lack of response to triptan therapy, and the absence of typical migraine symptoms all point to a diagnosis of cervicogenic headache.

Although cervicogenic headache is a controversial diagnosis with no clear agreement on its features, it likely originates from anatomic structures in the cervical spine. Depending upon the criteria used to diagnose cervicogenic headache, its prevalence in the general population ranges from 1% to 4.6%.

Diagnosis

Cervicogenic headache.

Tip

Nonpharmacologic approaches such as physical therapy, postural training, and attention to environmental triggers are first-line treatment measures for cervicogenic headache.

A man with frequent headaches interested in chiropractic treatment

Case

A 52-year-old man came to the office for evaluation of headaches which had been gradually worsening over the last four years. They were bilateral, posterior, aching or throbbing, moderate in severity, without associated features, and lasting up to several hours at a time. He thought they seemed worst when he woke up in the morning, and he had attributed this to sleeping in a bad position and thus straining his neck. He had tried several different pillows without any improvement. Imaging showed mild arthritic changes in the cervical spine. He was given a diagnosis of cervicogenic vs. tension-type headache and was offered medication, but he wanted to try nonpharmacologic treatments instead. He particularly wanted to know if chiropractic care would be an option as one of his friends had good success with chiropractic treatments for back pain.

Is spinal manipulation likely to help his headaches?

A recent systematic review of spinal manipulation for treatment of migraine included three randomized controlled trials, all of which had significant methodologic limitations. The study with the best methodology showed no benefit for spinal manipulative therapy, while one study showed benefit but was of poorer quality. An attempt to develop evidence-based guidelines performed by a group of chiropractors and not limited to randomized controlled trials found moderate or below level evidence. They concluded that spinal manipulation could be recommended for treatment of episodic or chronic migraine and for cervicogenic headache, and that no recommendations could be made for treatment of tension-type headache. The authors state that "adverse events were not addressed in most clinical trials; and if they were, there were none or they were minor." These two studies illustrate some of the differences between recommendations made by physicians and by chiropractors. In brief, there are no good quality studies suggesting benefit from spinal manipulation, and studies showing benefit are limited by methodologic weaknesses. In clinical practice, there are anecdotal reports of patients who have improvement in their headaches after spinal manipulation.

This patient was told that anecdotally some patients report improvement in their headaches with chiropractic treatments but that the studies have not supported it as a treatment.

What should he be told about risks associated with spinal manipulation?

Spinal manipulation has been associated with risks ranging from minor to major. In a prospective case series of patients treated with spinal manipulation, minor adverse effects were reported by 30–60% of patients and included neck pain, stiffness, headache, and fatigue. In retrospective and case–control studies, more dangerous outcomes included disc herniation, vertebral fracture, dural tear, and, perhaps of most concern, VAD. (Carotid artery dissection is reported much less frequently than VAD, likely because the carotid artery is not tethered in the cervical region and therefore moves more freely.)

Several case–control studies have shown a relationship between spinal manipulation, whether by chiropractors or other practitioners (orthopedic surgeons, shiatsu practitioners), and VAD. One case–control study showed that patients with VADs were more likely to report previously having chiropractic upper spinal manipulation than those with carotid artery dissection (6% vs. 30%). Dissection of both vertebral arteries was also linked to spinal manipulation. In another case–control study, the odds of developing a VAD were five times higher within one week after a chiropractor visit in patients under the age of 45. These cases with VAD were also five times more likely to have seen a chiropractor three or more times in the last month for a cervical diagnosis.

Other studies have suggested a possible alternative interpretation for these data, however. A large case–control and case-crossover study of the population of Ontario evaluated risk for VAD or vertebrobasilar stroke as a function of visits to the chiropractor or to the primary care physician. In this study, cases under the age of 45 were three times more likely to have visited their primary care physician and three times more likely to have visited a chiropractor in the month prior to the stroke. There was no association for cases over the age of 45.

The authors of this study and others note that VAD often presents with headache and neck pain. Because of this, patients may present to a chiropractor or to their primary care physician for these symptoms before they are finally diagnosed. It may therefore be difficult to assess whether the increased risk noted by the case–control studies is simply a reflection of usage of chiropractic care for a pre-existing condition, rather than the chiropractic care causing that condition. As one chiropractor summed up the results of this study: "You are no more likely to have a dissection walking out of my office than out of your primary care physician's office." Our practice is to educate patients about the risks of VAD associated with chiropractic treatment when the issue is discussed at an office visit.

Discussion

VAD has an incidence of about 1.5/100 000 and often presents with headache and neck pain. The concern about adverse effects from spinal manipulation was initially raised in the 1990s after reports of two deaths due to artery dissection after neck manipulation. Since these initial reports, the question of how much risk for cervical artery dissection is attributable to spinal manipulation has been hotly debated. VADs are more common in the cervical regions than carotid artery dissections. The vertebral artery is highly susceptible to trauma due to torsion particularly at the C1–C2 junction, where it wraps around the atlas prior to entering the cranium. VAD is caused by a hematoma in the vessel wall, and may be spontaneous or, more commonly, associated with trauma of some kind. VAD has been attributed to sudden neck movements associated with spinal manipulation, but also with sport activities such as volleyball, heavy lifting, dental examination, turning the head while driving, or a prolonged episode of coughing. There is also a case report of a patient who regularly "cracked" her neck due to neck pain and developed a VAD.

There are several mechanisms by which a VAD can lead to stroke or other neurologic deficits. The expanding intramural hematoma may occlude the lumen of the vertebral artery or one of its branches. If the hematoma expands outward, adjacent structures may be compromised. Lastly, dissection of the high cervical vertebral artery may also be associated with thrombosis leading to embolic infarcts. It is probably safe to say that data regarding the risks of VAD associated with spinal manipulation are conflicting, and given the significant degree of morbidity associated with VAD it is probably safest to avoid this treatment until more is known.

Diagnosis

Tension-type headache vs. cervicogenic headache.

Tip

Chiropractic treatments for headache and neck pain do not have proven efficacy and may be associated with increased risk for serious adverse events such as VAD. Patients should be educated about these risks.

A pregnant woman with cluster headaches

Case

A 26-year-old woman was seen in the headache clinic because of severe headaches that started two weeks ago. Three years ago she experienced a two-month episode of daily or near-daily headaches similar to her current headaches. The headaches were located behind the left eye and were extremely severe, although they lasted just 45 minutes to an hour. They recurred nightly, usually an hour or so after she fell asleep. Headaches were associated with tearing of the left eye and stuffiness of the left nostril. The patient had sought evaluation for these headaches. A CT scan of the head was normal with the exception of some bilateral mucosal thickening of the maxillary sinuses. She was treated with antibiotics and decongestants but the headaches had not improved. She was then scheduled for sinus surgery but cancelled the operation when the headaches spontaneously disappeared.

Two weeks ago these headaches began again, but instead of coming just once a day they were occurring up to four times a day. In the clinic, her neurologic and physical examinations were normal. She was in good health but was eight weeks pregnant and did not wish to use any medications. She added, however, that she was "desperate" and might consider terminating the pregnancy if medication treatment could not be avoided.

What is the diagnosis, and what nondrug treatments might be considered?

The history of severe, retro-orbital pain with associated autonomic features is consistent with a diagnosis of cluster headache. The patient's attacks lasted 45 minutes, which is well within the typical range of 15 minutes to 3 hours for cluster headache. Furthermore, they occurred at night shortly after she fell asleep, a time that coincides with the usual onset of rapid-eye-movement sleep. This "alarm clock" timing is characteristic of cluster headache, which is sometimes considered a parasomnia because of its common occurrence during this phase of sleep.

Individual attacks of cluster headache are usually treated with sumatriptan injections or inhalation of 100% oxygen at 7–12 liters using a nonrebreather face mask. For this patient, oxygen is an attractive nondrug approach to the management of individual headaches. It is somewhat cumbersome, however, and since this patient has four headaches a day it is also desirable to do something to try to prevent headaches or reduce their occurrence.

Nondrug approaches to cluster headache prevention include the use of implantable sphenopalatine ganglion stimulators or attempts at peripheral nerve blockade, typically blockade of the greater occipital nerve on the side of the headaches. Peripheral nerve blocks provide immediate analgesia of the territory supplied by the targeted nerve, but for unclear reasons they may also produce pain relief that persists for days or even weeks after the short-term effects of the nerve block wear off. Some speculate that this is due to inhibition of central sensitization when painful peripheral input into the central nervous system is interrupted. The effectiveness of greater occipital nerve blockade for the treatment of cluster headache is supported by results from two double-blind, randomized controlled trials.

How are greater occipital nerve blocks performed, and how often can they be repeated?

The greater occipital nerve supplies sensation to the posterior portion of the scalp, and is a branch of the second cervical nerve. Because it is relatively superficial and easy to access in the posterior portion of the head, greater occipital nerve blockade is not a technically challenging procedure. Most experts recommend that the position for the nerve block is localized by imagining a line running between two scalp landmarks: the occipital protruberance and the mastoid process. The greater occipital nerve is likely to lie approximately one-third of the distance from the occipital protruberance on this line. The occipital artery is usually located laterally to the nerve, so palpation is important to avoid intra-arterial injections.

Greater occipital nerve blockade may be done using only a local anesthetic such as lidocaine 1–2% or bupivacaine 0.25–0.5%, or a corticosteroid can be added to the local anesthetic. The volume of local anesthetic injected is usually 1–3 mL per injection. The Peripheral Nerve Block Special Interest Section of the AHS recommends that injections can be repeated

every 2–4 weeks depending upon patient response. In our practice, we use a 5 mL syringe with a 27 gauge needle and 2 mL of 1% lidocaine. We typically do not use corticosteroids unless patients do not have a response to local anesthetic used alone. In pregnant patients lidocaine is the local anesthetic of choice, since it has an FDA use-in-pregnancy rating of B (compared with C for the alternative choice of bupivacaine). We also recommend avoiding the use of corticosteroids in patients who are pregnant.

The patient in this case was given oxygen to use for individual attacks of headache, and treated with left greater occipital nerve block in an attempt to prevent headaches. After her first injection she was headache-free for ten days. The injection was then repeated, and her headaches did not recur.

Discussion

Cluster headache is more common in men, but it also occurs in women. Because it is less common in women, physicians may be more likely to assume that the headaches have other causes. In this case, the headaches were initially misdiagnosed as a sinus problem. Delayed and inaccurate diagnosis of cluster headache is common in patients of both sexes, however. Unfortunately, this patient's experience is not unusual. Cluster headache is often attributed to sinus problems, which may then lead to unnecessary and usually ineffective sinus surgery.

Pharmacologic management of cluster headaches is usually highly effective. Most patients respond well to subcutaneous sumatriptan, and verapamil or lithium treatment often completely eliminates attacks. Because these are the standard therapies for the disorder, it is easy to overlook nonpharmacologic treatment options.

There are good reasons in this patient to avoid the use of lithium and verapamil. She is in her first trimester of pregnancy, when organogenesis is occurring and teratogenic effects are most likely to occur. Lithium use during pregnancy has been associated with fetal cardiac malformations, and the high doses of verapamil necessary to treat cluster headache effectively would be likely to exacerbate pregnancy-related edema and constipation. Thus, nondrug preventive approaches to treatment such as the use of occipital nerve blocks are a first-line approach in pregnant patients with cluster headache.

"Bridging" therapy with high-dose corticosteroids is often used to bring cluster headaches under control quickly until preventive medications become effective, but the safety of such treatment in pregnancy is unknown. Likewise, although accumulated information about sumatriptan suggests it is probably safe in pregnancy, the number of reported pregnancy outcomes is too small to rule out completely any residual teratogenic risk of the drug. Oxygen inhalation, on the other hand, is likely to be safe and is therefore the preferred method of abortive cluster headache treatment in pregnancy.

Diagnosis

Episodic cluster headache during the first trimester of pregnancy.

Tip

Although cluster headache is usually treated pharmacologically, it is important to remember that effective acute and preventive nonpharmacologic treatment options exist. These are useful for patients who cannot or do not wish to take medications.

A woman with migraine aura who requests testing for a patent foramen ovale

Case

A 29-year-old woman was seen in the headache clinic with complaints of headaches associated with focal neurologic deficits. Her headaches had begun during her teenage years and increased in frequency and severity in her 20s. Headaches were described as throbbing and were associated with nausea. The patient typically experienced two or three headache days in an average month and they seemed to be especially common before the onset of menstruation. She treated individual attacks of headache with 5 mg of zolmitriptan. This was usually effective in eliminating the headache and she rarely needed to re-dose.

Six months prior to being seen in clinic, she began to experience typical visual and sensory aura symptoms consisting of numbness of her left hand and face. These symptoms were stereotyped and occurred before about a quarter of her headaches and never lasted more

than 40 minutes. An MRI scan of the brain showed rare punctuate foci of T2 hyperintensity in the deep frontal white matter regions bilaterally. She was on no medications.

Her neurologic symptoms were felt to be consistent with a diagnosis of migraine with typical aura, and no change in her treatment regimen was advised. Several days after her consultation, however, the patient contacted the headache clinic doctor. She had been reading about migraine with aura on the internet and had learned about a possible connection between this condition and patent foramen ovale (PFO). She wondered whether a PFO could be the cause of her problems and if she should undergo testing for a PFO. She had read that closure of a PFO could sometimes cure migraine, and she was excited about the possibility of a permanent "nondrug cure" for her migraine.

What is the relationship between migraine with aura and PFO?

PFO is a common cardiac anomaly in which there is an abnormal opening between the right and left atrial chambers of the heart. PFO is thought to occur during fetal life when the septal tissue between the two chambers does not completely fuse. The resulting opening is often quite small and is frequently covered by a flap of tissue. Under normal conditions pressure is higher in the left atrium than the right, and this holds the flap closed. The flap can open, however, when there is a sudden increase in pressure in the right atrium (for example, when people cough, sneeze, or strain). Under these circumstances blood from the right side of the heart can be shunted to the left atrium without first passing through the pulmonary circulation.

Autopsy studies suggest PFO occurs in roughly a quarter of the normal population. It rarely causes problems and usually does not come to medical attention. Since both PFO and migraine are common conditions, their frequent co-occurrence is not surprising. What has led to interest in their connection, however, is the fact that the prevalence of PFO appears to be increased in patients who have migraine with aura beyond what would be expected by chance alone. However, the magnitude and nature of the association between PFO and migraine with aura remain uncertain.

One possibility is that migraine and PFO share a common underlying cause, perhaps an inherited connective tissue abnormality that predisposes a person to both PFO and migraine. If that is the case, treatment of one problem would not be expected to have an effect on the other. Some investigators, however, have proposed that a PFO might actually cause migraine aura by allowing small emboli or vasogenic substances from the systemic circulation to pass directly into the cerebral circulation. Ordinarily these would be filtered when blood passes through the pulmonary circulation. According to this theory, these substances may then trigger aura and headache, and could also be responsible for small ischemic insults that lead to cerebral white matter changes.

Should patients who have migraine with aura be evaluated for a PFO and possible shunt closure?

Small case series and other observational studies suggested that closure of PFOs, usually performed percutaneously, produced substantial improvement of aura and headache. However, these studies had no control groups and were retrospective in nature. Additionally, most patients who underwent PFO closure were treated with aspirin or clopidogrel following the procedure. These things, along with the substantial placebo effects associated with a procedure, could have explained some or all of the apparent improvement in migraine and aura with PFO closure.

A randomized, sham-controlled trial performed in the United Kingdom evaluated the impact of PFO closure on migraine in 147 subjects who had migraine with aura refractory to at least two classes of prophylactic therapy. This study did not show a statistically significant difference between the sham or actual PFO closure for the primary endpoint of the trial, which was complete resolution of headaches. Only three patients in each group had complete resolution of headaches over the three months following the procedure. There were no major differences between the true and sham surgery groups for other prespecified secondary outcomes of the study. However, a post-hoc analysis that removed several subjects with a large number of headache days from the analysis showed that subjects who underwent PFO closure had a reduction of 2.2 headache days per month compared with a reduction of 1.3 headache days per month in those who underwent the sham procedure. This ambiguous result has left some experts interested

in further study of PFO closure for the treatment of migraine.

Discussion

In our view, available evidence clearly demonstrates an unfavorable balance between possible benefits and harms from PFO closure for migraine with aura. The UK randomized trial did not demonstrate convincing benefits of closure. In contrast, a number of adverse events occurred in the PFO closure group. These included cardiac tamponade, pericardial effusion, retroperitoneal hemorrhage, and atrial fibrillation. It is of concern that these events occurred in the context of a carefully conducted clinical trial in which PFO closure was performed by highly trained, expert interventional cardiologists in carefully selected, healthy patients with few comorbid conditions. It is likely that the complication rate would be higher if procedures were performed in the course of usual care in a broader range of patients.

Meanwhile, mounting evidence shows no clear correlation between the burden of white matter lesions on brain MRI and the presence of a PFO. This further weakens the argument that the presence of a PFO might lead to ischemic or embolic events that could produce aura or other lasting events. It is interesting to note that PFOs have also been suspected as a possible cause for ischemic stroke in young people with no other apparent reason for stroke. Yet a recent study failed to show any reduction in the risk of a second ischemic stroke in patients with PFO who underwent closure.

For all of these reasons, we do not recommend searching for a PFO in patients who have migraine with aura. In the case of the patient in the vignette, whose headaches are well controlled with abortive therapy alone, there is even less reason to pursue a workup for PFO.

Diagnosis

Migraine with typical aura.

Tip

Available evidence does not clearly support a causal link between PFO and migraine with aura, and the harms of PFO closure appear to outweigh the benefits. Patients with aura should not undergo testing for the presence of a PFO.

A young woman asking about migraine surgery

Case

A 23-year-old woman was seen in the headache clinic where she reported having headaches 20 or 25 days in a typical month. Her headaches had started when she was nine years old. They steadily worsened through high school and college. About 10–15 days in an average month the patient had dull, bilateral pain over her temples and forehead with no associated symptoms. This pain was rated 5 on a 0–10 pain scale. The rest of her headaches were more severe. These headaches began in the posterior occipital region of her head on the right side and radiated forward to the right temple. She also reported shock-like pain in her face, jaw, and cheek on the right. Headaches were associated with nausea and photo and phonophobia. She could not identify any clear triggers or relieving factors for her headaches. Examination and workup had been negative.

She was diagnosed with chronic migraine. Triptans were tried but were only partially effective for some headaches. Multiple trials of preventive medications including beta-blockers, tricyclic antidepressants, antiepileptic medications, and botulinum toxin injections had not been helpful or had produced intolerable side effects.

The patient had experienced difficulty forming successful long-term relationships with caregivers. She was bitter that doctors had not been able to cure her headaches. She was starting to miss work at a new job and was very concerned. At her visit she asked whether she would be a good candidate for the new "migraine surgery" she had heard about on the news.

What is the "migraine surgery" this patient is referring to?

Over the last decade the idea of a surgical "solution" to migraine has been popularized by plastic surgeons, reportedly inspired by headache improvement that was serendipitously noted in patients who underwent cosmetic "forehead rejuvenation" procedures. Because the plastic surgery procedures involved removal of muscles in the forehead, a plastic surgeon developed the idea that contraction of facial muscles might produce migraine by impinging on peripheral branches of the trigeminal nerve.

The procedures performed to reduce this "impingement" include resection of the corrugator supercilii muscle with the placement of fat grafts in the site. Some procedures involve dissection of the glabellar area. Transection of the zygomatical temporal branch of the trigeminal nerve is also often performed. In cases of posterior pain the semispinalis capitus muscle may be resected with placement of fat grafts in the area, with the aim of reducing pressure on the occipital nerve. Finally, some surgeons also perform nasal septoplasty or otherwise attempt to address possible intranasal trigger points.

The procedures involved are often referred to collectively as "migraine deactivation surgery" (MDS), although as described above a variety of surgical sites and procedures are involved. The approach to each patient is typically individualized, making it difficult to study outcomes objectively. Patients who fail to improve with surgery are often told that they need more surgery to deactivate other trigger points that were "missed" the first time around. Many plastic surgeons who do this form of surgery select patients for surgery on the basis of improvement in headaches with the injection of onabotulinumtoxinA and/or occipital nerve blockade, on the theory that response to such temporary procedures is proof of nerve impingement.

How strong is the evidence of benefit from migraine surgery?

Various uncontrolled observational studies have been published that report impressive success with MDS, and two randomized trials have been performed. Unfortunately, proponents of the surgery have performed all of these studies and nearly all were published in a single plastic surgery specialty journal. The two trials suffered from serious methodologic problems that limit the conclusions that can be drawn from them. Taken as a whole, the evidence base for MDS is remarkably weak.

Despite this MDS is becoming more common. A recent survey of members of the American Society of Plastic Surgeons found that 18% of respondents had performed migraine surgery. Of those who had not performed the surgery, 60% said they "would be interested if an appropriate patient was referred to them by a neurologist."

For these reasons, the AHS has issued a statement urging "patients, healthcare professionals and migraine treatment specialists themselves, to exercise caution in recommending or seeking such therapy." This statement went on to say that "In our view, surgery for migraine is a last-resort option and is probably not appropriate for most sufferers. To date, there are no convincing or definitive data that show its long-term value. Besides replacing the use of more appropriate treatments, surgical intervention also may produce side effects that are not reversible and carry the risks associated with any surgery. It also can be extremely expensive and may not be covered by insurance."

Discussion

Unfortunately, there are no cures for migraine and some patients with chronic migraine do not benefit from currently available treatments. It is easy to understand why the patient in this vignette is so interested in a potential nondrug, surgical approach to migraine treatment. However, surgical treatments for migraine have a long and undistinguished history and have not stood the test of time. "Migraine deactivation surgery" seems unlikely to be an exception to this pattern. In the early twentieth century some surgeons performed cervical sympathectomies for migraine, ligated the external carotid artery, or carried out various de-afferentation procedures on branches of the trigeminal nerves.

Despite unconvincing evidence of benefit and cautions from experts, MDS has received extensive and favorable coverage in the popular press, and anecdotal stories of patients with dramatic improvement in migraine are easy to find on the internet. Unfortunately, in our practice we have seen patients with poor outcomes following surgery, and reports of serious adverse events are also appearing online.

At this point it is difficult to predict who may have a good outcome from surgery for treatment of migraine and it remains experimental therapy. There are significant risks with any surgery, including cranial nerve injury and worsened long-term pain. The risks of MDS have not been well characterized or quantified by independent researchers. In our view, this surgery should only be performed in the context of a well-designed randomized sham-controlled trial. If this surgery turns out to have serious long-term complications, physicians who have referred patients for this treatment could face legal liability.

Diagnosis

Chronic refractory migraine.

Tip

Migraine deactivation surgery is not well studied as a treatment for migraine and remains experimental. Patients should be informed about the uncertain balance of benefits to harms and the potential for irreversible adverse effects.

Recommended reading

Food triggers for migraine

Panconesi A, Bartolozzi ML, Guidi L. Alcohol and migraine: what should we tell patients? *Curr Pain Headache Rep.* 2011;15(3):177–84.

Rockett FC, de Oliveira VR, Castro K, *et al.* Dietary aspects of migraine trigger factors. *Nutr Rev.* 2012;70(6):337–56.

Other triggers for migraine

Andress-Rothrock D, King W, Rothrock J. An analysis of migraine triggers in a clinic-based population. *Headache.* 2010;50(8):1366–70.

Martin PR. Behavioral management of migraine headache triggers: learning to cope with triggers. *Curr Pain Headache Rep.* 2010;14:221–7.

Martin PR, MacLeod C. Behavioral management of headache triggers: avoidance of triggers is an inadequate strategy. *Clin Psychol Rev.* 2009;29:483–95.

Nicholson RA, Buse DC, Andrasik F, Lipton RB. Nonpharmacologic treatments for migraine and tension-type headache: how to choose and when to use. *Curr Treat Options Neurol.* 2011;13(1):28–40.

Behavioral treatments

Andrasik F. What does the evidence show? Efficacy of behavioural treatments for recurrent headaches in adults. *Neurol Sci.* 2007;28:S70–7.

Campbell JK, Penzien DB, Wall EM. Evidence-based guidelines for migraine headaches: behavioral and physical treatments. 2000. Retrieved from http://www.aan.com/.

Nicholson RA, Buse DC, Andrasik F, Lipton RB. Nonpharmacologic treatments for migraine and tension-type headache: how to choose and when to use. *Curr Treat Options Neurol.* 2011;13(1):28–40.

Smitherman TA, Penzien DB, Rains JC. Challenges of nonpharmacologic interventions in chronic tension-type headache. *Curr Pain Headache Rep.* 2007;11:471–7.

Vitamins, supplements, and herbal treatments for migraine

Evans RW, Taylor FR. "Natural" or alternative medications for migraine prevention. *Headache.* 2006;46(6):1012–18.

Maizels M, Blumenfeld A, Burchette R. A combination of riboflavin, magnesium, and feverfew for migraine prophylaxis: a randomized trial. *Headache.* 2004; 44(9):885–90.

Mauskop A. Nonmedication, alternative, and complementary treatments for migraine. *Continuum (Minneap Minn).* 2012;18(4):796–806.

Physical therapy

Chaibi A, Russell MB. Manual therapies for cervicogenic headache: a systematic review. *J Headache Pain.* 2012;13:351–9.

Jull G, Trott P, Potter H, *et al.* A randomized controlled trial of exercise and manipulative therapy for cervicogenic headache. *Spine.* 2002;27(17):1835–43.

Sjaastad O, Bakketeig LS. Prevalence of cervicogenic headache: Vågå study of headache epidemiology. *Acta Neurol Scand.* 2008;117(3):173–80.

Chiropractic treatments for headache

Bryans R, Descarreaux M, Duranleau M, *et al.* Evidence-based guidelines for the chiropractic treatment of adults with headache. *J Manipulative Physiol Ther.* 2011;34(5):274–89.

Cassidy JD, Boyle E, Côté P, *et al.* Risk of vertebrobasilar stroke and chiropractic care: results of a population-based case-control and case-crossover study. *J Manipulative Physiol Ther.* 2009;32(2 Suppl):S201–8.

Ernst E. Adverse effects of spinal manipulation: a systematic review. *J R Soc Med.* 2007;100(7):330–8.

Posadzki P, Ernst E. Systematic reviews of spinal manipulations for headaches: an attempt to clear up the confusion. *Headache.* 2011;51(9):1419–25.

Nerve blocks

Ashkenazi A, Blumenfeld A, Napchan U, *et al.* Peripheral nerve blocks and trigger point injections in headache management – a systematic review and suggestions for future research. *Headache.* 2010;50(6):943–52.

Blumenfeld A, Ashkenazi A, Napchan U, *et al.* Expert consensus recommendations for the performance of peripheral nerve blocks for headaches – a narrative review. *Headache.* 2013;53(3):437–46.

PFO and migraine with aura

Davis D, Gregson J, Willeit P, *et al.* Patent foramen ovale, ischemic stroke and migraine: systemic review and stratified meta-analysis of association studies. *Neuroepidemiology.* 2013;40:56–67.

Dowson A, Mullen M, Peatfield R, *et al.* Migraine Intervention with STARRFlex Technology (MIST) trial: a prospective, multicenter, double-blind, sham-controlled trial to evaluate the effectiveness of patent foramen ovale closure with STARFlex septal repair implant to resolve refractory migraine headache. *Circulation.* 2008;117:1397–404.

Furlan AJ, Reisman M, Massaro J, *et al.* Closure or medical therapy for cryptogenic stroke with patent foramen ovale. *N Engl J Med.* 2012;366:991–9.

Tepper S, Cleves C, Taylor F. Patent foramen ovale and migraine: association, causation, and implications of clinical trials. *Curr Pain Headache Rep.* 2009;13: 221–6.

Migraine surgery

Gaul C, Holle D, Sandor PS, *et al.* The value of "migraine surgery". Overview of the pathophysiological concept and current evidence. *Nervenarzt.* 2010;81(4):463–70.

Guyuron B, Reed D, Kriegler JS, *et al.* A placebo-controlled surgical trial of the treatment of migraine headaches. *Plast Reconstr Surg.* 2009;124(2):461–8.

Kung TA, Pannucci CJ, Chamberlain JL, Cederna PS. Migraine surgery practice patterns and attitudes. *Plast Reconstr Surg.* 2012;129:623–8.

Chapter

10

Challenges and special situations in headache management

Dr. John R. Graham, who founded our headache center, wrote in 1955 that "The successful treatment of migraine is difficult but worth the effort. It taps every resource of the physician. Probably more hours of suffering are caused by migraine than by any other human affliction. Knowledge of its secrets is incomplete but increasing. For these reasons it presents a unique challenge." We find these words are as true today as when they were written, and they apply to all headache types, not just migraine. We devote the first part of this chapter to some of the more challenging situations that may arise in the care of a patient with headache. These include mismatches between patient and physician goals or expectations, requests for opioid treatment, refractory medication overuse, psychiatric comorbidities, and managing the many risk factors that can come together to worsen headache over time. At times it can be difficult to fully engage patients as active participants in their care, although a wealth of research shows that such a shared decision-making approach is the best treatment model for chronic conditions such as headache.

In all of these situations, there are steps physicians can take to increase the likelihood of a positive outcome. In this chapter, we aim to provide some suggestions about how to foster a therapeutic doctor–patient relationship, set clear boundaries, promote shared decision-making, and avoid some of the common pitfalls in managing these most difficult presentations of headache.

Lifelong migraine refractory to multiple treatments

Case

A 44-year-old man sought treatment for chronic headaches. He reported he has had headaches since he was a teenager and "I have tried everything and noth-

ing seemed to help a whole lot, although a couple of them worked for a year or so." Upon questioning, he could not recall the doses or duration of most of the medications he had used, although he was able to recall the names of many treatments. Records from his previous physician were handwritten and it is difficult to decipher the notes. After review of his history and neurologic examination, as well as the results of past testing, a diagnosis of chronic migraine was made. The physician suggested that as part of his treatment plan he should keep a record of the frequency and severity of his headaches and track his use of medication to treat individual headache attacks. The patient reported that he "used to keep a headache calendar but it was a lot of work and frankly, doc, I couldn't see the point. Trust me; I'll let you know when I'm doing better. I don't need a calendar to tell me that."

How is this patient's recall of headaches likely to compare with diary information?

Diagnostic and therapeutic decisions about headache treatment are made on the basis of information about headache frequency, intensity, and disability as well as medication response. Patient recall of headache activity is likely to be quite accurate over short periods of time. One study compared patient recall of headache frequency and intensity over a four-week period as recorded in a daily diary with their general recall of this information. Patient recall of headache frequency was accurate when compared with detailed diary information, but they recalled a higher intensity of headaches compared with diary information.

The authors of this study concluded that patient recall of headache intensity is not particularly good. The accuracy of headache information over a period of time longer than four weeks was not studied. It seems unlikely that patient recall of headaches that occurred in the distant past is particularly accurate, however.

This case illustrates the negative treatment implications of missing information about headache response to treatment.

Would headache calendars or diaries be helpful in headache diagnosis or treatment here? Would paper or electronic diaries be better?

One study evaluated the performance of a basic diagnostic headache diary for diagnosis of tension-type, migraine, and medication overuse headache in a number of European and Latin American countries. Subjects were randomized to receive the diary at least a month before their first visit to the headache center or to receive it at the first visit. In 98% of cases who received the diary before their first visit, information in the diary was complete and together with the clinical history was sufficient to make a definitive diagnosis. In contrast, among subjects who had not completed one month of diary recordings prior to the first visit, a diagnosis could be made in only 87% of cases. The authors concluded that a headache diary did improve diagnosis of headache.

Another study evaluated acceptance of and compliance with an electronic headache diary compared with a traditional paper headache diary in a group of headache patients diagnosed with medication overuse headache. At the onset of hospitalization for medication withdrawal, patients were asked to keep both an electronic and paper diary. Compliance with both was good but patients felt the electronic diary was easier to use.

However, another experiment assigned patients with chronic pain (not headache) to use either a paper diary with a hidden means of tracking use, or an electronic diary with time-stamped entries. Although the paper diaries submitted by participants were complete in 90% of cases, monitoring indicated that actual compliance with assigned timing of entries was only 11%, suggesting "a high level of faked compliance." The authors of this study concluded that their findings "call into question the use of paper diaries and suggest that electronic diaries with compliance-enhancing features are a more effective way of collecting diary information."

In this case, the patient was recommended to keep an electronic headache diary using a smartphone app. He was educated about the above studies and the physician also told him that it would be very difficult to make treatment decisions without numerical data to inform them. The patient agreed to keep the diary.

Discussion

An objective record of headache occurrence and medication use is important in order to follow the clinical course of headaches and evaluate the results of treatment. It is difficult to think of any other therapeutic situations in which global patient recall is accepted as the best way to monitor the natural history or treatment response of an illness.

While it is difficult to optimize headache treatment in the absence of sufficient information from a headache diary, there is also such a thing as too much information. Some patients present with color-coded spreadsheets with detailed information on headache activity, weather, diet, and other factors. In most cases it is beyond the ability of the physician – or the patient – to extract meaningful lessons from this "information overload." Overly detailed diaries also may draw needless attention to somatic symptoms, so we recommend that patients collect the minimum information necessary to make treatment decisions. We recommend keeping track of headache frequency (number of days a month with headache) and peak headache intensity. An ongoing record of medication intake is also helpful but can usually be very quickly compiled. One simple headache diary is shown in Figure 10.1.

There are of course elements of the patient experience that will not be captured in diary recordings, such as absence from work or social roles or the need to visit the emergency department for headache treatment. Diaries will never supplant a good physician interview, and it is important to corroborate diary findings with other signs that a patient is improving or worsening, including disability and absence from usual roles.

Diagnosis

Chronic migraine.

Tip

Accurate headache diagnosis and treatment planning depend upon an accurate and permanent record of headache activity and response to medication. In most cases, patient recall is inferior to carefully kept headache diaries.

HEADACHE CALENDAR

MONTH:

DAYS	MENSES	INTENSITY (1–3 Mild, 4–6 Mod, 7–10 Disabling)	ABORTIVE MEDICATION USED
ex	P	1 2 3 4 5 6 7 8 9 10	N + S
1		1 2 3 4 5 6 7 8 9 10	
2		1 2 3 4 5 6 7 8 9 10	
3		1 2 3 4 5 6 7 8 9 10	
4		1 2 3 4 5 6 7 8 9 10	
5		1 2 3 4 5 6 7 8 9 10	
6		1 2 3 4 5 6 7 8 9 10	
7		1 2 3 4 5 6 7 8 9 10	
8		1 2 3 4 5 6 7 8 9 10	
9		1 2 3 4 5 6 7 8 9 10	
10		1 2 3 4 5 6 7 8 9 10	
11		1 2 3 4 5 6 7 8 9 10	
12		1 2 3 4 5 6 7 8 9 10	
13		1 2 3 4 5 6 7 8 9 10	
14		1 2 3 4 5 6 7 8 9 10	
15		1 2 3 4 5 6 7 8 9 10	
16		1 2 3 4 5 6 7 8 9 10	
17		1 2 3 4 5 6 7 8 9 10	
18		1 2 3 4 5 6 7 8 9 10	
19		1 2 3 4 5 6 7 8 9 10	
20		1 2 3 4 5 6 7 8 9 10	
21		1 2 3 4 5 6 7 8 9 10	
22		1 2 3 4 5 6 7 8 9 10	
23		1 2 3 4 5 6 7 8 9 10	
24		1 2 3 4 5 6 7 8 9 10	
25		1 2 3 4 5 6 7 8 9 10	
26		1 2 3 4 5 6 7 8 9 10	
27		1 2 3 4 5 6 7 8 9 10	
28		1 2 3 4 5 6 7 8 9 10	
29		1 2 3 4 5 6 7 8 9 10	
30		1 2 3 4 5 6 7 8 9 10	
31		1 2 3 4 5 6 7 8 9 10	

Use P to indicate days of your menstrual period.

Use abortive medication abbreviations like T for Tylenol.

Combinations of medications like Naproxen and Sumatriptan can be written as N + S.

Figure 10.1 A simple headache calendar.

A patient with unrealistic expectations

Case

A 30-year-old female presented for evaluation of headache and was accompanied by her mother. At the start of the visit the patient stated "I've seen eight doctors; you are the last one." Her mother presented the physician with copious records and noted that her daughter had likely had her past medical care mishandled and was now "at the end of her rope." The patient had left school and work due to headache; she was now living at home and her major daily activity was confined to walking the dog. She had had mild depression in the past but was otherwise healthy.

At the end of the visit, the physician diagnosed chronic migraine and made some suggestions for treatment. Though she had extensive evaluation of her headaches in the past, she and her mother expressed their unhappiness that further testing was not suggested. Multiple treatment options suggested by the physician were rejected by the patient as having failed in the past or having caused unacceptable side effects or reactions. In some cases she had not tried the treatment but was afraid that it would cause intolerable side effects. At that point in the visit, she appeared to be losing confidence in the provider. She then asked the physician how she should treat her pain, as her prior provider had only given her enough analgesic medication to get her to this appointment. She was frustrated by the provider's response and both mother and daughter left the office clearly unsatisfied.

What elements of the visit predicted a suboptimal outcome?

While there is a great deal of variation in presentations of headache patients, and it can be difficult to predict how an individual patient will participate in their care, certain elements of this patient's presentation were potentially troubling. These "red flags" include the presence of a possibly codependent mother who tended to take over the interview and speak for the patient, multiple prior evaluations, and the comments suggesting the presence of unrealistic expectations on the part of the patient and family. While there are few data on this topic, our experience has been that unrealistic expectations for benefit from treatment can be one of the most significant barriers to effective care.

What could have been done to end this visit on a more positive note?

The establishment of an effective and therapeutic physician–patient relationship is the foundation for headache treatment. This is especially true in cases of refractory or particularly severe headache disorders, and also when psychopathology plays a role in the patient's presentation. Both of these elements seem to be at play in this case. Physicians can earn the trust of patients by practicing active listening and demon-strating empathy, eliciting patient goals for the visit and addressing them specifically, educating the patient about the nature of their diagnosis, being honest but positive about likely benefits from treatment, and setting boundaries. In this case, the patient and her mother may have been more reassured if their specific concerns were addressed.

Discussion

Addressing and managing patient expectations for treatment can be a very challenging aspect of headache medicine. While this issue is sometimes an afterthought or not included at all in headache education, this can make the difference between a successful treatment relationship and a dysfunctional one. Early recognition and management of unrealistic expectations can at times change the outcome of a visit.

One challenge is that headache seems uniquely suited to self-diagnosis, with some patients insisting that their headaches are caused by food disorders, sinus disease, or an allergy condition, for example. In the headache clinic, we also encounter patients fixated on the idea that there is an as-yet undiscovered structural problem underlying their headaches, which the "right" test will reveal. Unless these concerns are managed, patients are at high risk to be noncompliant with suggested therapy, because in their view the treatment does not address the cause of their symptoms. Patients sometimes decline headache medications because they do not want to mask pain until the underlying cause is found. Other management challenges include medication-seeking behavior and the presence of comorbid psychiatric conditions, primarily personality disorder. One particularly difficult scenario is the patient who insistently asks for help for their pain, but refuses all recommendations for treatment.

When the problem is recognized early on, it may sometimes be useful to dispense with the remainder of the medical history and instead explore with the patient their assumptions, expectations, and fears. When the provider is clearly unable to change the course of the illness, messages that express the provider's wish that things could be different can be supportive while simultaneously setting limits on what the provider can offer. Concerning developments in the history (e.g. overreliance by the patient on one diagnosis) can be highlighted by the provider expressing worry about the situation, but not blame (e.g. "I worry that your focus on your sinus condition could end up leaving another condition out of the picture."). The result can be the forging of the basics of a therapeutic relationship upon which the headache problem can be further addressed. Lastly, the importance of referring patients for psychiatric evaluation and treatment when indicated cannot be overstated. This suggestion is more likely to be positively received in the context of a good therapeutic relationship.

Diagnosis

Chronic migraine.

Tip

Failure to consider and address patient expectations in every interaction, or to recognize and if possible manage unrealistic expectations up front, may lead to suboptimal outcomes.

Chronification of migraine in a patient lost to follow-up

Case

A 24-year-old woman presented to the headache clinic for evaluation of headaches meeting criteria for migraine without aura. Headache onset was at age 14, and at the time of her initial evaluation she was having about seven headaches per month. She was given oral sumatriptan and an antiemetic for symptomatic therapy. At her follow-up appointment she reported increased headache frequency to 11 headaches per month, each treated with sumatriptan, and she was started on amitriptyline for preventive therapy. Despite recommendations to return to clinic in six months, she was lost to follow-up for the next two years, and when she next presented to the clinic her headaches were now occurring 25 days per month.

What may have contributed to the increased frequency of this patient's headaches?

Patients with high frequency episodic migraine (10–14 headache days per month) are at higher risk of transitioning to chronic migraine than those with low frequency episodic migraines, as might be expected. This patient was therefore at higher risk for transitioning

Table 10.1. Risk factors for migraine chronification

Medical conditions
- Obesity
- Sleep disorders and snoring
- Depression
- Anxiety
- History of head or neck trauma

Lifestyle and habits
- Caffeine intake
- Poor response to life stress
- Medication overuse
- Headache-specific factors
- Frequent headache
- Presence of cutaneous allodynia

Non-modifiable factors
- Female sex
- Genetic predisposition
- Low educational level
- Low socioeconomic status
- Younger age

to chronic migraine. She had several other risk factors, however, including medication overuse, female sex, and younger age. Upon further questioning, she also revealed poor sleep which she had attributed to ongoing anxiety, but her boyfriend had also told her she snored. The risk factors for transition to chronic migraine are listed in Table 10.1. Medication overuse is a significant risk factor, as described elsewhere in this book.

What could have been done to prevent the transition to chronic migraine?

This case illustrates the importance of scheduling frequent follow-up appointments while treatments are being optimized. If the physician had been able to track the increased frequency of headaches, a more aggressive preventive regimen could have been initiated. In patients with high frequency episodic migraine, specifically evaluating risk factors for transition to chronic migraine is appropriate. Some risk factors, including age and sex, are not modifiable but may be informative in determining risk. Treatment of modifiable risk factors may help prevent transition to chronic migraine. The appropriate intervention is specific to the risk factor. In this case, the patient could have been referred to a sleep specialist to evaluate for possible sleep apnea. Anxiety can be specifically addressed with cognitive behavioral therapy, or with appropriate medication.

Discussion

About 3% of patients with episodic migraine, defined as fewer than 15 headache days per month, transition to chronic migraine, or having 15 or more headache days per month, each year. Some risk factors for transition cannot be modified, but many risk factors can be reduced or eliminated. The treatments are specific to the risk factors. Stress and psychiatric diagnoses may respond to behavioral therapy or biofeedback. Obstructive sleep apnea is one of the easiest comorbidities to treat once the diagnosis has been made. Although obesity, on the other hand, is notoriously difficult to treat, patients can be referred for nutrition and exercise programs to support weight loss. Emerging data from small prospective samples suggest that gastric bypass may improve migraine. Dietary triggers, including caffeine use, can be reduced.

Because medication overuse is such a strong risk factor for migraine chronification, close monitoring of headache frequency and symptomatic medication use is important. When patients transition from low frequency episodic migraine to high frequency episodic migraine, active measures to reduce headache frequency are in order. These can include starting a preventive pharmacologic agent, lifestyle modification, complementary and alternative treatments, and biofeedback. Patients should also be counseled on the factor leading to transition to chronic migraine and invited to be active partners in reducing headache frequency.

Because of the need to monitor symptomatic medication use, headache frequency, and risk factors for transition to chronic migraine, we recommend regular follow-up for all patients taking prescription medications for migraine. While there are no guidelines established, our practice is to see patients every 6–12 months while we are writing prescriptions. At these follow-up visits, we assess these risk factors and try to address any potentially problematic issues that arise.

Diagnosis

Chronic (transformed) migraine.

Tip

Transition from episodic to chronic migraine is more common in patients with high frequency episodic migraine. Some risk factors for transformation are modifiable and should be addressed in at-risk patients.

A patient requesting early refills

Case

A 37-year-old man with chronic migraine called the office on a Friday afternoon to request a prescription for oxycodone/acetaminophen tablets. He had last been seen for an office visit a month prior. At that visit his preventive medications were adjusted, he was asked to keep a headache diary to monitor headache frequency and medication use, and he was given a prescription for 18 zolmitriptan tablets (with 3 refills) to treat individual attacks of headache. He was also given 30 tablets of hydrocodone to use as rescue medication for attacks of headache that did not respond to zolmitriptan. The physician reviewed the concept of medication overuse headache with him and asked him to limit treatment of individual attacks to no more than two or three days a week. He was also told that the 30 tablets of hydrocodone were to be used conservatively and should last for at least six months, and that the practice did not refill opioid prescriptions outside of regular office visits.

At his follow-up visit the patient said that he had used up the hydrocodone tablets he was given. The zolmitriptan was effective but he had run out of it and "the pharmacy won't give me any more unless you call to say it is okay." He admitted that he had been taking these medications on a daily basis, but insisted that he had many important things going on at work and could not afford to have a headache. He pleaded for the physician to prescribe oxycodone/acetaminophen "just this once" because he believed it would more effectively treat his pain. He added that he finds it hard to believe anyone should have to suffer so much given all of the strong medications that are available to treat pain.

Are this patient's treatment goals realistic?

This patient is clearly overusing his short-acting headache medications, and is not compliant with previously agreed limits on medication use. The treatment imperative that most patients feel when faced with severe pain, when paired with daily or near-daily headaches, is probably the biggest management challenge in headache medicine. Disagreement about the amount and type of medication allowed for acute episodes of pain can be an ongoing source of tension between doctor and patient. Despite this, one of the most important duties in managing patients with chronic headache disorders is to set safe and appropriate limits on treatments used for individual headaches.

The need to limit use of short-acting pain relief medications is the main point of difference between the treatment of patients who have infrequent headache attacks and those who have daily or near-daily headaches. In patients whose attacks of headache are relatively infrequent – typically less than one attack a week – it is reasonable to expect that acute treatment will return the patient to their baseline level of function and eliminate pain. Early, aggressive treatment of individual attacks of headaches, sometimes using powerful medications, is the strategy most likely to achieve these goals.

These objectives, however, are not realistic in patients who have frequent headaches. In fact, overuse of medications that produce good short-term pain relief may paradoxically lead to worsening headache over time, a situation known as medication overuse headache. In patients with frequent headache, treatment goals for individual headache attacks typically must be adjusted: complete pain relief may not be possible and return to baseline function may not be achievable in all attacks. Instead, it is necessary to balance the desire for short-term pain relief with the longer-term goal of preventing disease progression and complications. Patients with frequent attacks may have to pick and choose which attacks they treat aggressively. Less convenient but more effective non-oral medications with a higher short-term side effect burden may be needed.

What are reasonable limits on medication use? How much medication is "too much" or "too frequent" when it comes to treating individual attacks of headache?

The exact amount and type of medication that can produce medication overuse headache is unclear. There is no definite evidence of an amount below which no one will have problems and above which everyone will. Rather, the susceptibility to medication overuse headache probably exists on a continuum. Because we do not know what the threshold is to produce medication overuse headache in an individual patient, we err on the side of conservative recommendations. A typical rule of thumb is that medications to treat individual headaches – whether they be triptans, nonsteroidal anti-inflammatory drugs (NSAIDs), opioids, or other

drugs – should not be used more than two or three days a week. That's days of use, not doses.

Particularly in specialty practice, there may be situations where deviation from this limit is defensible or the best that can be accomplished, but this is a decision to make only after usual attempts at treatment have been tried.

What is the best way to handle this patient's request for medication?

Whatever rules are in place, not all patients will adhere to them. Quickly and firmly addressing the matter will help reduce misaligned expectations. Regular review and reinforcement of medication limits will have a longer-lasting impact. Doctors and patients who plan regular follow-up visits to monitor medication use will likely fare better than those who leave this to chance or individual motivation.

The best response to this patient's request is therefore to remind him of agreements about medication use and ask him to schedule an office visit where you might discuss alternative ways to treat his headache. One strategy that may help defuse tension is to consider a trial of medications that probably do not cause medication overuse headache even when used frequently. Some examples are listed in Table 10.2. Even if these strategies are not effective for extremely severe headaches, they may satisfactorily treat less severe headaches and thus "spare" more potent and problematic drugs for less frequent use.

Discussion

Treatment of chronic headache conditions is frequently characterized by a tension between the desire to relieve individual headaches and a need to prevent the development of medication overuse headache. We use the term "treatment imperative" to refer to the compulsion to treat severe pain that most headache patients experience. Even in the presence of substantial side effects and long-term harms from the overuse of symptomatic medications, patients and their doctors often continue to pursue aggressive treatment of individual headache episodes. It can be difficult for a physician to enforce reasonable limits on medication use, however, as doctors naturally feel an obligation to administer some sort of treatment to relieve pain and suffering.

Table 10.2. Options for acute treatment of headache with a low risk of causing medication overuse headache

Treatment	Sample doses and formulations
Baclofen	10–20 mg orally up to three times daily
Diphenhydramine	Orally or 25–50 mg IM or IV up to three times daily
Hydroxyzine	25–50 mg orally up to three times daily
Lidocaine nasal drops	½– 1 mL of 4% lidocaine via dropper in one or both nostrils every two hours as needed
Neuroleptics (e.g. promethazine, chlorpromazine)	These drugs are useful parenterally in the emergency department; on an outpatient basis we prefer rectal administration, e.g. promethazine suppositories 25 mg per rectum up to three times daily
NSAIDs	Indomethacin as a rectal suppository is often remarkably effective for severe headaches. We use 50 mg per rectum up to three times daily. Gastrointestinal side effects make long-term use problematic. Ketorolac is available for oral use but also available as a nasal spray and in preloaded syringes for IM administration
Occipital nerve blocks	
Steroids	Use must be limited, but to abort prolonged headache we use 4 mg orally twice daily for three days or 15 mg IV (one time dose)
Tizanidine	2–6 mg orally up to three times daily
Trigger point injections	

Chronic headache disorders, however, are conditions of long duration that are not amenable to cure. Expectations must be adjusted in patients with very frequent headaches. The same self-care rehabilitative philosophy applied to other chronic pain conditions is relevant in headache: immediate pain relief is not the goal in management of chronic pain, and patients should be helped to realize that "hurt does not mean harm." In some cases the problem is compounded by patient inability to tolerate any level of pain or distress. The stark urgency of an individual headache, which is reducible with medication, means that the standard of practice is to focus on individual headaches. Unfortunately, for patients with frequent headaches this misguided approach can lead to the ever-escalating use of stronger and stronger medications for individual headaches, with the paradoxical result that over time headaches become worse and more difficult to manage.

It is difficult to say to suffering patients that they must limit the use of medications that effectively treat an individual headache in order to obtain long-term benefits. Still, it is important that everyone involved realize that the patient will need to pick and choose which headaches they treat, and may need to accept partial rather than complete pain improvement.

Diagnosis

Medication overuse headache; chronic migraine.

Tip

Failure to set and enforce limits on the amount and type of medication used to treat individual attacks of headache is a common cause of poor treatment outcomes in patients with frequent headaches.

A woman requesting treatment with opioids

Case

A 34-year-old woman consulted a physician about a 20-year history of frequent, disabling migraine headaches that have not responded well to treatment. She had relocated from out of state and was establishing medical care. She brought past medical records that document prior unsuccessful treatment trials with a large number of preventive drugs for migraine. The doses and duration of these trials appeared to have been adequate, but headaches continued to be disabling. She was allergic to triptans and had been told she could not use NSAIDs because of gastric bypass surgery. She reported that oxycodone was helpful for headaches and that her prior physician provided her with a prescription for 120 tablets a month. Her neurologic examination was normal. Neuroimaging done in the last year was also normal. She requested that the physician continue her oxycodone prescription.

Should the physician continue her oxycodone prescription? What important information is missing in this case?

We lack information about whether this patient has risk factors for opioid misuse or has displayed previous behaviors consistent with opioid addiction or dependence. Problematic behaviors include such things as unauthorized escalation of prescribed doses of opioids, requests for early refills, or instances of lost prescriptions. A conversation with her previous prescribing physician would be very useful in identifying whether any of these things have been problems in the past.

It is also unclear whether the use of opioids has improved the patient's headache problem or her ability to function. Frequent use of symptom-relieving medications such as opioids or triptans is associated with paradoxical worsening of headache in some cases, a situation known as medication overuse headache. Pain relief is an important goal of headache therapy, but so is return to normal activities, including work. If this patient's ability to function has not improved or has worsened, then continued use of opioids may not be a good treatment choice.

How can a patient's risk for opioid misuse, addiction, or dependence be assessed?

There is no completely reliable way to determine if patients will misuse opioids or develop addiction or dependence syndromes. It is possible, however, to identify patients who are at high risk of developing problematic drug-related behaviors in the future. One commonly used tool, which is validated for use in pain patients, is the Opioid Risk Tool. Based on self-report about personal and family history of substance abuse, sexual abuse, sex, age, and psychiatric comorbidity, patients are identified as low, medium, or high risk to develop problems with opioid treatment.

In this case, a telephone call to the patient's prior prescribing physician revealed that the patient had a long history of daily headache that had responded poorly to treatment, and there had been no apparent worsening of headaches after oxycodone treatment was started. The physician reported, though, that he had become increasingly uncomfortable prescribing opioids for this patient. He noted that despite several increases in the amount of oxycodone the patient was allowed to use on a monthly basis, she remained on social security disability for headache and sought emergency department treatment for headaches several times a month. Additionally, when screened with the Opioid Risk Tool this patient reported a prior personal history of alcohol abuse, depression, and sexual abuse at age five by a stepfather.

Discussion

This patient reported a long history of migraine headaches refractory to numerous appropriate attempts at treatment. Refractory migraine is a common and vexing problem, and not all patients respond to aggressive attempts at treatment. Research is limited about the use of maintenance opioid therapy to treat such patients, but suggests that only a minority of patients achieve long-lasting benefit. Meanwhile, evidence is emerging to suggest that long-term opioid therapy can be associated with harms such as the development of opioid-induced hyperalgesia.

The main considerations with this patient are whether there is sufficient evidence of meaningful clinical benefit from maintenance opioid therapy to warrant continuation of that treatment, and whether she is at risk for the development of abuse or dependence syndromes. The conversation with her prior prescribing physician shows there has been no meaningful improvement in function with the regular use of opioids. Her score on the Opioid Risk Tool also indicated that she is at high risk of opioid abuse. Thus, this patient is probably best managed using non-opioid therapies.

Diagnosis

Chronic migraine.

Tip

It is possible to identify patients at high risk of misusing controlled substances.

A patient with recurrent medication overuse headache

Case

A patient returned to the headache clinic after being lost to follow-up. One year ago, he had been able to discontinue his long-term use of a butalbital-containing compound. He was taking six to nine tablets a day and had relied on the drug for years, during which his headaches had worsened. He had been diagnosed with medication overuse headache. The patient followed a weaning schedule and was started on amitriptyline for prevention of headaches. He used eletriptan 20 mg to treat up to two bad headaches a week. His previously daily headaches were then recognizable as episodic migraine. When he did not come back for subsequent visits, it was assumed that his headaches were so much improved that he no longer required specialty care.

The patient returned to the clinic one year later accompanied by his wife. She said that since last year his headache frequency had slowly increased and that he had returned to the use of butalbital-containing medication to treat his headaches. He then discontinued amitriptyline since it did not seem to be working. The butalbital was helpful at first but over time he had needed more and more to keep his headaches under control. He admitted that his primary care physician had been prescribing the medicine for the last four months but "she's worried about how much I'm taking and won't prescribe it any more. She gave me just enough medicine to make it to this appointment." He was advised to discontinue daily use of butalbital again and resume preventive therapy. He replied, "Oh doctor, with my schedule and the pressure at my work, I just can't afford to do that and have a headache!" His wife interrupted and said that if he did not have his medicine, he would be unable to work.

What additional diagnosis is suggested by this patient's presentation?

This patient meets criteria for medication overuse headache. He has a pre-existing headache disorder that has worsened in the context of daily use of a medication known to produce medication overuse headache. Furthermore, previous treatment has established that his headaches improve when this medication is withdrawn. However, this patient *also* displays features consistent with dependence on medication, including tolerance to the effects of the drug, taking the drug in larger amounts than intended, failed attempts to reduce drug use, and continued use despite the presence of a medical condition that is likely to be related to drug use.

In this case, the patient's dependence is likely due to the interaction of a genuine medical problem (migraine) with behavioral features that may signal the presence of a complicating psychiatric disorder. Behavioral dynamics that contribute to relapse in patients with medication overuse headache include overreliance on drugs as the only way to handle headaches, medication use in anticipation of pain, and the use of medication to treat emotional distress or anxiety. Joel Saper and colleagues have suggested that medication overuse headache "is not a unitary phe-

Table 10.3. Warning signs that a patient's care will be challenging

- Blaming others for their problems or misuse of medications
- Noncompliant with treatment recommendations
- Discrepancy between pain ratings and observable behavior or demeanor
- Enlistment of others to endorse requests for medication

nomenon." They distinguish between simple (type 1) and complex (type 2) medication overuse headache. The latter term refers to patients whose medication overuse headache is associated with comorbid psychiatric disorders and a history of relapse.

What additional clinical features suggest that management of this patient will be challenging?

It is not always possible to identify patients whose care will be challenging, but certain warning signs and indications should be heeded. Table 10.3 lists a number of warning signals that should be heeded, several of which are present in this case. The patient has demonstrated disagreement with treatment recommendations through his nonadherence to prescribed therapy and follow-up care. His wife, who speaks for the patient, is overly solicitous and blames the doctor rather than the headaches or medication misuse for the possibility that the patient might miss work.

Discussion

Most patients with headache problems are eager to get better and are compliant with treatment recommendations. Others, however, are challenging to care for. Their personal or medical situations are often complex, with the result that they may not benefit from or adhere to treatment. Some of the conditions that make patients difficult to care for include drug or alcohol dependence, personality disorders, or family problems. It is not always possible to identify patients whose management will turn out to be difficult, but the signs and signals discussed here can sometimes provide an opportunity to intervene early to prevent later problems.

In our experience, patients such as the one in this case need a team approach. Their care is too much for a single doctor, and ongoing psychiatric treatment is important to maximize the chances that treatment will be successful. Firm limit-setting is important, as is confrontation about inappropriate behavior.

We often find it useful to remember and act on the wise advice of Joel Saper and his colleagues at the Michigan Head Pain and Neurological Institute in Ann Arbor. His staff has years of experience dealing on an inpatient basis with challenging and refractory headache patients who are referred from around the country. In their chapter on inpatient strategies for refractory migraine in the book *Refractory Migraine*, Saper and colleagues suggest an approach such as the following:

'Your behavior is part of the problem.' (Give examples). 'It is a barrier to effective therapy. You reject our recommendations and battle us for control. This behavior is counterproductive and undermines the basic trust that is required in order to help you. Medical care is voluntary on both sides. Quite frankly, I don't have to be your physician if this unpleasant behavior continues, and you don't have to be my patient if you don't choose to be. If we can't agree that I am in charge of your case and you will be respectful, communicative, and compliant, I will discontinue care.'

Diagnosis

Migraine complicated by medication overuse headache, drug dependence, and family dysfunction.

Tip

Be alert for signs or signals of problem patients. Pursue a consistent, firm approach to treatment and insist that the patient be involved in psychiatric care as a condition of treatment.

Medication agreements

Case

A 65-year-old female presented, accompanied by her husband, for management of her chronic migraine. Migraines had been episodic and rare for many years and were well controlled with a butalbital-containing medication. About ten years prior the headaches escalated in frequency and butalbital use also slowly escalated over time. At the time of the visit, she was using four to five tablets daily and on this regimen had 15–20 headache days per month. No other headache medications had been tried as she was able to function well

while taking butalbital. Medical history was significant only for a family history of alcoholism.

She was given a diagnosis of chronic migraine and medication overuse headache and options for management were discussed with her. She voiced clear understanding of the need to change her current method of treating her headaches but was apprehensive about reducing the dosage of butalbital. She nonetheless agreed to a modest reduction as part of the overall plan, in addition to starting topiramate for prevention of headaches. At follow-up, however, she reported minor cognitive side effects and had not increased the dosage of topiramate as requested. She had also run out of the butalbital tablets that had been prescribed. She did not view this as a problem; instead, she and her husband both repeatedly commented that she was suffering, that she was entitled to an early refill of butalbital and that she should not be left without it. They repeatedly refocused the discussion away from traditional management and sought assurance that her access to butalbital would not be restricted.

Could a different approach to initial management have led to a better outcome?

The patient and her husband initially appeared to be motivated to treat her headache problem and readily agreed to the treatment plan. Apart from a family history of alcoholism, no other risk factors for substance abuse or misuse were identified. There was no indication of visits to multiple practitioners, multiple emergency department visits, or history of misuse of prior medications. For many patients like this, the problem of medication overuse simply "goes away" when they are provided with more effective and appropriate treatment for headaches.

Because the physician initially thought that the patient's prognosis for improvement was good, he had not asked the patient to sign a medication agreement. In hindsight, this was probably a mistake. A written treatment agreement, completed at the initial visit, would have served as a clear record of the physician's expectations about medication use, and outlined the conditions under which treatment would occur. This might have led to a better outcome.

What is the best management at this point?

At the follow-up visit, the patient appeared to be medication seeking, and her husband appeared to be

Table 10.4. Features of a typical medication agreement or contract

Outlines patient responsibility to comply with recommended doses and limits on medication

Documents discussion of the potential harms of treatment

Describes the fact that treatment goals are relief but not elimination of pain

Summarizes the details of monitoring that will be used, for example random urine drug testing

Lists the ways in which the patient should contact the office to request refills

Specifies expected behavior, for example no abusive language or behavior towards staff, compliance with referral for behavioral or psychologic evaluation

Identifies the circumstances under which treatment will be discontinued

codependent in her medication overuse. In this challenging setting, several options for treatment might be pursued. One option is to recommend abrupt cessation of butalbital as a condition of continued treatment. Another approach might be to formulate a treatment agreement that outlines the responsibilities of the patient and physician. These agreements are often particularly helpful when prescribing medications with high potential for abuse or dependence.

Although agreements are not legal contracts they do serve as a record of expected behavior and consequences contingent upon these behaviors. The objective is to help ensure adherence to agreed-upon limits of the medication with the goal of preventing misuse, abuse, or diversion. Most experts recommend that these agreements be used routinely whenever potentially abusable medications are prescribed, because it can be very difficult to determine in advance which patients are at high risk for aberrant drug-related behavior. In this situation, a medication agreement would put the patient "on notice" that infractions could jeopardize her access to care and focus attention on the management plan. It also makes it easier for the caregiver to refuse any request to deviate from the plan. Components of a medication agreement are described in Table 10.4.

Discussion

Medication agreements have long been employed when opioids or other chronic treatments with abuse potential are used to treat headache or other nonmalignant pain syndromes. Prototype agreements are widely available on the internet and can be adapted to suit an individual practitioner's or patient's situation.

Agreements have been criticized as paternalistic and unduly restrictive. Some feel that agreements contribute to the undertreatment of pain or stigmatize the patient. On the other hand, although these agreements are not legal contracts enforceable in a court of law, they may protect physicians from legal liability in the event of adverse events or claims of negligent management, although evidence to support that view is lacking. Given widespread concern over the increase in opioid prescribing, however, many healthcare systems recommend the use of agreements as part of a care plan for patients who require these drugs. Medication agreements can be a useful part of efforts to systematize and coordinate patient care. It is certainly the case that clear written policies and procedures can help clarify management.

Specific issues, especially the possibility of medication overuse headache, arise when dependence-inducing drugs are used chronically to treat headache conditions. Some experts have suggested that treatment should be reserved for compliant, reliable patients with moderate to severe pain, and prescribed by an experienced provider who knows the patient well. Relative contraindications to such therapy for headache include major psychiatric disorders such as psychosis, personality disorder, or somatoform disorder; prior addiction disorders; past legal issues related to prescription drug abuse or diversion; or an at-risk family environment that might be associated with an increased risk of drug diversion.

Diagnosis

Chronic migraine; medication overuse headache.

Tip

Medication agreements in headache management can benefit all parties and should be considered when potentially dependence-inducing medications are in use. It can be difficult to predict in advance when an agreement will be required and agreements are likely underused.

Further reading

Headache diaries

Allena M, Cuzzoni MG, Tassorelli C, Nappi G, Antonaci F. An electronic diary on a palm device for headache monitoring: a preliminary experience. *J Headache Pain.* 2012;13(7):537–41.

Jensen R, Tassorelli C, Rossi P, *et al.*; Basic Diagnostic Headache Diary Study Group. A basic diagnostic headache diary (BDHD) is well accepted and useful in the diagnosis of headache. a multicentre European and Latin American study. *Cephalalgia.* 2011;31(15): 1549–60.

McKenzie JA, Cutrer FM. How well do headache patients remember? A comparison of self-report measures of headache frequency and severity in patients with migraine. *Headache.* 2009;49(5):669–72.

Nappi G, Jensen R, Nappi RE, *et al.* Diaries and calendars for migraine. A review. *Cephalalgia.* 2006;26(8):905–16.

Stone AA, Shiffman S, Schwartz JE, Broderick JE, Hufford MR. Patient compliance with paper and electronic diaries. *Control Clin Trials.* 2003;24(2):182–99.

Migraine chronification

Scher AI, Stewart WF, Buse D, Krantz DS, Lipton RB. Major life changes before and after the onset of chronic daily headache: a population-based study. *Cephalalgia.* 2008;28(8):868–76.

Scher AI, Stewart WF, Ricci JA, Lipton RB. Factors associated with the onset and remission of chronic daily headache in a population-based study. *Pain.* 2003;106(1–2):81–9.

Schulman E, Levin M, Lake AE, Loder E, eds. *Refractory Migraine.* New York, NY, Oxford University Press, 2010.

Medication agreements

Arnold RM, Han PK, Seltzer D. Opioid contracts in chronic nonmalignant pain management: objectives and uncertainties. *Am J Med.* 2006;119(4):292–6.

Saper JR, Lake AE. Borderline personality disorder and the chronic headache patient: review and management recommendations. *Headache.* 2002;42:663–74.

Saper JR, Lake AE 3rd, Bain PA, *et al.* A practice guide for continuous opioid therapy for refractory daily headache: patient selection, physician requirements, and treatment monitoring. *Headache.* 2010;50(7):1175–93.

Medicolegal pitfalls in headache management

The legal aspects of caring for patients, and fear of malpractice suits or other legal entanglements, are understandably matters of great concern for all physicians. This chapter reviews topics of relevance to legal aspects of headache management, including areas of actual and potential malpractice liability. Several features of headache influence the type of legal issues that may arise and their likelihood. Although most chronic headache disorders are not life threatening, some secondary causes of headache are. In certain types of headache, such as cluster headache, the intensity of the pain makes medical treatment imperative, not optional, for almost all patients and creates a degree of desperation seen in few other pain disorders. In unusual headache conditions, diagnosis and appropriate treatment may be delayed. Current treatments for most primary headache disorders are not curative, and not always effective, increasing the chance that patients will seek disability status or require off-label, experimental, or nonvalidated therapy. In addition, there are serious risks associated with certain headache treatments.

One legal area that is almost certain to involve the headache practitioner is that of disability determination. Headache practitioners frequently receive patient requests for information to claims for disability payments through Social Security Disability Insurance (SSDI) or other programs.

There is much confusion about this topic and almost no formal training is given to medical care providers about disability determination. Disability is essentially a legal, not a medical, concept. It is defined differently depending on the rules that apply in a particular situation. These range from Social Security disability rules, Workers' Compensation laws, the Family and Medical Leave Act (FMLA), Veterans Association guidelines, to requirements of private insurance policies. Table 11.1 lists some common disability benefit programs that require medical support of claims.

Medical leave and disability determination: when to make the call?

Case

A 45-year-old information systems technician for a large company presented for an initial visit with a past history of clearly documented migraine without aura that had, over the past two years, evolved to chronic migraine. He had struggled to remain at work over the past 18 months, using the majority of his sick time as well as some of his vacation time to rest. His supervisor had discussed the possibility that the FMLA might cover his absences. Box 11.1 outlines the key features of the FMLA. The patient asked the physician to fill out paperwork to help him qualify for FMLA protection. He also asked whether the physician would support him if he decided to apply for SSDI payments.

Congress enacted FMLA in order to protect workers who are ill or who have caregiving responsibilities for children or other family members and need to take time away from work for these reasons. The law applies only to employers, including state agencies and schools, with 50 or more workers. Employees are eligible for up to 12 weeks of unpaid FMLA leave in any calendar year if they have been employed for 12 months out of the preceding 7 years, worked at least 1250 hours during those 12 months, and worked at or near a location with at least 50 employees.

The FMLA law allows employers to require physician certification of a serious medical condition, and recertification every six months for a chronic ongoing medical problem. FMLA requires that covered workers are entitled to return to their job or an equivalent job when they return from leave and that they are entitled to maintain health insurance coverage while they are on leave. One useful feature of FMLA is that employees are allowed to take small amounts of leave time, for example a single day at a time, and on an

Table 11.1. Some benefit programs that require medical provider support for claims

Program	Funding agency	Jurisdiction	Beneficiaries	Benefits	Restrictions	Comments
Social Security Disability Insurance (SSDI)	Social Security Tax	Federal	Employees; 7.7 million (2009) disabled workers	Wage replacement and medical care	Long-term permanent disability only	Prior work history, waiting period
Workers' Compensation	Employer Tax	Individual states	Employees; 126 million (2002) disabled workers	Wage replacement and medical care	Work-related illness or injury only	In force from day one (limited liability for employer in return)
Family Medical and Leave Act (FMLA)	US Dept of Labor	Federal	Employees of at least one year	12 weeks unpaid leave per year for specific reasons	Employer must have 50 or more employees	Job is protected
Private Insurance	Private	Private, may be mandatory or optional to employees	Employees injured in the workplace. Temporary disability programs protect employees, owners, and professionals for injury or illness at or away from the workplace	Wage replacement and medical care	May offset the amount received from Social Security	Does not compete with workers' compensation coverage
Veterans Administration Disability	Veterans Administration budget	Federal	Veterans; 3.1 million claimants (2009)	Compensation only	Honorable discharge or left the service under less than "dishonorable" terms.	

intermittent basis. Some patients may use FMLA leave to attend office visits related to their medical condition, for example.

Among other things, FMLA leave can be granted for employees who have a serious health condition that makes them unable to perform the functions of their job, or if they need to care for a spouse, child, or parent with a serious health condition. If the health condition requiring FMLA leave is "foreseeable" (e.g. an elective surgical procedure) an employee must give 30 days' notice of the leave. For unforeseeable events, only "practicable" notice is required.

In this case, the physician explained that he was happy to support the patient's request for FMLA protection so that the patient could attend office visits and remain at his job despite headache-related absences. In response to the patient's request for SSDI, however, his opinion on this first visit was that the patient's condition had not yet been aggressively treated and he expected the patient would improve with such treatment. Thus, he did not feel that he could support an application for SSDI. The remainder of the visit was devoted to a discussion of the proposed management. Two weeks later the physician received a letter from a lawyer requesting a statement of disability for this patient.

Did the physician respond appropriately to this patient's request for disability?

A request for support of a disability application need not always be met with a "yes" or "no" answer. If a review of the patient's medical information fails to support a decision one way or the other, then a brief note to that effect is appropriate. In this situation, the physician has seen the patient only once and thinks it is likely that he will improve with treatment. He is not in a position to reach a firm conclusion about disability and may simply note that the patient remains under care. Thus, the physician's response to this patient's disability request seems appropriate.

Discussion

Physicians who treat patients with serious headache disorders should be familiar with the provisions of FMLA. It is a very useful way for patients to remain employed despite severe headaches and also makes it

Box 11.1. Medical certification for the Family and Medical Leave Act (FMLA)

Provides: Unpaid, job-protected leave, up to 12 work-weeks in a 12-month period for a number of reasons, including a serious health condition that makes the employee unable to perform the essential functions of his or her job. Pertinent to migraine, employees may at times take intermittent leave.

Medical certification for a serious health condition: The employer may require *complete and sufficient certification* in support of the leave from a healthcare provider. The employee is responsible for paying for the cost of the medical certification and for making sure the certification is provided to the employer. The employer may not request *additional* information but may ask the provider for clarification. The employer may also request a recertification periodically and may request a fitness-for-duty certification when the leave is complete.

Requested information:
- Medical facts about the condition
- Indication that the employee cannot perform the essential functions of the job
- Estimated frequency and duration of expected incapacity

Optional forms (e.g. WH-380-E) can be downloaded for use in documentation of an employee's serious health condition.

Adapted from US Dept of Labor website: http://www.dol.gov/whd/fmla/

Box 11.2. Functional capacity information needed for disability determination

Diagnosis, symptoms, physical findings, and test results leading to disability (include all physical findings):

Will/Has disability or impairment last/lasted one year or more?

Does the disability or impairment prevent the patient from standing/sitting for six to eight hours? Yes/No

If yes, what is the reason?

Does the disability or impairment require the patient to lie down during the day?

Estimate the part-time or reduced work schedule the employee needs, if any:

<> hour(s) per day; <> days per week from <> through <>.

Will the condition cause episodic flare-ups periodically preventing the employee from performing his/her job functions? Yes/No.

Is it medically necessary for the employee to be absent from work during the flare-ups? Yes/No

If so, explain:

Estimate the frequency of flare-ups and the duration of related incapacity that the patient may have over the next six months (e.g. one episode every three months lasting one to two days):

Frequency: <> times per <> week(s)/month(s) Duration: <> hours or <> day(s) per episode.

Describe any other restrictions (what the patient is advised not to do) or limitations (what the patient cannot do), e.g. reaching and fine motor movements:

possible for patients to take time off to receive needed treatment. With regard to disability determination, most requests for physician information will request a determination of patient impairment and functional capacity. Box 11.2 lists information that is commonly needed to fill out these requests. Physicians may wish to maintain a template in the medical record to facilitate collection of information about functional capacity and objective findings likely to be of interest to the disability examiner. Providers who routinely document this information may often simply submit their clinical notes in support of a patient's disability claim.

Diagnosis

Chronic migraine with possible disability.

Tip

The Family and Medical Leave Act provides useful job protection for workers with serious health conditions such as chronic headache. Physicians should not feel pressured to make disability determinations in the absence of sufficient information.

Is the patient really disabled?

Case

A 32-year-old diesel mechanic presented for evaluation of headache after an injury. There was no past or family history of migraine and no history of prior injury. He reported that he slipped in the shop while working and struck his right temple, with a resulting laceration requiring medical attention but with no loss of consciousness. The next day he reported headache, nausea, photophobia, and tinnitus. He was diagnosed, by another physician, with a concussion and treated with simple analgesic medications. An MRI of the brain was normal. Headache and tinnitus were exacerbated by noise exposure at work and the patient said he had been unable to return to work because of the noisy work environment. A neurologist added gabapentin and metoclopramide and referred the patient to an otolaryngologist, who found no abnormalities on examination. The patient was advised to wear earplugs to limit exposure to noise at work but he objected to this solution on the grounds that this would interfere with his personal safety.

When evaluated in the headache clinic four months after the injury, symptoms had improved but he continued to report episodic disabling headaches that occurred three to five times per week. He had not returned to work and had an open worker's compensation case. His work history and level of activity were not documented in detail, however, since the headache specialist felt that his post-traumatic headaches were likely to improve and expected that he would ultimately return to work.

Further improvement was noted at a follow-up visit several months later. The patient had begun to take some college courses and was generally more active. Despite this, he had not returned to work. He had refused an offer of a job modification designed to protect him from noise at work because it was associated with reduced pay. He also noted other problems, such as a long commute, that he felt prevented a return to work.

After this follow-up visit, his physician received a request from the workman's compensation insurer for written certification of disability.

How should the physician respond to this request for a determination of disability?

The patient's employer has attempted to accommodate this patient's disability. The patient has rejected the proposed accommodations and has additional reasons not to return to work. However, he is taking col-

lege courses and his headaches are improving. The medical record documents this improvement in pain and function. The most reasonable course of action for the physician in this case is to advise the patient that there is no clear medical reason to avoid returning to work. Although uncomfortable, such a conversation and approach is preferable to either ignoring the disability request altogether or acquiescing to the request to support the patient's application for disability compensation.

Discussion

To avoid future strain on the therapeutic relationship, physicians should respond frankly to patients who request disability certification that the physician feels is not warranted. Any disability determination by a physician should reflect the facts and be able to withstand close scrutiny in a legal system that is adversarial by design.

Diagnosis

Post-traumatic headache with unusual and persistent symptoms.

Tip

A seemingly routine return-to-work situation can quickly become complicated and leave the unwary provider awash in a swirl of legal and ethical questions. Prior training and preparation are key to handling these situations effectively.

Shouldn't someone help?

Case

A 44-year-old female was evaluated for refractory chronic migraine present since childhood and unassociated with psychiatric comorbidities. "I've had headache as long as I can remember. Over the years I've had multiple treatments and nothing has ever worked." She had been followed in several different university clinic settings and had been compliant with multiple different therapies but could not recall any sustained period of headache control.

Further progression of headache had been noted in the months before the current evaluation, with worsening of baseline headache and superimposed episodes of more severe pain that could last days at a time. She was an unemployed nurse and was receiving some unemployment compensation but had never considered or applied for disability payments.

After almost six months of intensive outpatient management, the patient was unimproved. She had moved back in with her mother because she was unable to afford rent and reported that she was receiving no outside financial support of any kind. Despite her symptoms, she was looking for work in order to be able to pay for her private health insurance plan.

Should this patient be advised to seek disability?

Often the tone of disability discussions reflects suspicion of a patient's motives. On occasion, however, physicians encounter patients who are too reluctant to seek disability status. The patient in this case seems never to have been aware of or considered outside help, but could benefit from it, especially if by receiving assistance she is able to maintain her health insurance coverage. In this setting, the provider could advise the patient of the availability of assistance programs and provide a referral if necessary, for example to social services, to further guide the patient.

Discussion

Most headache experts would agree that a portion of their patient population is disabled, some permanently so. In fact, many studies of migraine-related disability suggest that the disability associated with chronic headache disorders such as migraine is underreported and underestimated. Measures of medically determined disability may not, however, always meet legal or administrative standards for disability determination. From a legal perspective, disability determination usually is based upon objective medical findings. Since migraine is not typically associated with objective findings, the physician's opinion as to the basis of disability becomes especially important.

Diagnosis

Chronic migraine.

Tip

Physicians are an important resource for disabled patients who may be unaware of available forms of financial assistance.

A patient who asks to record his office visit

Case

A 70-year-old retired psychologist presented alone for evaluation of headache. Without any discussion he produced a tape recorder and said he wished to record the interview because he had memory problems that make it difficult for him to remember what doctors tell him. He was a vague and tangential historian who lived alone and reported a pattern of headache that was consistent with chronic tension-type headache. He also had many other somatic complaints. He was a frequent user of medical services and had several comorbid conditions, including anxiety. Other providers had indicated in their records that they allowed the patient to tape record medical visits.

Is the request to record the visit reasonable and should it be allowed?

Although mildly unsettling, under most circumstances such a practice is probably benign, and in this case the physician allowed it. He viewed it as similar to situations in which other patients took written notes during a visit, or an accompanying family member typed on a laptop during a visit. These activities usually take place without specific advance permission and generally represent a desire to make sure that medical information and recommendations are understood and available for reference. If the patient's intention is simply to aid recall of the visit the activity is probably benign and might even be useful. Advantages of recording could include retention and reinforcement of complex information and recommendations as well as reassurance for concerned family members who could not attend the visit.

Although likely to be a reasonable request in this situation, it is understandable that similar requests by other patients and under other circumstances might provoke anxiety in medical providers. The ubiquity of smartphones and other devices makes recording visits easy to do, and such requests are likely to become more common in the future.

What are the potential pitfalls or harms associated with recording of medical visits?

Potential pitfalls associated with tape recordings of medical visits include the possible compromise of privacy. Even if they instigated the taping, patients might be concerned that others in their family will gain access to the tapes, and be more guarded in the history they provide to the physician. Similarly, physicians concerned about the future use of the tape, or about the possibility that remarks might be taken out of context, may become more guarded in their discussion and take a more defensive attitude towards treatment.

In this case, the patient requested permission to record a visit, but surreptitious recording is certainly possible. If this comes to light later on, physicians might understandably feel that the behavior indicates a lack of trust in his or her recommendations or worry that the patient is litigious. Although records of medical conversations are generally considered to be protected health information, if the material is under the voluntary control of the patient typical legal restrictions do not apply. Patients are free to share their health information with whomever they wish; it is medical providers and healthcare entities that are subject to privacy rules.

If providers feel uncomfortable about a patient request to record a medical visit, there are several possible courses of action. The request could be denied and the patient told that the practice seems intrusive and will limit opportunities for a frank discussion. If the request is refused, it may be prudent to inquire about the reason for the request, since this might be addressed in other ways. It could be, for example, that a patient seeking to record a visit would be satisfied with a more detailed set of written recommendations, a copy of the finished visit note, or a call by the physician to a concerned spouse to explain things the patient feels he or she will not be able to recall. As part of this discussion it may be helpful for the provider to state what he or she suggests be done to improve the problem while not necessarily simply agreeing to a patient's request, for example by saying "I'm sorry I can't allow _ but am happy to _ instead."

Discussion

Since it seems likely that technologic advances will increase the frequency of patient requests to record medical visits, physicians may want to institute policies about the use of various technologies during the office visit. If recording will not be allowed, it is prudent to consider giving notice of this policy, for example a sign in the waiting room might indicate, "no audio or video recording is allowed in this office."

Diagnosis

Chronic tension-type headache.

Tip

Discussion about office policies about audio or video-taping of medical visits can help prevent confusion and delay when such requests arise.

Overreliance on steroids in cluster headache

Case

A 43-year-old man described a 23-year history of 90-minute daily or twice-daily headaches that met criteria for cluster headache. The headaches were unilateral, behind his left eye, and associated with ipsilateral nasal stuffiness and ptosis. For many years the patient experienced only one or two bouts of cluster headache a year, often in the spring and fall. These periods of headache susceptibility would typically last two months, during which headache attacks occurred one to several times a day. During cluster bouts the patient managed individual headaches with sumatriptan. After two months headaches would remit and he was completely headache-free until the next bout.

Three years ago he developed chronic cluster headache and his new insurance company would not provide him with sufficient sumatriptan to treat all of his attacks. Preventive treatment with verapamil at a dose of 80 mg twice daily was ineffective. He was then placed on prednisone 60 mg a day and reported he only had headaches "when I forget to take it or some fool doctor tries to take me off." He was in good health but had a hip replacement last year because of osteonecrosis of the hip. He was told this was probably caused by his steroid treatment, but responded, "if steroids are the only thing that works, what am I supposed to do?" The patient was on 60 mg of prednisone a day and asked to have the prescription refilled.

What is the role of corticosteroids in the treatment of cluster headache?

In our practice we think of cluster headache (sometimes known as "suicide headache") as a true headache emergency. Most patients, like the one described here, are desperate for rapid, reliable relief from the agonizing, unpredictable attacks. Injectable sumatriptan or oxygen is typically effective for treatment of individual headaches, but relying solely on symptomatic treatment of attacks is impractical and forces patients to endure short periods of intense pain while waiting for treatment to take effect. Thus, most cluster headache patients should be offered daily preventive medicine, which is given with the aim of reducing or eliminating the headaches.

A short course of oral corticosteroid treatment – often referred to as "bridging therapy" – can suppress cluster headaches during the week or so it may take preventive treatment to become effective. Patients usually are grateful to find that steroids work quickly, and steroids may seem to have few side effects, at least initially. The mild euphoria steroids produce also may relieve the dread associated with severe, unpredictable episodes of pain.

Unfortunately, repeated or long-term treatment with corticosteroids can cause serious side effects such as osteonecrosis of the hip. Occasionally even relatively short courses or low doses of steroids can produce serious problems. Most doctors in a headache specialty practice have seen patients like this who are steroid dependent and have suffered serious medical consequences as a result.

How can steroid dependence and complications be avoided?

The use of corticosteroids to treat cluster headache, though off-label, cannot be completely avoided, but the drugs should be used with caution, in the smallest doses for the shortest period of time necessary to allow a transition to other, safer treatments. The mainstays of preventive treatment for cluster headache are verapamil and lithium, either alone or in combination.

The dose of verapamil necessary to control cluster headache may be very high, and heart block or constipation pose important safety and tolerability problems. These problems are reversible, however, and can often be prevented or caught early with careful monitoring. Lithium is perceived to be highly effective for chronic cluster headache, but patients may prefer to avoid a drug they associate with bipolar disorder. Blood tests and electrocardiograms are needed to monitor treatment and can be inconvenient. For the patient described in this case, attacks finally came under control on a preventive regimen of 240 mg of sustained release verapamil twice daily, along with 300 mg of lithium carbonate three times daily. He was slowly weaned from steroids over several months.

Discussion

The off-label use of steroids for cluster headache has not been carefully studied, owing to the rarity of the disorder. Many patients, however, report that steroids help temporarily but over the long run seem to make headaches worse. Some even suspect that steroid treatment may prolong bouts of cluster headache. Many seasoned cluster headache veterans believe that the short-term benefits of steroid treatment are not worth the problems they can cause when used repeatedly over many bouts of cluster headache.

A frank discussion with patients prior to any prescription of corticosteroids is important, and it may be appropriate to provide written information about potential side effects and harms. It is not uncommon for patients who have suffered serious steroid-related complications from cluster headache treatment to say that they were not warned about side effects when the drugs were prescribed. In one review of medicolegal aspects of cluster headache, adverse events from steroid treatment, particularly osteonecrosis of the hip, were identified as a cause of several large malpractice liability payments.

There are few published guidelines or protocols to help the clinician decide on a weaning schedule for patients who are steroid dependent, but patients who have become steroid dependent must be weaned from steroids carefully to avoid precipitating adrenal insufficiency. Patients remain at risk of acute adrenal insufficiency during periods of critical illness for up to a year after discontinuation.

One weaning strategy, developed for patients with inflammatory bowel disease, is to switch patients taking prednisone to an equivalent dose of dexamethasone, assuming that 0.75 mg of dexamethasone is equivalent to 5 mg of prednisone. Using 0.5 mg tablets of dexamethasone, reductions of 0.5 mg can be made every few weeks until the patient is off steroids.

Diagnosis

Chronic cluster headache with steroid dependence.

Tip

Short-term "bridging therapy" with oral corticosteroids can bring rapid relief to patients with cluster headache, but repeated courses of steroid treatment can cause serious harm and exposure of the physician to legal risk. Corticosteroids should be used cautiously and for short periods of time.

A request for medical marijuana to treat migraine

Case

A 24-year-old woman with transformed migraine and medication overuse presented for initial evaluation at a headache clinic. Her fiancé accompanied her. The patient met criteria for a diagnosis of chronic migraine. She reported that she was taking amitriptyline prescribed by her primary care physician but that her symptoms were not fully controlled. She used ibuprofen and a triptan for individual attacks of headache and these medications provided some relief. She had also tried vaporized marijuana and found it very helpful for the headaches. In fact, she reported that it was as effective as her triptan. She also reported that it improved the quality of her sleep. She asked whether the physician would provide a letter of medical necessity supporting her use of medical marijuana. Voters in the state had recently approved a ballot question that allowed patients with "debilitating medical conditions" to obtain and use marijuana for medical reasons. The physician declined the patient's request and suggested alternative combinations of standard abortive and preventive medications. However, the patient's fiancé repeatedly interrupted the discussion and insisted the physician provide a letter allowing the patient to obtain medical marijuana.

What are the legal implications of supporting a patient's request for medical marijuana?

Voters in many states have approved ballot questions that allow the use of marijuana for medical purposes. Although marijuana is a Schedule I controlled substance under US federal law and remains unavailable by prescription, providers can write letters certifying the medical necessity for such treatment for serious medical conditions, including headache. Patients are then able to purchase marijuana from approved medical marijuana dispensaries. In Massachusetts, qualifying patients are allowed to possess a 60-day supply (10 ounces) of marijuana for personal use.

Although straightforward on one level, there are potential medicolegal pitfalls for physicians who certify patients for the use of medical marijuana. In the situation described in this case there is the additional possibility of coercion based on the behavior of the patient's fiancé. It is possible that he wishes to grow and use (or possibly distribute) marijuana under an umbrella of legal protection provided by the physician and in the name of the patient.

This is certainly a less well-defined situation than is the routine prescribing of a pharmaceutical grade medication for a patient. Determining the true intentions of a patient seeking a letter supporting the use of medical marijuana may at times be difficult or impossible.

What advice should be given to this patient about the harms and benefits of marijuana in headache treatment?

Marijuana has not been carefully studied as a treatment for migraine or other headache conditions, even though descriptions of marijuana-based treatments for headache date far back in history. In the 1850s, for example, Sir William Osler advocated daily marijuana use as a treatment for migraine. Endogenous cannabinoids act as neurotransmitters through a series of receptors throughout the brain and other organs and may produce antinociceptive and neuroprotective effects, and reduced levels of endogenous cannabinoids have been found in the spinal fluid of chronic headache subjects.

Although it is plausible that medical marijuana could be an appropriate therapy for some forms of headache, there are as yet no guidelines as to when and how to use this therapy in the headache patient. There also is no high quality evidence supporting the efficacy of marijuana in headache management but there is some evidence suggesting potential harms. Marijuana use has been associated with the development of reversible cerebral vasoconstrictive syndromes, and it is possible that patients with migraine are particularly susceptible to this problem. Regular use of marijuana in the migraine patient, especially in combination with selective serotonin reuptake inhibitor drugs, has been associated with the development of the reversible cerebral vasoconstrictive syndrome with headache worsening and focal MRI changes. Other potential adverse effects relevant to migraine management include mood changes and memory dysfunction.

Discussion

Although marijuana use remains illegal under federal law, a growing number of states* have legalized medical marijuana and physicians can expect to encounter patients requesting medical marijuana with increasing frequency. The landscape is changing rapidly but unfortunately information is scarce about the potential associated medical and legal dangers for physicians and patients. Careful documentation of advice given to patients about this matter is important and likely to be protective for all involved.

*AK, AZ, CA, CO, CT, DC, DE, HI, MA, ME, MI, MT, NV, NJ, NM, OR, RI, VT, and WA.

Diagnosis

Chronic migraine.

Tip

The harm-to-benefit balance of marijuana as a treatment for headache disorders is uncertain. In the absence of firm evidence of benefit and given the possibility of serious adverse events related to use, physicians should be cautious about certifying patients for medical marijuana, as they would be in recommending the use of other treatments whose effects are poorly understood.

Risks associated with prescribing off-label medication

Case

A 35-year-old female with high frequency episodic migraine presented for evaluation. Her neurologic examination and vital signs were normal. After discussion, she was advised to consider preventive therapy to decrease the frequency of headaches. Because she was planning to become pregnant, the physician recommended avoiding divalproex or topiramate. Instead, the patient was prescribed a low dose of metoprolol with plans for a slow upward titration of the dose. Two weeks into her treatment, the patient reportedly became dizzy and fainted at work, sustaining a scalp laceration that required sutures. She was advised to stop the metoprolol.

At her next visit her husband accompanied her. He was a lawyer, and was concerned because he had learned that metoprolol was used to treat heart and blood pressure problems and was not approved by the US Food and Drug Administration (FDA) for use in migraine. He wondered why this medication had been prescribed in a headache clinic and why his wife had not been informed that it was an unapproved treatment.

Did the provider do anything wrong?

Although not every headache expert would have prescribed metoprolol as first-line treatment for this particular patient, it was certainly a reasonable treatment choice. Although the drug does not have an FDA indication for migraine treatment, it is in the same therapeutic beta-blocker medication class as two other drugs that are approved to treat migraine: propranolol and timolol. In addition, several placebo-controlled studies support metoprolol as an effective treatment for migraine. On the basis of this evidence, metoprolol received the highest rating (Level A) in the recent joint American Headache Society/American Association of Neurology migraine prevention guidelines. Many other migraine preventives recommended by that guideline also do not have FDA approval for migraine prevention.

Although physicians are understandably concerned about the legal risks associated with prescribing off-label medications, one paradox of current practice is that most third-party payers will not reimburse for treatment of chronic migraine with onabotulinumtoxinA unless patients have previously failed to obtain benefit from a number of other drugs. These include many that are not FDA approved for migraine treatment.

How can this situation best be handled?

Providers may become accustomed to prescribing what they view as standard therapy and neglect to discuss the off-label nature of recommended treatments with patients. Some may consider such disclosure to be an unimportant matter. As the husband's question in this case makes clear, however, this view is unlikely to be shared by patients, especially if they suffer an adverse event related to the medication. The further a therapy is outside the mainstream and the more potential risk involved, the more important it probably is to fully discuss and document patient understanding and acceptance of an off-label therapy before initiation of treatment.

In general, informed consent requires that a patient be provided with enough information about the benefits and risks of a proposed treatment in order to make an informed decision. Material risks that could be of significance to the patient should be disclosed and discussed. Assent is implied if the patient accepts the plan and voices no dissent, and currently the use of off-label drugs in a clinical setting requires no special written consent. It is noteworthy, however, that written consent *would* be required of participants in a drug trial for a new indication of an established drug because the drug's risks and benefits would have yet to be proved (for the purposes of FDA approval). Whether the off-label use of medication constitutes a separate risk over and above risks of the same medication for an indicated use is uncertain given the level of evidence supporting many off-label medications for headache, but this should be considered carefully when less is known about a treatment. Finally, physicians should prescribe medications only for indications that they believe are in the best interest of the patient on the basis of the most credible available evidence.

In this case, the physician first expressed her distress about the patient's experience by saying "I am sorry that this happened to you." She then spent time explaining her choice of medication to the patient and her husband. The patient's husband, who had not been at the original visit, said that he accepted the physician's explanation for the treatment with metoprolol, and understood that although his wife's experience had been an exception, overall this had not been a particularly unusual or risky treatment.

Discussion

A review of off-label prescribing in migraine concluded that it was not only common but an integral part of headache practice and, at least for commonly used drugs, within the standard of care. For a number of headache disorders there are no FDA-approved therapies. For example, there are no FDA-approved preventive treatments for cluster headache, but good quality evidence supports the use of verapamil and lithium and essentially all headache physicians routinely employ these medications for that purpose. Similarly, there are no approved treatments for other trigeminal autonomic cephalgias, some of which are even defined by their response to an off-label therapy (e.g. the indomethacin responsive-headache syndromes). Many commonly used pediatric therapies are off-label since relatively few medications are tested in pediatric populations prior to marketing.

US Food and Drug Administration approval of a medication for a specific indication implies that, when used in accordance with label instructions, the drug meets a minimum set of efficacy and safety standards. The testing process to gain FDA approval for individual indications or dosing regimens is cumbersome and expensive. Because of this manufacturers often choose not to obtain approval for all possible uses of a drug. Thus, the label for any particular drug will not list all potential medical uses, even some for which there is good clinical trial or other evidence of efficacy. This distinction between FDA approval and scientific validation of a drug's usefulness is an important one. In recognition of this distinction the FDA notes that "accepted medical practice includes drug use that is not reflected in approved drug labeling" and that "once a drug has received FDA approval for any indication, physicians may prescribe it for other conditions, in other doses, or for different populations than those listed in approved labeling."

Although off-label medication use is clearly common and defensible, there is no clear definition of what constitutes acceptable off-label medication use. The use of metoprolol in this case seems acceptable. Less acceptable uses might include prescribing an off-label medicine based on only anecdotal evidence of benefit in a patient who has not had previous trials of standard therapy, especially if this is done without a clear discussion about the nature of use.

Diagnosis

High frequency migraine without aura; syncope related to medication-induced hypotension.

Tip

Minimize the legal risks of off-label drug use by providing patients with clear and relevant information about the benefits and harms of any proposed therapy.

Further reading

Disability and the Family and Medical Leave Act

Buse DC, Manack AN, Fanning KM, *et al.* Chronic migraine prevalence, disability, and sociodemographic factors: results from the American Migraine Prevalence and Prevention Study. *Headache.* 2012;52:1456–70.

Doyle HA. Sound medical evidence: key to FECA claims. *Monthly Labor Review.* September 1991, 26–28.

Holmes WF, MacGregor EA, Sawyer JP, Lipton RB. Information about migraine disability influences physicians' perceptions of illness severity and treatment needs. *Headache.* 2001;41:343–50.

Leonardi M, Raggi A, Ajovalasit D, *et al.* Functioning and disability in migraine. *Disabil Rehabil.* 2010;32(S1): S23–32.

United States Department of Labor. Leave Benefits. Family and Medical Leave Act. http://www.dol.gov/dol/topic/benefits-leave/fmla.htm.

Overreliance on steroids

Byyny RL. Withdrawal from glucocorticoid therapy. *N Engl J Med.* 1976;295:30–2.

Loder E, Loder J. Medicolegal issues in cluster headache. *Curr Pain Headache Rep.* 2004;8(2):147–56.

Murphy SJ, Wang L, Anderson LA, *et al.* Withdrawal of corticosteroids in inflammatory bowel disease patients after dependency periods ranging from 2 to 45 years: a proposed method. *Aliment Pharmacol Ther.* 2009; 30:1078–86.

Weinstein RS. Glucocorticoid-induced osteoporosis and osteonecrosis. *Endocrinol Metab Clin North Am.* 2012; 41(3):595–611.

Zhao FC, Li ZR, Guo KJ. Clinical analysis of osteonecrosis of the femoral head induced by steroids. *Orthop Surg.* 2012;4(1):28–34.

Medical marijuana

An Act for the Humanitarian Medical Use of Marijuana. http://www.malegislature.gov/Laws/SessionLaws/Acts/2012/Chapter369.

Chen SP, Fuh JL, Wang SJ. Reversible cerebral vasoconstriction syndrome: current and future perspectives. *Expert Rev Neurother.* 2011;11:1265–76.

Ducros A, Boukobza M, Porcher R, *et al.* The clinical and radiological spectrum of reversible cerebral vasoconstriction syndrome. A prospective series of 67 patients. *Brain.* 2007;130:3091–101.

McGeeney BE. Cannabinoids and hallucinogens for headache. *Headache.* 2013;53(3):447–58.

Off-label drug use in headache

Loder EW, Biondi DM. Off-label prescribing of drugs in specialty headache practice. *Headache.* 2004;44: 636–41.

Mithani Z. Informed consent for off-label use of prescription medications. *Virtual Mentor.* 2012; 14(7):576–81.

Wittich CM, Burkle CM, Lanier WL. Ten common questions (and their answers) about off-label drug use. *Mayo Clin Proc.* 2012;87(10):982–90.

Index

Note: page numbers in *italics* refer to figures and tables, those in **bold** refer to boxes